全国中医药行业高等教育“十四五”创新教材
National Traditional Chinese Medicine Industry Higher Education “14th Five-Year Plan” Innovative Textbooks

中医学基础（汉英对照）
Fundamentals of Traditional Chinese Medicine（Chinese-English）

（供临床医学专业用）
（For Majors of Clinical Medicine）

主　编　　付耕南　冯　健　张宁苏
Editors-in-Chief　Fu Gengnan　Feng Jian　Zhang Ningsu

全国百佳图书出版单位
中国中医药出版社
·北　京·

China Press of Traditional Chinese Medicine
Beijing

图书在版编目（CIP）数据

中医学基础：汉英对照 / 付耕南，冯健，张宁苏主编 . 北京：中国中医药出版社，2024. 12.（2025. 1 重印）--（全国中医药行业高等教育“十四五”创新教材）.

ISBN 978-7-5132-9207-8

Ⅰ. R22

中国国家版本馆 CIP 数据核字第 202417GY83 号

中国中医药出版社出版

北京经济技术开发区科创十三街 31 号院二区 8 号楼

邮政编码　100176

传真　010-64405721

北京盛通印刷股份有限公司印刷

各地新华书店经销

开本 787×1092　1/16　印张 19.5　字数 676 千字

2024 年 12 月第 1 版　2025 年 1 月第 2 次印刷

书号　ISBN 978－7－5132－9207－8

定价　85.00 元

网址　www.cptcm.com

服务热线　010-64405510

购书热线　010-89535836

维权打假　010-64405753

微信服务号　zgzyycbs

微商城网址　https://kdt.im/LIdUGr

官方微博　http://e.weibo.com/cptcm

天猫旗舰店网址　https://zgzyycbs.tmall.com

如有印装质量问题请与本社出版部联系（010-64405510）

全国中医药行业高等教育“十四五”创新教材

《中医学基础》（汉英对照）编委会

主　编　付耕南　冯　健　张宁苏

主　译　谢　群　刘子宁

副主编　林　非　李国峰　张　璐　田　露　潘嘉祥
李　越　刘立明

编　委（以姓氏笔画为序）

于志峰　王　邈　华声瑜　刘佳林　闫　琪
孙　牧　孙　峰　李英冬　李晓康　杨福双
陈　怡　周禄荣　赵宏杰　崔沐群　葛骁欧
潘　森　戴永娜

National Traditional Chinese Medicine Industry Higher Education "14th Five-Year Plan" Innovative Textbooks

Editorial Board for *Fundamentals of Traditional Chinese Medicine*(Chinese–English)

编写说明

中医药是中华优秀传统文化的重要载体，在促进文明互鉴、维护人民健康等方面发挥着重要作用。中医药以其在疾病预防、治疗、康复等方面的独特优势，受到许多国家民众的广泛认可。中医药具有独特的生命观、健康观、疾病观、防治观，不仅为中华民族繁衍昌盛作出了卓越贡献，也对世界文明进步产生了积极影响。本教材由长春中医药大学牵头组织，各中医药高等院校专家共同编写，供全国医学高等院校临床医学专业来华留学生及爱好传统医学的外国人士学习使用。

本教材创新性地运用中英双语对照的形式，凝练地阐述了中医学理论、知识与技能的精髓，可供来华学习临床医学的国外留学生作为学习中医学的教材，使其通过学习，掌握中医学的基本理论、基本知识和基本技能，掌握中医学理、法、方、药的基本原则，为今后治病行医奠定基础。此外，本教材可作为通识读本，供爱好传统医学的外国人士阅读，指导其培养养生保健的意识，建立良好的生活习惯与行为。

本教材紧扣中医思维培养的目标，内容专业、翔实、全面，立足实用性，充分考虑临床医学的专业背景和留学生的特殊身份，言简意赅，难易适度，形式多样，集文、图、表多种知识呈现形式，便于学习记忆和知识点之间的横向比较，有利于学生理解和掌握。

本教材共分为十二章，编写分工如下：第一章为中医学的源流与特点，由田露、潘淼编写；第二章为中医学的哲学基础，由林非、王邈编写；第三章为人体的基本物质，由王邈、李国峰、孙牧编写；第四章为脏腑与经络，由刘立明、李晓康编写；第五章为常见病因，由华声瑜、赵宏杰编写；第六章为基本病机，由崔沐群、华声瑜编写；第七章为养生与防治原则，由张璐、李晓康编写；第八章为中医诊断疾病的方法，由戴永娜、杨福双编写；第九章为中医常用的辨证方法，由于志峰、孙峰编写；第十章为中药基本知识，由李英冬、葛骁欧、闫琪编写；第十一章为方剂基本知识，由陈怡、李越、刘佳林编写；第十二章为针灸基本知识，由周禄荣、潘嘉祥编写。全书由付耕南、冯健、张宁苏负责统稿。

在教材编写过程中，长春中医药大学校领导和国际交流合作处领导给予了大力支持，同时也得到中国中医药出版社本教材责任编辑的精心指导和严格把关，在此一并表示感谢。

本教材全体编委会成员反复研究、探讨国际交流合作教材的编写模式，虽竭尽所能，但仍有不足之处，敬请各位同仁不吝赐教。

《中医学基础》编委会

2024 年 7 月

Writing Instructions

Traditional Chinese medicine is an important carrier of China's excellent traditional culture and plays an important role in promoting mutual learning among civilizations and safeguarding people's health. Traditional Chinese medicine is widely recognized by people in many countries for its unique advantages in disease prevention, treatment and rehabilitation. Traditional Chinese medicine has a unique view of life, health, disease and prevention, which has not only made outstanding contributions to the prosperity of the Chinese nation, but also exerted a positive impact on the progress of world civilization. This textbook is led by Changchun University of Traditional Chinese Medicine and jointly compiled by experts from Chinese medicine colleges and universities. It is used by overseas students majoring in clinical medicine in medical colleges and universities across the country and foreigners who are interested in traditional medicine.

The essence of TCM theory, knowledge and skills is innovatively expounded in this textbook using a bilingual form of Chinese and English. It can be used as a textbook for foreign students who come to China to study clinical medicine to help them grasp the basic theories, knowledge and skills of traditional Chinese medicine, as well as understand the basic principles of TCM diagnosis, treatment principles, prescriptions and herbs, laying a foundation for their future medical practice. In addition, this textbook can be used as a general reading material for foreigners who are interested in traditional medicine, and guide them to cultivate their awareness of health care and establish good living habits and behaviors.

This textbook closely follows the goal of cultivating traditional Chinese medicine thinking, with professional, detailed and comprehensive content that is practical and takes into account the professional background of clinical medicine and the special identity of international students. The content is concise and comprehensive, with moderate level of difficulty, diverse forms, and various knowledge presentation methods such as text, pictures, and tables. This facilitates learning, memory retention, and horizontal comparison between knowledge points, which helps students understand and master the material.

This textbook is divided into twelve chapters, and the division of labor is as follows: Chapter 1 is about the origin and characteristics of Traditional Chinese Medicine, written by Tian Lu and Pan Miao; Chapter 2 is the philosophical basis of traditional Chinese medicine, written by Lin Fei and Wang Miao; Chapter 3 is the essential substances of the human body, written by Wang Miao, Li Guofeng, and Sun Mu; Chapter 4 is the zang-fu viscera and meridians, written by Liu Liming and Li Xiaokang; Chapter 5 is about common etiological factors, written by Hua Shengyu and Zhao Hongjie; Chapter 6 is the basic pathogenesis, written by Cui Muqun and Hua Shengyu; Chapter 7 is the principles of health preservation and prevention and treatment, written by Zhang Lu and Li Xiaokang; Chapter 8 is the methods of diagnosing diseases in traditional Chinese medicine, written by Dai Yongna and Yang Fushuang; Chapter 9 is the syndrome differentiation methods commonly used in traditional Chinese medicine, written by Yu Zhifeng and Sun Feng; Chapter 10 is the basic knowledge of Chinese medicine, written by Li Yingdong, Ge Xiaoou, and Yan Qi; Chapter 11 is the basic knowledge of prescriptions, written by Chen Yi, Li Yue, and Liu Jialin; Chapter 12 is the basic knowledge of acupuncture and moxibustion, written by Zhou Lurong and Pan Jiaxiang. Fu Gengnan, Feng Jian, and Zhang Ningsu are responsible for final compilation and editing.

During the compilation of the textbook, we received strong support from the leaders of Changchun University of Traditional Chinese Medicine and the International Exchange and Cooperation Office. Additionally, we benefited from careful guidance and strict quality control provided by the responsible editor at China Traditional Chinese Medicine Press for this textbook. We extend our sincere gratitude to all parties involved.

All members of the editorial board of this textbook have repeatedly studied and discussed the compilation mode of international exchange and cooperation textbooks. Although we have tried our best, there are still shortcomings. We sincerely ask for your valuable advice.

Editorial Board of *Fundamentals of Traditional Chinese Medicine*

July 2024

目 录

第一章　中医学的源流与特点
Chapter 1　Origin and Characteristics of Traditional Chinese Medicine

中医学，是以中医药理论与实践经验为主体，研究人类生命活动中健康与疾病的转化规律及其预防、诊疗、康复的综合性科学。中医学兼具自然科学和社会科学的属性，是综合性的医学科学知识体系。

Traditional Chinese medicine (TCM) is a comprehensive science which takes the theory and practical experience of TCM as its mainstay and studies the transformation between health and disease as well as its prevention, diagnosis, treatment and rehabilitation in human life. It integrates the attributes of natural sciences and social sciences and is a comprehensive medical science system.

第一节　中医学的形成与发展
Section 1　Formation and Development of Traditional Chinese Medicine

中医学历史悠久，源远流长。从原始社会医药知识的逐步积累，到中医学理论体系的确立，再经后世补充、完善，经历了漫长的发展过程。

TCM has a long history. From the accumulation of medical knowledge in primitive society, to the establishment of its theoretical system, and then to the supplementation and perfection by later generations, TCM has developed for a long time.

一、中医学理论体系的形成
1 Formation of the theoretical system of TCM

（一）中医学理论体系形成的条件
1.1 Conditions for the formation of the theoretical system of TCM

中医学理论体系形成的条件包括医疗实践的积累、厚植的中国传统文化底蕴、社会科学和自然科学知识的渗透、丰富而合理的哲学渊源。

These conditions include: the accumulation of medical practice, profound traditional Chinese culture, the infiltration of social sciences and natural sciences and rich and reasonable philosophical origin.

（二）中医学理论体系形成的标志

1.2 The symbol of the formation of the theoretical system of TCM

战国至秦汉时期《黄帝内经》《难经》《伤寒杂病论》《神农本草经》四部医学经典著作的问世，形成了集中医学的理、法、方、药（针）为一体的独特的医学理论体系。

From the Warring States Period (403 BC–221 BC)to Qin and Han Dynasties (221 BC–AD 220), the publication of four TCM classics, namely *Huangdi Neijing (Inner Canon of Huangdi)*（黄帝内经）, *Nan jing (Classic of Questioning)*（难经）, *Shanghan Zabing Lun (Treatise on Cold pathogenic and Miscellaneous Diseases)*（伤寒杂病论）and *Shennong Bencao Jing (Shennong's Classic of Materia Medica)*（神农本草经）, marked the formation of a unique medical theoretical system integrating the principles, methods, formulae and medicines (acupuncture) of TCM.

二、中医学理论体系的发展概况

2 The development of the theoretical system of TCM

中医学在汉代以后进入全面发展时期。魏晋南北朝、隋唐至五代是中国医学发展史上承前启后的重要时期。学科分化日趋成熟，出现了众多名医名著。宋金元时期，流派纷呈，百家争鸣，中药学、方剂学、针灸学、临床各科学等发展迅速，医药著作大量刊行。明清时期，中医学理论深化发展，标志性成果是命门理论的发展、温病理论的创新。近现代时期，中医学理论在自身发展的同时，逐步结合西医学，走上了新的发展道路。

TCM entered an all–round development period after the Han Dynasty (202 BC–AD 220). The period of Wei, Jin, Southern and Northern, Sui, Tang and Five Dynasties (AD 220–AD 960) are important periods of inheriting the past and ushering in the future. At that time, discipline differentiation became increasingly mature, and many famous physicians and works emerged. During the Song, Jin and Yuan Dynasties (AD 960–AD 1368), numerous schools of TCM flourished and contended. Chinese materia medica, prescription, acupuncture and moxibustion, and various clinical specialties developed rapidly, and a large number of medical works were published. During the Ming and Qing Dynasties (AD 1368–AD 1912), TCM theory advanced deeply with the symbolic achievements of the Mingmen (life gate) theory and the innovation of the theory on epidemic febrile diseases. In modern times, in addition to developing itself, TCM theory integrates with Western medicine and embarks on a new development path.

第二节　中医学的基本特点
Section 2　Basic Characteristics of Traditional Chinese Medicine

中医学的理论体系有两个基本特点，一是整体观念，二是辨证论治。

The theoretical system of TCM has two basic characteristics. One is the holism concept, and the other is treatment based on syndrome differentiation.

一、整体观念
1 The holism concept

整体观念，是关于人体自身的完整性及人与自然和社会环境的统一性的认识，是整体思维方法在中医理论中的体现，并贯穿中医学理论和实践始终。

The holism concept is the understanding of the integrity of human body and the unity of man, nature and society and the embodiment of holistic thinking method in TCM theory, running through TCM theory and practice all the time.

（一）人体自身是一个整体
1.1 The human body itself is a whole

中医学认为，人体是一个以心为主宰，五脏为中心，通过经络“内属于脏腑，外络于肢节”联系的有机整体。

According to TCM, the human body is an organic whole with the five zang viscera as the center, the heart as the master, and connected by meridians which travel through the zang-fu viscera inside and the limbs outside.

（二）人与环境的整体关联
1.2 The overall relationship between man and the environment

1. 人与自然环境　人的生命依靠天地之气和水谷精微之气，并伴随着四时寒热温凉、生长化收藏的规律及地理环境的变迁而存在。自然界的变化都对人体产生直接或间接影响，产生一系列生理或病理的变化。

Man and the natural environment　Human life depends on the qi of heaven and earth and the qi of food essence, and exists with the law of warm, hot, cool and cold and birth, growth, transformation, harvest and storage in the four seasons, as well as the change of the geographical environment. Thus, changes in nature have direct or indirect effects on human body, resulting in a series of physiological or pathogenic changes.

2. 人与社会环境　人与人组成了社会。人在生活社会之中，社会环境、生活习性、文化背景的不同，都会造成人们身心功能上的诸多差异，人自身的心理状态也随时影响着人体。

Man and the social environment People form societies. People live in various societies, so different social environments, living habits and cultural backgrounds will all cause many differences in people's physical and mental functions, and people's own psychological states also affect the human body at any time.

二、辨证论治

2 Treatment based on syndrome differentiation

辨证论治，是中医学诊断和治疗疾病的主要方式。辨证，是将四诊所搜集的症状、体征等信息，在中医理论指导下，辨清其原因、性质、部位、邪正关系，概括、判断为某种性质证候的识病方法。论治，是根据辨证的结果，确定相应的治疗方法。

Treatment based on syndrome differentiation is the main way to diagnose and treat diseases in TCM. Syndrome differentiation is a disease recognition method that identifies the symptoms, signs and other information collected by the four diagnostic methods and distinguishes their cause, nature, location and the relationship between vital qi and pathogenic qi, and then summarizes and judges them as a certain syndrome. And the determination of corresponding treatment methods is based on the results of syndrome differentiation.

辨证是确定治疗方法的前提和依据，论治是辨证的目的。

Syndrome differentiation is the premise and basis for determining treatment methods, and treatment is the purpose of syndrome differentiation.

第三节　中医学的主要思维特点

Section 3　Main Thinking Characteristics of Traditional Chinese Medicine

中医思维，是中医学理论体系构建过程中理性的认识方法，是中华优秀传统文化在生命科学领域中的体现。

TCM thinking is rational cognitive methods in the process of constructing the theoretical system of TCM and the embodiment of excellent traditional Chinese culture in the field of life sciences.

一、取象思维

1 The analogy thinking

取象思维，是根据两个（或两类）对象之间在某些方面的相似或相同而推断它们在其他方面也可能相似或相同的一种逻辑方法。中医学常以自然界和社会的事物与人体内在的事物相类比，以探索和论证人体生命活动的规律、疾病的病理变化及疾病的诊断防治等问题，对中医学理论体系的形成和发展发挥了重要的方法学作用。

The analogy thinking is a logical method of deducing that two (or two kinds of) objects may be similar or identical in other aspects according to their similarity or identity in some certain aspects. TCM often draws analogies from the things in nature and society to those in human body to explore and demonstrate the laws of human life activities, pathological changes of diseases, and diagnosis, prevention and treatment of diseases, etc., which plays an important methodological role in the formation and development of the theoretical system of TCM.

二、整体思维
2 The holism thinking

整体思维，是指世界一切事物都广泛联系的思维方法。中医学注重从整体上来认识和分析人体正常生命活动和疾病变化，既注重人体解剖结构、内在脏腑器官的客观存在，又重视各脏腑组织器官之间的功能联系，更强调人体自身内部及人与环境之间的协调统一关系。

The holism thinking refers to the thinking method of considering everything in the world is widely connected. TCM sets great store by understanding and analyzing the normal life activities and disease changes of human body as a whole, paying attention not only to the objective existence of anatomical structure of human body and internal zang–fu viscera and organs, but also to the functional connection between zang–fu viscera, organs and tissues, and emphasizing the coordination and unity within human body and between human and environment.

三、中和思维
3 The neutralization thinking

中和，是中国古代哲学重要的思维方式。中，即不偏不倚的平衡状态；和，是指一切有内在联系的事物之间的和谐状态。中医学认为，人体的阴阳、气血、脏腑功能处于相对平衡状态，就意味着健康；反之，则生疾病。此思想不仅对中医学理论体系的构建起到关键作用，且对养生、诊疗均具有重要意义。

Zhong he (neutralization) is an important way of thinking in ancient Chinese philosophy. “Zhong” (medium) means an impartial and balanced state; while “he” (harmony) refers to the harmonious state among all things with internal relations. TCM believes that if yin and yang, qi and blood and zang–fu viscera functions of human body are in a relatively balanced state, then the person is healthy; if not, diseases will arise. This thought not only plays a key role in the construction of the theoretical system of TCM, but is of great significance to health preservation, disease diagnosis and treatment.

第二章　中医学的哲学基础

Chapter 2　The Philosophical Basis of Traditional Chinese Medicine

中医学在探索人体生命运动规律时，以中国古代先进的哲学理论气一元论、阴阳学说和五行学说作为思维方法，并将其与医学理论相熔铸，使之成为中医学理论体系的重要组成部分。

When exploring the laws of human life movement, TCM takes the advanced ancient Chinese philosophical theories of qi monism, yin–yang theory and five elements theory as its thinking methods, and fuses them with medical theories to incorporate them as an important part of the theoretical system of TCM.

“气－阴阳－五行”的逻辑结构贯穿理、法、方、药各个层面，用以阐释生命的起源和本质，探究生命运动的基本规律，认识并分析疾病的发生发展规律，有效地指导着疾病的诊断、治疗和养生防病。气的相关内容在人体的基本物质章节论述，本章主要介绍阴阳学说及五行学说。

The logical structure of “qi–yin–yang–five elements” runs through all levels of principles, methods, formulae and medicines, which is used to explain the origin and essence of life, explore the basic laws of life movement, understand and analyze the laws of disease occurrence and development, and effectively guide the diagnosis, treatment, health preservation and disease prevention. The related content of qi are included in the chapter of “Essential Substances of the Human Body”. This chapter mainly focuses on yin–yang theory and five elements theory.

第一节　阴阳学说
Section 1　Yin–Yang Theory

一、阴阳的概念与归类
1 The concept and classification of yin and yang

（一）阴阳的概念
1.1 The concept of yin and yang

阴阳是中国古代哲学的基本范畴。气一物两体，分为阴阳。阴阳是自然界的根本规律，标示事物或现象相互对立又相互关联的属性。如明与暗、表与里、寒与热、动与静、内与外等。

Yin and yang are the basic categories of ancient Chinese philosophy. Qi is one thing, but it can be divided into two aspects, that is, yin and yang. Yin and Yang are the fundamental laws of nature, marking the opposite and interrelated attributes of things or phenomena. Such attributes include: bright and dark, exterior and interior, cold and heat, moving and static, inside and outside, etc.

事物或现象的阴阳属性具有普遍性、相对性和关联性。阴阳的普遍性是指阴阳的对立统一是天地万物运动变化的总规律。由于阴和阳之间可以发生相互转化及阴阳的无限可分性，具体事物的阴阳属性并不是绝对的，而是相对的。阴阳的关联性指阴阳所分析的事物或现象应是在同一范畴、同一层次，即相关的基础之上。

The yin and yang attributes of things or phenomena are universal, relative and related. The universality of yin and yang means that the unity and opposition between yin and yang is the general law of the movement and change of all things in the world. Because of the mutual transformation between yin and yang and the infinite separability of yin and yang, the yin and yang attributes of specific things are not absolute, but relative. The correlation between yin and yang means that the things or phenomena analyzed by yin–yang theory should be in the same category and at the same level, namely, they are correlated.

（二）阴阳属性的归类
2.2 The classification of yin and yang attributes

中医学以水火作为阴阳的征象，来划分事物、现象的阴阳属性。凡属于运动的、外向的、上升的、温热的、明亮的、功能的……属于阳的范畴；凡属于静止的、内在的、下降的、寒凉的、晦暗的、物质的……属于阴的范畴。

TCM takes water and fire as the manifestations of yin and yang, and accordingly divides the yin and yang attributes of things and phenomena. Anything featuring sportive, extroverted, rising, warm, bright, functional ... belongs to the category of yang; while anything that featuring static, inner, falling, cool, dull, material ... belongs to the category of yin.

二、阴阳学说的内容
2 The content of yin-yang theory

（一）阴阳对立
2.1 Opposition of yin and yang

阴阳对立，是指阴阳双方的属性相反、互相制约。例如水能灭火，火能烤干湿衣服。阴与阳相互制约和相互斗争的结果须达到动态平衡，事物才能正常发展变化，人体才能维持正常的生理状态。

The opposition of yin and yang means that the yin and yang attributes are opposite and restrict each other. For example, water can extinguish fires, and fire can dry wet clothes. The result of mutual restriction and struggle between yin and yang must be in dynamic balance for things to develop and change normally and human body to maintain normal physiological state.

（二）阴阳互根
2.2 Mutual rooting of yin and yang

阴阳互根，指相互对立的事物之间的相互依存、相互依赖，任何一方都不能脱离另一方而单独存在。如没有下之属阴，也就无所谓上之属阳；没有昼之属阳，就无所谓夜之属阴。

The mutual rooting of yin and yang refers to the interdependence and reliance between mutually opposing things. Neither side can exist independently without the other. For instance, without the lower part belonging to yin, there would be no upper part belonging to yang; without the day belonging to yang, there would be no significance of the night belonging to yin.

（三）阴阳消长
2.3 Waning and waxing of yin and yang

阴阳消长，是阴阳对立双方的增减、盛衰、进退的运动变化。其表现为互为消长和皆消皆长两种形式，是阴阳双方对立斗争、依存互根的必然结果。

The waning and waxing of yin and yang is the increase and decrease, rise and fall, advance and retreat of yin and yang. It is manifested in two forms: mutual waning and waxing as well as both waning or waxing, which is the inevitable result of the opposition and struggle as well as interdependence and mutual rooting between yin and yang.

（四）阴阳转化
2.4 Mutual convertibility of yin and yang

阴阳转化，是指阴阳对立的双方在一定条件下可以相互转化，阴可以转化为阳，阳可以转化为阴。阴阳的转化必须具备一定的条件，这种条件中医学称为“重”或“极”。

The mutual convertibility of yin and yang means that the opposite sides of yin and yang can transform into each other under certain conditions, that is, yin can be transformed into yang and vice versa. In TCM, these certain conditions are called “heavy” or “extreme”.

三、阴阳学说对中医理论的指导
3 The guidance of yin-yang theory to TCM theory

（一）作为思维方法
3.1 As a thinking method

阴阳可用以说明人体的组织结构和生理功能。就人体部位来说：人体的上半身属阳，下半身属阴；背部属阳，腹部属阴；体表属阳，脏腑属阴。人体生理活动的基本规律可概括为阴（物质）与阳（功能）的对立统一运动。人体的生理活动（阳）是以物质（阴）为基础的，没有阴精就无以化生阳气，而生理活动的结果又是不断地化生阴精。

Yin and yang can be used to explain the structure and physiological function of human body. As for parts of human body, the upper part belongs to yang while the lower part belongs to yin; the back belongs to yang while the abdomen pertains to yin; body surface belongs to yang and zang-fu viscera belong to yin. The basic law of human physiological activities can be summarized as the opposition and unity between yin (material) and yang (function). The physiological functions of human body (yang) are based on material (yin). Without yin essence, yang qi cannot be generated, and physiological activities are constantly generating yin essence.

（二）作为具体学术内容
3.2 As specific academic content

中医学在分析病机变化及治疗疾病时，阴阳又作为具体学术内容而被应用。如阴阳失调病机包括阴阳偏盛、阴阳偏衰等病理变化。而调整阴阳，损其有余、补其不足是中医学最重要的治疗法则之一。

When analyzing pathogenesis and treatment methods in TCM, yin and yang are applied as specific academic content. For example, the pathogenesis of yin-yang imbalance includes pathological changes such as excess of either yin or yang and deficiency of either yin or yang.

And regulating yin and yang by damaging its surplus and making up its deficiency is one of the most important treatment principles of TCM.

第二节 五行学说
Section 2 Theory of the Five Elements

一、五行的概念与归类
1 The concept and classification of the five elements

（一）五行的概念和特性
1.1 The concept and characteristics of the five elements

五行是指木、火、土、金、水五类事物及其属性，以及其运动和变化。木具有生长、升发的特性，火具有发热、温暖、向上的特性，土具有载物、生化的特性，金具有沉降、肃杀、收敛、变革的特性，水具有滋润、下行、闭藏的特性。

The five elements refer to five things and attributes of wood, fire, earth, metal and water, as well as their movements and changes. Wood has the characteristics of growth, rise and dispersion; fire has the characteristics of heating, warmth and moving upward; earth is characterized by loading, generation and transformation; metal is characterized by descending, chilliness, convergence and changing; and water is characterized by moistening, moving downward, closing and storing.

（二）五行属性的归类
1.2 The classification of the attributes of the five elements

根据五行的特性，与自然界的各种事物或现象相类比，运用归类和推演等方法，将其最终分成五大类（表 2–1）。

According to the characteristics of the five elements, and using methods of analogy, classification and deduction, all things or phenomena in nature can be divided into five categories (Table 2–1).

表 2-1 自然界事物与人体五行属性归类

Table 2-1 Classification of the Five Elements Attributes of Things in Nature and Human Body

自然界 Nature						五行 Five Elements	人体 Human body					
五味 Five Flavors	五色 Five Colors	五化 Five Transformations	五气 Five Qi	五方 Five Directions	五季 Five Seasons		五脏 Five Zang Viscera	六腑 Six Fu Viscera	五官 Five Organs	形体 Five Tissues	情志 Five Emotions	五液 Five fluids
酸 Sour	青 Blue	生 Birth	风 Wind	东 East	春 Spring	木 Wood	肝 Liver	胆 Gallbladder	目 Eye	筋 Tendon	怒 Anger	泪 Tear
苦 Bitter	赤 Red	长 Growth	暑 Summer Heat	南 South	夏 Summer	火 Fire	心 Heart	小肠 Small Intestine	舌 Tongue	脉 Vessels	喜 Joy	汗 Sweat
甘 Sweet	黄 Yellow	化 Transformation	湿 Dampness	中 Center	长夏 Late Summer	土 Earth	脾 Spleen	胃 Stomach	口 Mouth	肉 Muscles	思 pensiveness	涎 Thin Saliva
辛 Pungent	白 White	收 Harvest	燥 Dryness	西 West	秋 Autumn	金 Metal	肺 Lung	大肠 Large Intestine	鼻 Nose	皮毛 Skin and Hair	悲 Sorrow	涕 Nasal Discharge
咸 Salty	黑 Black	藏 Storage	寒 Cold	北 North	冬 Winter	水 Water	肾 Kidney	膀胱 Bladder	耳 Ear	骨 Bone	恐 Fear	唾 Thick Saliva

二、五行学说的内容

2 The content of the five elements theory

（一）五行的正常调节机制

2.1 The normal regulation mechanism of the five elements

五行的生克制化是在正常状态下五行系统所具有的自我调节机制。

The generation, restraint, control and transformation among the five elements is a self–regulating mechanism of the five elements system under normal conditions.

1. 相生规律 相生即递相资生、助长、促进之意。五行相生的次序是木生火，火生土，土生金，金生水，水生木。

The law of mutual generation Mutual generation means mutual birth, support and promotion. The sequential engendering relationships among the five elements are, wood generates fire, fire generates earth, earth generates metal, metal generates water and water generates wood.

2. 相克规律 相克即相互制约、克制、抑制之意。五行相克的次序是木克土，土克水，水克火，火克金，金克木。

The law of mutual restraint Mutual restraint means mutual restriction, control and inhibition. The sequential restraining relationships among the five elements are, wood restrains earth, earth restrains water, water restrains fire, fire restrains metal, and metal restrains wood.

3. 制化规律 制化是五行生克关系的结合。没有生，就没有事物的发生和成长；没有克，就不能维持正常协调关系下的变化与发展。因此，必须生中有克（化中有制），克中有生（制中有化），相反相成。如木克土，土生金，而金克木；木生火，火生土，木又克土。具体规律见图 2–1。

The law of mutual control and transformation Mutual control and transformation is the combination of the mutual generation and mutual restraint among five elements. Without generation, there will be no birth and growth of things; without restraint, we can’t maintain the change and development under the harmonious condition. Therefore, there must be restraint in generation (control in transformation) and generation in restraint (transformation in control), making their relationships opposite and complementary. For example, wood controls earth with earth generating metal, but metal controls wood; wood generates fire with fire generating earth, but wood controls earth. Figure 2–1 illustrates these specific rules.

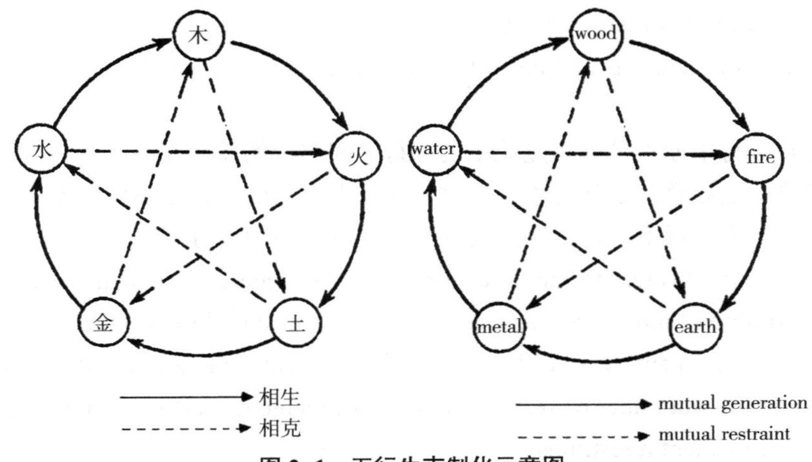

图 2-1　五行生克制化示意图

Figure 2-1.　Generation, Restraint, Control and Transformation among the Five Elements

（二）五行的异常

2.2 The anomaly of the five elements

1. 母子相及　母子相及是五行间不正常的相生现象，包括母病及子和子病及母两个方面。母病及子与相生次序一致，子病及母则与相生的次序相反。如水行不足，影响木行，可引起木也不足，为母病及子；火行太旺，导致木行消耗过快，属于子病及母。

Mutual affecting between mother and child　The mutual affecting between mother and child is abnormal phenomena in the process of mutual generation among the five elements, including mother viscera passing illness to the child one and child's illness affecting the mother. The sequential relationships of mother's illness affecting the child are of the same as those of mutual generation, and the sequential relationships of child's illness affecting the mother are in the same order. For instance, if the water element is so insufficient that it affects the wood element, the wood can also be insufficient, and this is one kind of child's illness affecting the mother; too much fire consumes wood too fast, which belongs to child's illness affecting the mother.

2. 相乘相侮　相乘即相克太过，超过正常制约的程度，使事物之间失去了正常的协调关系。五行之间相乘的次序与相克一致，但被克者更加虚弱。可由五行中任何一行不足或太过导致。如正常情况下，木克土，但若土本身不足（衰弱），或木行太过，两者之间则会失去原来的平衡状态，发生木乘土的变化。

Over-restraint and counter-restraint　Over-restraint means one element restrains the other one so excessive, making things lose their coordinated relationship. The sequential engendering relationships among the five elements are the same as those of the mutual restraint, but the difference is that those that are restraint are made weaker. The reasons can either be insufficiency or excess of any one of the five elements. For example, under normal circumstances, wood restrains earth, but if earth itself is insufficient (too weak), or wood is excessive, the initial balance will be lost , and that's when the wood over–restraining earth occurs.

相侮是指五行中原本具有相克关系的两行之间出现的反向克制。同样可由五行中任何一行不足或太过导致。如某行本身太过，使原来克它的一行，不仅不能去制约它，反而被它所克制；或某行不及，使原本我克一行反过来制约本行。

Counter–restraint refers to the reverse restraint between two elements which originally have the relationship of mutual restraint which can also be caused by insufficiency or excess of any one of the five elements. If one element itself is excessive, the element that restrains it can no longer restrain it, but rather be restrained; or if one element itself is insufficient, it becomes restrained by the element it restrains.

五行的相乘和相侮可同时发生，如木有余可过度克制其所胜之土，同时恃己之强反去克制其“所不胜”的金。

The over–restraint and counter–restraint of the five elements can happen at the same time. For example, if wood is excessive, it will over–restrain earth, and at the same time, it will also counter–restrains metal.

三、五行学说对中医理论的指导

3 The guidance of the five elements theory to TCM theory

（一）构建天人一体的五脏系统

3.1 Building a five zang viscera system integrated with nature

五行学说将人体的内脏分别归属于五行，以五行的特性来说明五脏的部分生理功能。在此基础上，又以类比的方法，根据脏腑组织的性能、特点，将人体的组织结构分属于五行。同时也将人体的五脏、六腑、五体、五官等，与自然界的五方、五季、五味、五色等相应，这样就把人与自然环境统一起来。

The five elements theory classifies the internal organs of the human body into five elements, and explains some of their physiological functions with the characteristics of the five elements. On this basis, it also divides the tissue structure of the human body into five elements according to the property and characteristics of tissue structure as well as the analogy method. In addition, five zang viscera, six fu viscera, five tissues and five senses corresponds to five directions, five seasons, five flavors and five colors in nature, thus unifying man and the natural environment.

（二）说明五脏病变的传变规律

3.2 Explaining the transmission law of diseases of five zang viscera

1. 相生关系传变 包括“母病及子”和“子病及母”两个方面。如水不涵木，主要由于肾阴虚不能滋养肝木，其临床表现为：肾阴不足，多见耳鸣、腰膝酸软、遗精等；肝之阴血不足、肝阳偏亢，多见眩晕、消瘦、乏力、肢体麻木，或手足蠕动，甚则震颤抽搐等。

The transmission through the mutual generation sequence It includes "mother viscera passing illness to the child one" and "child's illness affecting the mother". If water fails to nourish wood, it is mainly due to deficient kidney yin failing to nourish liver wood. Its clinical manifestations are kidney yin deficiency, such as tinnitus, soreness and weakness of waist and knees, spermatorrhea, etc. as well as deficiency of yin and blood in liver, hyperactivity of liver yang, vertigo, emaciation, fatigue, numbness of limbs, wriggling of limbs, and even tremor and spasm.

2. 相克关系传变 包括"相乘"和"相侮"两个方面。如中医学中脾属土，负责运化水湿，脾虚之人容易出现眼睑、下肢等部位水肿，属于土虚水侮的表现。

The transmission through the mutual restraint sequence It includes "over–restraint" and "counter–restraint". For example, in TCM, spleen belongs to earth, which is responsible for transporting and transforming water and dampness. People with spleen deficiency are prone to have edema in eyelids, lower limbs and other parts, which is a manifestation of water counter–restraining earth because of earth deficiency.

（三）指导疾病的诊断、治疗

3.3 Guiding the diagnosis and treatment of diseases

诊断方面，可从本脏所主之色、味、脉来诊断本脏之病，亦可通过五行关系推断脏腑病变的传变趋势。

In terms of diagnosis, we can diagnose the diseases of the internal viscera from their color, taste and pulse and infer the transmission trend of viscera diseases from the relationships among the five elements.

五行学说在治疗上的应用，体现于药物、针灸、精神等疗法之中。中药以色味为基础，以归经和性能为依据，按五行学说加以归类，如青色、酸味入肝，赤色、苦味入心。针灸医学将手足十二经四肢末端的穴位分属于五行，即井、荥、输、经、合五种穴位分属于木、火、土、金、水。临床根据不同的病情以五行生克乘侮规律进行选穴治疗，也可利用情志的相互制约关系来达到治疗的目的，如"怒伤肝，悲胜怒""喜伤心，恐胜喜"等。

The application of the five elements theory in treatment is reflected in medicine, acupuncture and moxibustion, psychotherapy and other therapies. According to the five elements theory, Chinese herbal medicines are classified basing on color and taste as well as meridian tropism and property, such as blue and sourness enter the liver while red and bitterness enter the heart. Acupuncture and moxibustion divides the acupoints at the ends of the limbs of the twelve regular meridians into five elements, that is, the five kinds of acupoints of Jing–well points, Ying–spring points, Shu points, Meridian points and He–sea points respectively belong to wood, fire, earth, metal and water. According to different conditions, And the acupoints are selected for treatment according to the law of the generation, restraint, over–restraint and counter–restraint of the five elements and different disease conditions. What's more, the mutual restraint of emotions can also be used for treatment, such as "excessive anger damaging the liver and sadness prevails over anger", "excessive joy damages the heart and fear prevails over excess joy", etc.

第三章　人体的基本物质
Chapter 3　Essential Substances of the Human Body

气、精、血、津液既是人体脏腑功能活动的产物，又是脏腑功能活动的物质基础。

Qi, essence, blood and fluid are not only the products, but also the material basis of the functions and activities of zang–fu viscera.

第一节　气
Section 1　Qi

一、气的概念与生成
1 The concept and generation of qi

（一）气的概念
1.1 The concept of qi

气是人体内运动不息的精微物质，是构成人体和维持生命活动的基本物质。天地二气交感化生万物，人同样禀受天地之气而生。

Qi is a subtle substance that moves endlessly in human body, and it is one of the essential substances that constitute human body and maintain life activities. Everything is born by the interaction of yin qi and yang qi, and human beings are also born by it.

（二）气的生成
1.2 The generation of qi

人体一身之气由三部分构成：①肾藏精，源于父母的先天之精是肾精的主体。先天之精化生元气，是人体之气的根本，故肾为生气之根。②饮食水谷在脾胃作用下化生水谷之精，再化生水谷之气，为人出生后一身之气的最主要来源，故脾为生气之源。③肺主气，参与宗气的生成，被称为生气之主。

The qi of human body is composed of three parts: ① Kidney stores essence, with the congenital essence originating from parents as its main part. Congenital essence generates primordial qi which is the fundamental of the qi of human body, so kidney is the root of qi. ② With the function of spleen and stomach, water and food are transformed into the essence of water and food, then into the qi of water and food, which is the most important source of qi after birth, so spleen is the source of qi. ③ Lungs govern qi and participate in the generation of pectoral qi, so it is called the master of qi.

二、气的运动与功能

2 The movement and functions of qi

（一）气的运动

2.1 The movement of qi

人体之气有升、降、出、入四种运动形式，是人体生命活动的根本，一旦停息则生命终止。

There are four movement forms of qi, namely, ascending, descending, exiting and entering, which are the foundation of human life activities. Once qi movement stops, life will end.

（二）气的功能

2.2 The functions of qi

1. 推动作用 推动作用指气的激发、兴奋和促进等作用，可激发和促进人体的生长发育与生殖，各脏腑经络的生理功能，精、血、津液的生成及运行，兴奋精神。

Promoting function It refers to the functions of stimulating, exciting and promoting of qi. It means qi can stimulate and promote the growth and reproduction of human body, the physiological functions of various viscera and meridians and the generation and circulation of essence, blood and fluid, as well as exciting the brain.

2. 温煦作用 指阳气温暖周身的作用。如维持体温稳定；温煦脏腑经络、形体官窍，以及精、血、津液等生命物质，维持其正常的生理活动。

Warming function It refers to the functions regarding yang qi warming the whole body, such as maintaining body temperature; warming viscera, meridians, body constituents and orifices, as well as essence, blood, fluid and other substances to maintain their normal physiological activities.

3. 防御作用 指抵御外邪的入侵及祛邪外出。气的防御功能正常，邪气不易侵入；即便侵入，发病亦多轻浅，易于治愈。

Defensive function It refers to resisting the invasion of external pathogenic factors or dispelling them. If the defensive function of qi is normal, the pathogenic qi is not easy to invade; even if it invades, the condition is mild and the location is superficial, so it's easy to cure.

4. 固摄作用 指气对体内液态物质的固护、统摄作用。

Securing function It means qi can secure and astringe fluid substances in the human body.

三、气的分类

3 The classification of qi

（一）分类依据

3.1 The classification basis

气因来源、部位及功能不同而分类，共包含三个层次：第一层次是人身之气，亦称一身之气；第二层次是元气、宗气、营气、卫气；第三层次是脏腑之气、经络之气。

The classification of qi includes three levels with different basis of sources, positions and functions: the first level is the human qi, also known as the whole body qi; the second level is primordial qi, pectoral qi, nutrient qi and defense qi; and the third level is qi of zang-fu viscera and qi of meridians.

（二）具体类别

3.2 Specific categories

元气，指主要由先天精气所化生，赖后天充养的气，是人体最根本、最重要的气。

Primordial qi refers to the qi mainly produced by congenital essence and nourished by acquired essence, which is the most fundamental and important qi of human body.

宗气，指自然界清气与水谷精气融合化生并聚于胸中之气，具有行呼吸、行气血和资先天三个方面的作用。

Pectoral qi refers to the qi merged with clear qi in nature and qi of water and food and gathered in the chest. It has three functions: controlling breathing, circulating qi and blood, and supplementing congenital essence.

营气，指由水谷精微中精专柔和部分所化生的气，行于脉内，具有化生血液、营养周身的功能。

Nutrient qi refers to the qi generated by the subtle and soft parts of food essence, which travels in the vessels and has the functions of generating blood and nourishing the whole body.

卫气，指由水谷精微中剽悍滑疾部分所化生的气，行于脉外，具有温煦机体，司汗孔开合，卫护肌表、抗御外邪的功能。

Defense qi refers to the qi generated by the fierce and slippery part of food essence, traveling outside the vessels and has the functions of warming the body, opening and closing sweat pores, defending muscle surface and resisting external pathological factors.

脏腑之气与经络之气支撑各脏腑经络的功能活动。

Qi of zang-fu viscera and qi of meridians support the functions and activities of each zang-fu viscera and meridians.

第二节 精
Section 2 Essence

一、精的概念与生成
1 The concept and generation of precision

（一）精的概念
1.1 The concept of essence

精是构成和维持人体生命活动的最基本物质。广义之精是气、血、津液等人体一切精微物质的统称，狭义之精专指生殖之精。

Essence is the most the essential substances that constitute human body and maintain life activities. In its broad sense, essence is the joint name of all subtle substances of human body, including qi, blood and fluid. But broadly speaking, essence refers to the essence of reproduction.

（二）精的生成
1.2 The generation of essence

人体之精由禀受于父母的先天之精及来源于吸入清气与水谷精微的后天之精相融合而生成。

The essence of human body is generated by the integration of congenital essence from parents and acquired essence from inhaled clear qi and food essence.

二、精的功能
2 The functions of essence

1. 繁衍生命 生殖之精具有繁衍生命的功能。男女媾精，阴阳调和，胎孕方成。

Reproducing life The essence of reproduction has the function of reproducing life. Men and women have sex with each other, so yin and yang are interacted, and pregnancy is achieved.

2. 濡养作用 精能濡养滋润一身之脏腑、形体、官窍。

Moistening and nourishing Essence can moisten and nourish the zang-fu viscera, body constituents and orifices.

3. 化气、化血、化神作用 精是气血生成的重要来源，先天之精化生元气，后天之精化生谷气，与肺吸入自然界清气相结合，构成一身之气。肾精与肝血同源，相互资生、转化，精足则血旺，精亏则血虚。精又能够化神，是神产生的物质基础。

Transforming into qi, blood and spirit Essence is an important source of qi and blood. Congenital essence generates primordial qi while acquired essence generates food qi, and these two kinds of qi are combined with clear qi in nature inhaled by lungs to form the whole body qi. Kidney essence and liver blood share the same source and they can generate and transform into each other. Sufficient essence lead to hyperactivity of blood, while essence deficiency causes blood deficiency. Essence can transform into spirit, serving as the material basis for the generation of spirit.

4. 抗邪作用 精具有保卫机体、抵御外邪入侵的功能。

Resisting pathological factors Essence has the function of protecting the body and resisting the invasion of pathological factors.

5. 生长发育 人体之精是机体生长发育的物质基础，具有推动和促进人体生长发育的作用。

Promoting growth and development The essence of human body, the material basis of the growth and development of the body, has the function of promoting the growth and development of human body.

三、精的分类

3 The classification of essence

从来源上，精可分为先天之精与后天之精。前者指源于父母，构成胚胎的原始物质；后者是指脾胃运化生成的水谷精微。

Essence can be divided into congenital essence and acquired essence according to the source. The former refers to the initial substance that originates from parents and forms embryo while the latter refers to the food essence transported and transformed by the spleen and stomach.

从功能上，精可分为脏腑之精与生殖之精。前者指脏腑所藏的具有濡养、滋润作用的精华物质；后者是由先天之精在后天之精的充养和天癸的激发下形成的，具有繁衍后代的功能。

Essence can be divided into essence of zang–fu viscera and essence of reproduction according to the function. The former refers to the essence substance with nourishing and moistening functions stored by zang–fu viscera; the latter is formed by the congenital essence nourished by the acquired essence and stimulated by tian gui (sex promoter), and has the function of reproducing offspring.

第三节 血
Section 3 Blood

一、血的概念与生成
1 The concept and generation of blood

（一）血的概念
1.1 The concept of blood

血即血液，是行于血脉之中，循环于全身，具有营养和滋润作用的红色液态物质。

Blood is a red fluid substance that runs in the blood vessels, circulates throughout the whole body and has the functions of moistening and nourishing.

（二）血的生成
1.2 The generation of blood

水谷精微和肾精是血液化生的基础物质。在脾、胃、心、肺、肾等脏腑的共同作用下，化生为血液。

Food essence and kidney essence are the basic substances of blood generation. They can be transformed into blood with the joint action of spleen, stomach, heart, lungs, kidneys and other zang–fu viscera.

二、血的功能
2 The functions of blood

1. 濡养作用 血液具有营养和滋润全身的功能。血液充盈，则面色红润，肌肉壮实，皮肤毛发润泽，肢体感觉灵敏，运动自如。

Moistening and nourishing Blood has the function of nourishing and moistening the whole body. When the blood is sufficient, the person will have ruddy complexion, strong muscles, moist skin and hair, and sensitive and flexible limbs.

2. 化神作用 血液是人体精神活动的主要物质基础。若血液充盛，则精神充沛，神志清晰，感觉灵敏，活动自如。若血亏、血热，或内有瘀血，则可出现多种精神情志方面的病证。

Transforming into spirit Blood is the main material basis of human mental activities. If the blood is sufficient, then untiring energy, clear mind, sensitive feeling and flexible movement can be seen. Blood deficiency, blood heat or blood stasis can cause a variety of mental and emotional disorders.

三、血与气的关系
3 The relationship between blood and qi

血与气的关系体现在：一为血能养气，对气具有化生作用；二为血能载气，血液是气的载体，气存于血中，依附血液而不致散失。同时，血液的运行有赖于气的推动、温煦和固摄作用。气的推动作用，是血液运行的根本动力。气的温煦作用，也是维持血液正常运行的重要因素。气的固摄作用，保障了血液行于脉中而不逸出脉外。

The functions of blood on qi is are as follows. First, blood can nourish qi, having the function of generating qi; second, blood can carry qi, which means that blood is the carrier of qi, making qi exists in blood without dissipating. In the meantime, the circulation of blood depends on the promoting, warming and securing functions of qi. The promoting function of qi is the fundamental driving force of blood circulation. The warming function of qi is also an important factor to maintain the normal circulation of blood. The securing function of qi ensures that blood travels in the vessels without escaping out of the vessels.

第四节 津 液
Section 4 Fluid

一、津液的概念与生成
1 The concept and generation of fluid

（一）津液的概念
1.1 The concept of fluid

津液，是人体一切正常水液的统称，包括脏腑、形体、官窍的内在液体及其正常的分泌物，分为津与液。

Fluid is a joint name for all normal fluid in human body, including the internal fluid of zang-fu viscera, body constituents and orifices and their normal secretion, and it is divided into clear fluid and turbid fluid.

（二）津液的生成
1.2 The generation of fluid

津液来源于饮食水谷，在脾胃运化及有关脏腑的共同参与下生成。胃主受纳腐熟，参与将饮食水谷转化为精微及津液的过程。小肠主液，吸收肠中大部分津液。大肠主津，可吸收食物残渣中的津液，促使糟粕成形为粪便。胃、小肠、大肠所吸收的津液，均依赖脾的运化功能而得以生成，并通过脾气的转输及肺气的宣发肃降作用布散到全身。

Fluid comes from water and food, which is generated under the joint effort of spleen and stomach and other related zang–fu viscera. The stomach governs receiving, holding and decomposition, and participates in the process of transforming water and food into essence and fluid. The small intestine governs thick fluid and absorbs most fluid in the intestine. The large intestine governs thin fluid, and can absorb fluid in food residues and promote them to form feces. The fluid absorbed by stomach, small intestine and large intestine is generated depending on the transportation and transformation function of spleen, and is distributed to the whole body through the transportation function of spleen qi and the purification and descending function of lung qi.

二、津液的功能

2 The functions of fluid

1. 滋润濡养　津的性状较清稀，主要布散于皮毛、肌腠，以及目、口、鼻、耳等官窍，起滋润作用；液的性状较为稠厚，灌注于脏腑、骨髓、脑脊髓及关节，起濡养作用。

Moistening and nourishing　The thin fluid is clear and thin, mainly existing in skin and hair, muscles and interstices, eyes, mouth, nose, ears and other orifices, and play a moistening role; The thick fluid is relatively thick and perfuses into zang–fu viscera, bone marrow, brain marrow, spinal cord and joints, and plays a role in nourishing.

2. 充养血脉　津液可以渗入血脉，并化生血液。津液和血液都来源于水谷精微，两者之间又能够相互渗透和转化。

Nourishing blood vessels　Fluid can penetrate into blood vessels and transform into blood. Fluid and blood both come from the food essence, and they can penetrate and transform into each other.

三、津液与气、血的关系

3 The relationship between fluid and qi and blood

气行则津行，津液在气的作用下，向上、向外输布至人体上部和体表，向下、向内滋养其他脏腑并输布至膀胱。津液与血液同源化生，且能相互转化，故有津血同源之说。

With the promoting function of qi, fluid is transported upward and outward to the upper part and surface of human body, and transported downward and inward to nourish zang–fu viscera and enter the bladder. Fluid and blood share the same source and can transform into each other, so it is said that fluid and blood are homologous.

第四章 脏腑与经络

Chapter 4 Zang-fu Viscera and Meridians

脏腑是人体内脏的总称。经络是联通人体脏腑和外周的通道。

The term zang-fu viscera is the general name of human internal organs. Meridians are the channels connecting zang-fu viscera and periphery of human body.

在哲学思想的指导下，古代中医对内脏的研究偏重功能而略于解剖。根据功能特点的不同，脏腑被分为五脏、六腑和奇恒之腑三类。

Under the guidance of philosophy, the study of internal organs in ancient Chinese medicine focused on their functions rather than anatomy. According to different functions, zang-fu viscera are divided into five zang viscera, six fu viscera and extraordinary fu-viscera.

五脏，即心、肺、脾、肝、肾，它们的共同功能特点是化生和贮藏精气。六腑，即胆、胃、小肠、大肠、膀胱、三焦，它们的共同功能特点是传化食物。奇恒之腑，即脑、髓、骨、脉、胆、女子胞，它们的功能与五脏类似，形态却多与六腑相似。

The five zang viscera, namely, heart, lungs, spleen, liver and kidneys, all have the function of generating and storing essence and qi. Six fu viscera, namely, gallbladder, stomach, small intestine, large intestine, bladder and sanjiao, all have the function of transmitting and transforming food. Extraordinary fu-viscera, namely, brain, marrow, bone, vessels, gallbladder and uterus, have similar functions to the five zang viscera, but their shapes are more similar to the six fu viscera.

第一节 五 脏

Section 1 Five Zang Viscera

一、心

1 Heart

心位于胸腔。心为阳中之阳，五行属火。心通过经脉与小肠构成阴阳相配的关系。

The heart is located in the thoracic cavity. It is yang within yang, and belongs to fire in terms of five elements. The heart and the small intestine form a pairing relationship of yin and yang through meridians.

（一）心的主要功能

1.1 The main functions of the heart

1. 心主血脉 心的阳气是心跳的动力，能推动和温煦血液，从而将富有营养的血液推送到全身。心的阴气负责制约阳气，避免心阳亢进而心跳过速。

The heart governs the blood and vessels The yang qi of the heart is the driving force of the heartbeat, which can promote and warm the blood, thus pushing the nutritious blood to the whole body. The yin qi of the heart is responsible for restricting yang qi, thus avoiding fast heartbeat due to hyperactivity of heart yang.

2. 心主神明 《素问·灵兰秘典论》载："心者，君主之官也，神明出焉。"心具有主管生命和精神活动的功能。广义的神是生命活动的综合体现，包括生理和心理活动，可以从面色、眼神、言语、应答、肢体姿态等观察。狭义的神是指人的意识活动、思维和情绪。这些活动都由心主宰。

The heart governs the mind and spirit *Suwen Ling Lan Mi Dian Lun*（素问·灵兰秘典论）records: "The heart is the viscus similar to the monarch and is responsible for spirit and mental activity." The heart has the function of governing life and mental activities. Broadly speaking, spirit is the comprehensive embodiment of life activities, including physiological and psychological activities, which can be observed from complexion, eyes, words, responses, postures and so on. In a narrow sense, it refers to people's conscious activities, thoughts and emotions. These activities are all dominated by the heart.

（二）心的外应内合

1.2 The external manifestations of the heart

1. 心在体合脉 心连通血脉，血脉随心的跳动而搏动，配合完成推动血液行于全身的功能。心气充足则脉象正常。

The vessels are the outer aspect of the heart The heart connects the blood vessels which throbs with heartbeat, and they work together to complete the function of pushing blood to the whole body. If the heart qi is sufficient, the vessels condition will be normal.

2. 心其华在面 华指外在的光彩。五脏精气血的盛衰可表现于体表的不同部位。心的气血运行可以从面部加以了解。心的气血充足且运行无阻，则面色红润有光泽；心神正常，则面部表情自然。

The lustre of the heart shows in the face Lustre refers to the external brilliance. The sufficiency or deficiency of essence, qi and blood of the five zang viscera can be manifested in different parts of the body surface. And the circulation of qi and blood in the heart manifests on the face. If the qi and blood of the heart are sufficient and run unimpeded, the complexion is ruddy and shiny; If the mind is normal, the facial expression will be natural.

3. 心开窍于舌 舌位于口腔，具有感受味觉、辅助进食和发音等功能。心与舌有络脉相连，舌的颜色、运动、味觉与心主血脉和主神志有关。

The heart opens into the tongue The tongue is located in the mouth and has the functions of receiving taste, and assisting eating and pronunciation. Heart and tongue are connected by collaterals, and the color, movement and taste of tongue are related to heart's functions of governing blood vessels and spirit.

4. 心在液为汗 汗是阳气蒸发阴津从汗孔排出而成，即汗为津液转化，而血液与津液可相互转化，心主血脉，所以汗的产生与心有一定关系。

The fluid of the heart is sweat Yin fluid evaporated by yang qi discharges from sweat pores to form sweat, which means sweat is transformed from fluid. Blood and fluid can transform into each other, and the heart governs blood vessels, so the generation of sweat has a certain relationship with the heart.

5. 心在志为喜 喜，是满足、放松、愉快的情绪。心的功能正常，则较易欢喜，有利于健康；反之，如果喜乐过度，则可使心神涣散，甚至导致心气暴脱而亡等。

The emotion of the heart is joy Joy is a feeling of satisfaction, relaxation and happiness. If the function of the heart is normal, it is easier to be happy, which is beneficial to health; on the contrary, if the joy is excessive, it can cause mind distraction, and even lead to death caused by sudden collapse of heart qi.

6. 心应夏 夏季是一年之中炎热的季节，属阳中之阳的太阳。心为火脏，阳气最盛，同气相求，故与夏季相通应。

The season of the heart is summer Summer is the hottest season of the year, which belongs to the yang within yang, namely, taiyang. The heart is the viscus of fire and has the most abundant yang qi, which accounts for its correspondence to summer.

二、肺
2 Lungs

肺位于胸腔，左右各一，通过气道与自然界相通。肺为阳中之阴，五行属金。肺通过经脉与大肠构成阴阳相配的关系。

The lungs are located in the thoracic cavity, one on the left and one on the right, and connect with nature through the airway. Lungs are yin within yang, and belong to metal in terms of five elements. The lungs and the large intestine form a pairing relationship of yin and yang through meridians.

（一）肺的主要功能
2.1 The main functions of the lungs

1. 肺主呼吸，生成宗气 肺主管呼吸运动，是清浊之气的交换场所。肺吸入的清气是人体之气的来源之一，宗气就是由肺所吸入的清气和脾运化的水谷精气结合而生成的。肺气旺盛，呼吸正常，则有利于全身的气升降协调，从而维持人体生命活动的正常进行。

The lungs govern breathing and the generation of pectoral qi The lungs govern respiratory movement, serving as the exchange place of clear qi and turbid qi. Clear qi inhaled by lungs is one of the sources of human qi, and pectoral qi is generated by the combination of clear qi inhaled by lungs and qi of water and food transported and transformed by spleen. Exuberant lung qi and normal breathing are conducive to the coordination of qi ascending and descending of the whole body, thus maintaining the normal human life activities.

2. 肺朝百脉，助心行血 肺朝百脉是指肺中有众多血脉，而且肺与心相通，经过肺的气体交换，将含清气的血液由心主导输送至全身。如果肺气虚弱，呼吸功能减弱，血中浊气多而清气少，则不利于心主血脉功能，可表现为胸中憋闷胀痛、咳喘、心悸和唇舌青紫等症。

The lungs preside over all vessels and helps the heart to circulate blood The lungs preside over all vessels, which means that there are many blood vessels in the lungs. The lungs connect with the heart and through the qi exchange of the lungs, the blood containing clear qi is transported from the heart to the whole body. If lung qi is weak, breathing is weakened, and there is more turbid qi in blood and less clear qi. All this is not conducive to the function of heart governing blood and vessels, which can be manifested as chest tightness and distending pain, cough and asthma, palpitation, blue lips and tongue, etc.

3. 肺通调水道，促进水行 水液代谢平衡需要多个脏腑的共同合作。肺气能宣发和肃降，可将津液输布于全身各脏腑器官与皮毛、肌腠，以发挥津液滋养作用，也有利于汗液的形成。

The lungs regulate water channels and promotes the circulation of water The balance of fluid metabolism requires the cooperation of multiple viscera. Lung qi governs upward and outward diffusion as well as descent and purification, distributing fluid to all viscera, skin, hair, muscles and interstices of the whole body, so as to play the nourishing function of fluid and promote the formation of sweat.

（二）肺的外应内合

2.2 The external manifestations of the lungs

1. 肺在体合皮 肺气宣发，将卫气、津液和水谷精微布散至体表，以护卫、温养和润泽皮肤。

The outer aspect of the lungs is the skin Lung qi governs upward and outward diffusion, and distribute the defence qi, fluid and food essence to the body surface to protect, warm and moisten the skin.

2. 肺其华在毛 毫毛生长于皮肤，肺宣发津液在润泽皮肤时也使得毫毛获得养分。肺的功能异常时，可见皮毛枯槁稀疏。

The lustre of the lungs shows in the hair Hairs grow on the skin. Lungs promote the upward and outward diffusion of fluid to moisten the skin, also making hair get nutrients in this process. When the lung function is abnormal, it can be seen that hair is withered, yellow and sparse.

3. 肺开窍于鼻　鼻为呼吸道的最上端，肺的呼吸生理功能与鼻的关系密切。外邪常从口鼻而入，进一步引起肺的功能失常。

The lungs open into the nose Nose is the uppermost part of respiratory tract, and the respiratory function of lungs is closely related to nose. Exogenous pathogens often enter through the nose and mouth, further causing malfunctioning lungs.

4. 肺在液为涕　鼻涕湿润鼻腔，有清洁和保护鼻腔的作用。由于鼻为肺窍，肺的病证常可见鼻涕的分泌和色质异常改变。

The fluid of the lungs is nasal discharge Nasal discharge moistens the nasal cavity and has the function of cleaning and protecting it. Because the nose is the orifice of the lungs, the abnormal changes of the secretion, color and property of nasal discharge can often be seen in lung diseases.

5. 肺在志为悲　悲是人的低沉消极情绪，过度的悲伤能耗伤肺气，导致呼吸短促、少气懒言、体倦乏力等肺气虚证。

The emotion of the lungs is sorrow Sorrow is a person's low and negative emotion. Excessive sorrow consumes hurts lung qi, which leads to syndrome of deficiency of lung qi, including such symptoms as shortness of breath, panting, no desire to speak, tiredness and fatigue.

6. 肺应秋　秋为阳中之阴的太阴，人体肺气清肃下降，同气相求，与秋季相通应。

The season of the lungs is autumn Autumn belongs to yin within yang, namely, shaoyin. The lung qi of human body governs descent and purification, which is similar to the qi movement in autumn, so the lungs correspond to autumn.

三、脾
3 Spleen

脾位于左上腹内。中医学所指的“脾”不同于西医学的脾脏。脾为阴中之至阴，五行属土。脾通过经脉与胃构成阴阳相配的关系。

The spleen is located in the left upper abdomen. The spleen in TCM is different from that in western medicine. Spleen is yin within yin, and belongs to earth in terms of five elements. The spleen and the stomach form a pairing relationship of yin and yang through meridians.

（一）脾的主要功能
3.1 The main functions of the spleen

1. 脾主运化　运化即转运、消化和吸收。小肠进一步消化吸收的过程需要脾的主导，脾进一步将精微物质上输于心肺，化生为气血，以营养全身；脾也直接将精微物质布散至附近的脏腑组织而发挥其营养作用。

The spleen governs transportation and transformation Transportation and transformation refers to transportation, digestion and absorption. The process of further digestion and absorption of the small intestine needs the leading role of the spleen which further transports subtle substances to the heart and lungs and transforms them into qi and blood to nourish the whole body; spleen also directly distributes subtle substances to nearby viscera to play their role in nourishing the viscera.

脾气运动以升为主：一方面将消化吸收的水谷精微上输于心肺及头面五官，通过心肺的作用化生为气血，营养全身；另一方面，脾气具有托举内脏，使其维持相对恒定位置的作用。

Spleen qi mainly ascends. On the one hand, it distributes the digested and absorbed food essence to the heart, lungs, head, face and five organs of the head and face, and transforms it into qi and blood through the action of the heart and lungs to nourish the whole body; on the other hand, spleen qi has the function of lifting viscera and maintaining them in a relatively constant position.

2. 脾统血 脾气具有控制血液在脉管内流行而防止血逸出脉外的功能，这实际上是气的固摄作用。脾气虚则不能统血，可导致皮下出血、便血、尿血、月经过多等。

The spleen contains blood The spleen qi has the function of controlling the blood to circulate within vessels and preventing it from escaping out of the vessels, which actually belongs to the securing function of qi. Deficiency of spleen qi causes failure in controlling blood, which can lead to subcutaneous hemorrhage, hemafecia, hematuria, menorrhagia and so on.

（二）脾的外应内合

3.2 The external manifestations of the spleen

1. 脾在体合肉 全身尤其是四肢肌肉的丰满与否，是由精微的多少决定的。如果脾气虚，人体产生和吸收的精微物质不足，则四肢肌肉消瘦无力。

The outer aspect of the spleen is the muscles The fullness of the whole body, especially the muscles of the limbs, is determined by the sufficiency of essence. If the spleen qi is deficient, the subtle substances produced and absorbed by the human body will be insufficient, and so the muscles of the limbs will be emaciated and weak.

2. 脾其华在唇 脾的功能正常与否影响唇的色泽。脾气健运，气血生成充足，则口唇红润光泽；脾气虚则可致气血虚，唇色淡白。

The lustre of the spleen shows in the lips The spleen's function affects the color and lustre of lips. If the spleen qi functions well, the qi and blood will be sufficient, and so the lips will be ruddy and lustrous; deficiency of spleen qi can lead to deficiency of qi and blood, and the lips will turn pale.

3. 脾开窍于口 口腔是消化道的开端，口腔辨食物滋味与脾的运化功能密切相关。脾气健运，则口味良好，食欲正常；反之则食欲不振，口淡无味。

The spleen opens into the mouth Mouth is the first organ of the digestive tract, and the differentiation of food taste in mouth cavity is closely related to the transportation and transformation function of the spleen. If the spleen qi functions well, taste and appetite will be normal; on the contrary, poor appetite and bland taste in the mouth will occur.

4. 脾在液为涎 涎具有湿润食物，使其易于吞咽的作用。脾气健旺，运化水液功能正常，则水液上行润口；如脾气虚而不摄津，涎液可自口角流出。

The fluid of the spleen is thin saliva Thin saliva has the function of moistening food and making it easy to swallow. If the spleen qi is sufficient, and the function of transporting and transforming fluid is normal, the fluid will go up and moisten the mouth; if the spleen qi is too deficient to control blood, thin saliva can flow out from the corners of the mouth.

5. 脾在志为思 脾气健运则气血旺盛，有利于血养神。过度思虑则导致脾气结滞，运化功能失常，出现不思饮食、腹胀等；久则气血生成不足，导致形体消瘦。

The emotion of the spleen is pensiveness If the spleen qi functions well, qi and blood will be exuberant, which is beneficial for blood to nourish the mind. Excessive pensiveness leads to stagnation of spleen qi and dysfunction of transportation and transformation, including such symptoms as poor appetite, abdominal distension and so on; if it lasts for a long time, the qi and blood will be insufficient, resulting in emaciation.

6. 脾应长夏与脾主四时 关于脾主时有两种学说。一种学说认为脾与长夏相通应，因脾属土，土生万物，长夏为气候炎热，万物华实，故脾与长夏同气相求而相通应。另一种学说认为脾主四时，因脾属土，居中央，主四时，以四季之末各十八日统领其他四脏。

The season of the spleen is late summer and the spleen governs the four seasons There are two theories about spleen governing seasons. One is that spleen corresponds to late summer. The spleen belongs to the earth which generates everything, and the late summer is hot and everything is prosperous in this season, so the spleen is similar to the late summer and corresponds to it. The other is that the spleen governs the four seasons. Because the spleen belongs to the earth and locates in the center, it governs the four seasons as well as the other four zang viscera by commanding eighteen days at the end of each season.

四、肝
4 Liver

肝位于右上腹腔之内，肝为阴中之阳，五行属木。肝通过经脉与胆构成阴阳相配的关系。中医学以木性升发、条达舒畅来类推肝脏的特性和生理功能。

The liver is located in the upper right abdominal cavity. It is yang within yin, and belongs to wood in terms of five elements. The liver and the gallbladder form a pairing relationship of yin and yang through meridians. In TCM, the characteristics and physiological functions of the liver are analogized by the wood's ascending, dispersing, free will and refreshing characteristics.

（一）肝的主要功能

4.1 The main functions of the liver

1. 肝主疏泄 肝能疏通调畅全身的气机，这有利于以下各方面功能的顺利进行。

The liver governs the free flow of qi The liver can maintain free flow of qi over the entire body, which is conducive to the following subdivided functions.

（1）维持血的运行 血液需要气的推动才能运行，肝主疏泄功能正常，则各脏腑气机调畅，血液能正常在脉中运行，从而发挥濡养作用。

Maintaining the circulation of blood Blood needs the promotion of qi to circulate. If the liver can govern the free flow of qi, the qi movement of each zang–fu viscera will be smooth, and the blood can run normally in the pulse, thus playing a nourishing role.

（2）调畅情志 肝主疏泄功能正常，有助于血养神，从而维持情志的正常反应。

Regulating emotion The liver's function of governing the free flow of qi helps blood to nourish spirit, thus maintaining the normal reaction of emotion.

（3）促进饮食消化 肝可以协助脾的升清和胃的降浊；肝可以分泌胆汁，帮助食物消化。

Promoting digestion The liver can help the spleen to ascend the clear and the stomach to descend the turbid; it can also secrete bile to help digest food.

（4）协助水液代谢 水液的运行需要各脏腑之气的推动作用，肝能促进各脏腑气机调畅，这有利于维持水液正常的输布与排泄。

Assisting the metabolism of fluid fluid requires the promotion of qi in zang–fu viscera, and the liver can promote the free flow of qi in each viscus, which is conducive to maintaining the normal distribution and excretion of fluid.

（5）调节生殖功能 肝的疏泄作用能促进女子的排卵和月经，也能促进男子的排精。

Regulating reproduction This function means the liver can promote ovulation and menstruation of women as well as spermiation of men.

2. 肝藏血 肝内贮藏有一定的血液，除了濡养自身，还有助于以下生理活动。

The liver stores blood There is a certain amount of blood stored in the liver, which not only nourishes the liver itself, but also contributes to the following physiological activities.

（1）制约肝阳，防止其上亢 由于阴阳有互相制约的关系，肝的阴血可以制约肝的阳气，这有助于维持肝的正常疏泄功能。

Restricting liver yang and preventing its hyperactivity Because yin and yang can control each other, yin blood of liver can control its hyperactive yang qi, which is helpful to maintain the normal function of governing the free flow of qi.

（2）涵养魂　魂是神的一种，与做梦等意识活动相关。血可藏神，所以肝血充足，则魂能安居于肝血中而不妄动。

Cultivating the soul　Soul is a kind of spirit, which is related to consciousness activities such as dreaming. Blood can store spirit, so sufficient liver blood can maintain the soul stored in liver blood without reckless stirring.

（3）调节血流量　当人休息时，肢体等部位对血液的需要量减少，多余的血液就归于肝；当人体活动时，肝将所贮藏的血液通过血脉送到头面和四肢。

Regulating blood flow　When people rest, the demand for blood in limbs and other parts decreases, and excess blood is stored in the liver; when people move, the liver sends the stored blood to the head, face and limbs through blood vessels.

（4）防止出血　是指肝气具有固摄血液的作用，可防止血液逸出脉外。

Preventing bleeding　It means that liver qi has the function of securing blood and preventing blood from escaping out of the vessels.

（二）肝的外应内合

4.2 The external manifestations of the liver

1. 肝在体合筋　全身筋的运动需要肝血的滋养。肝血充足，则肢体活动自如有力。

The outer aspect of the liver is the tendons　Tendons of the whole body needs the nourishment of liver blood. If liver blood is sufficient, limbs can move freely and forcefully.

2. 肝其华在爪　爪甲为筋的衍生，即“爪为筋之余”。肝血在濡养四肢远端筋肉时，也能濡养爪甲，爪甲的色泽正常与否可以反映肝血的盛衰。

The lustre of the liver shows in the nails　Nails are the derivative of the tendons, that is, “Nails are the extension of the tendons”. In addition to nourishing the tendons and muscles at the distal end of limbs, liver blood can also nourish nails. Whether the color and lustre of nails is normal or not can reflect the sufficiency and deficiency of liver blood.

3. 肝开窍于目　肝的经脉连目系（眼球连于脑的组织），视觉有赖于肝血对眼球的滋养。

The liver opens into the eyes　The liver meridian connects the eye system (the tissue that connects eyeball and brain), so vision depends on the nourishment of liver blood to the eyeball.

4. 肝在液为泪　泪由肝的阴液上于目所化生。

The fluid of the liver are tears　Tears are generated from the yin fluid of the liver ascending to the eyes.

5. 肝在志为怒　如肝气郁滞或升发太过，就难以维持情志的稳定，人容易急躁发怒；而强烈的不满也可反过来使肝气不舒，导致两胁胀痛等病症，即大怒伤肝。

The emotion of the liver is anger　Stagnation or excessive ascending and dispersing of liver qi leads to difficulty in maintaining emotional stability, and people are prone to impatience and rage. And huge dissatisfaction can in turn suppress liver qi, resulting in symptoms such as distending pain in both hypochondrium, which is the so called , great anger damages the liver.

6. 肝应春　春季阳气始生，万物欣欣向荣，属阴中之阳的少阳。人体肝气生发、疏泄，肝喜条达，恶抑郁，故与春气相通应。

The season of the liver is spring　Yang qi comes into being and everything is thriving in spring which belongs to yang within yin (shaoyang). The liver qi ascends and disperses and the liver likes free will and hates to be suppressed, so it corresponds to spring.

五、肾

5 Kidneys

肾位于腰脊内部两旁，左右各一。肾为阴中之阴，五行属水。肾通过经脉与膀胱构成阴阳相配的关系。

The kidneys are located on both sides of the lumbar spine, one on each side. Kidneys are yin within yin, and belong to water in terms of five elements. The kidneys and the bladder form a pairing relationship of yin and yang through meridians.

（一）肾的主要功能

5.1 The main functions of the kidneys

1. 肾藏精，主管生长发育与生殖　肾藏先天之精和后天之精。人出生之后，后天之精培养先天之精，共同主导人体的生长发育。

The kidneys store essence and governs growth, development and reproduction The kidneys store congenital essence and acquired essence. After a person is born, the acquired essence cultivates the congenital essence and they jointly dominates the growth and development of the human body.

（1）主管生长发育　人体自幼年开始，肾中精气逐渐充盛，儿童迅速生长，七八岁时换乳牙；青壮年时肾中精气处于充盛状态，表现为智齿生长，筋骨强健；此后肾精逐渐衰减，表现为头发变白、脱发、牙齿松动、腰弯背驼等。

Governing growth and development　Since childhood, kidney essence has been gradually filled, and children grow rapidly. When they are seven or eight years old, they shed their deciduous teeth; when they become young adults, kidney essence is in a sufficient state, which is characterized by wisdom teeth cutting and strong bones and muscles; after that, the kidney essence gradually decayed, showing symptoms like gray hair, alopecia, loose teeth, bent waist, kyphosis, etc.

（2）主管生殖　随着肾中精气的不断充盛，人体在青春期产生促进和维持生殖功能的精微物质——天癸。这种物质使生殖器官发育成熟，女子则月经按时来潮，男子则能排泄精液，从而具备了生殖能力。当人进入老年时期，肾精渐少，天癸耗竭，生殖功能也随之下降乃至丧失。

Governing reproduction With the kidney essence becoming more sufficient during puberty, the human body produces a subtle substance – tian gui which promotes and maintains reproductive function. This substance makes reproductive organs mature, so that women's menstruation comes on time, while men can excrete semen, thus having reproductive capacity. When people enter the old age, the kidney essence is gradually reduced, with tian gui exhausted, and the reproductive function is also declined or even lost.

（3）主管一身阴阳 肾精可化为无形的肾气，运动到全身，对各脏腑组织发挥作用。受阴阳学说的影响，肾气的作用在理论上被分为肾阴和肾阳两种，对脏腑组织具有滋养和宁静作用的称为肾阴，对脏腑组织具有温煦和推动作用的称为肾阳。肾阴和肾阳调节全身阴和阳，肾阴为全身阴气的根本，肾阳为全身阳气的根本，二者相互制约，相互为用。

Governing yin and yang over the entire body Kidney essence can be transformed into invisible kidney qi which travels through the whole body and plays roles in zang–fu viscera and tissues. According to the yin–yang theory, kidney qi can be divided into kidney yin and kidney yang. The kidney qi having the function of nourishing and tranquilizing zang–fu viscera and tissues is called kidney yin; and that with the function of warming and promoting is called kidney yang. Kidney yin and kidney yang regulate yin and yang of the whole body, with kidney yin being the root of yin qi of the whole body and kidney yang the root of yang qi. And they control and utilize each other.

2. 肾主水液 肾具有主持和调节水液代谢的功能。肾阳能温煦和促进肺、脾、三焦、膀胱等，使其各自发挥推动水液代谢的生理功能。肾阳还具有蒸腾水液的作用，大量的水液被推送上达周身，重新被利用；其余的水液经肾的气化，变为尿液下输膀胱。

The kidneys govern fluid The kidneys have the function of presiding over and regulating fluid metabolism. Kidney yang can warm and promote lungs, spleen, sanjiao, bladder, etc., so that they can respectively play their physiological functions of promoting fluid metabolism. Kidney yang also has the function of transpiring fluid, making large amount of fluid pushed up to the whole body and reused; the rest of the fluid, with the qi transformation of the kidneys, is turned into urine and delivered to the bladder.

3. 肾主纳气 肺的呼吸运动需要其他脏腑的支持，肾精充足有利于肺正常呼吸，维持呼吸深度，保证气体正常的交换，所以有“肾主纳气，为气之根”的说法。

The kidneys govern qi reception The respiratory movement of the lungs needs the support of other zang–fu viscera. Sufficient kidney essence is beneficial to the normal breathing of the lungs, maintaining the breathing depth and ensuring the normal gas exchange. Therefore, there is a saying that “The kidneys govern qi reception and serve as the root of qi”.

（二）肾的外应内合

5.2 The external manifestations of the kidneys

1. 肾在体合骨 骨髓为肾精所化生。骨髓可充养骨骼。如果肾精不足，则骨髓虚少，骨骼的养分不足，导致小儿骨骼生长迟缓，或老年人骨质疏松。此外，“齿为骨之余”是指牙齿是骨骼的衍生。牙齿的生长和脱落与肾中精气的盛衰密切相关。

The outer aspect of the kidneys is the bone Bone marrow is generated by kidney essence, and can nourish bones. Insufficient kidney essence causes bone marrow deficiency and bone nutrient will be deficient, leading to bone growth retardation in children or osteoporosis in the elderly. In addition, the saying “Teeth are the extension of the bone” means that teeth are the derivative of the bones. The growth and loss of teeth are closely related to the sufficiency and deficiency of kidney essence.

2. 肾其华在发 “发为血之余”，头发的生长有赖于血提供营养。而肾精能化血，精与血旺盛，则头发生长正常。所以发为肾精充足与否的外候。

The lustre of the kidneys shows in the hair “Hair is the extension of the blood”, and the growth of hair depends on blood to provide nutrition. The kidney essence can transform into blood, and if the essence and blood are sufficient, the hair will grow normally. That’s why hair is one external manifestation of the kidneys.

3. 肾开窍于耳及二阴 肾精与耳的听力密切相关。老年人听力减退是肾精亏虚的表现。二阴，即前阴和后阴。前阴是指外生殖器和尿道口，其生殖与排尿功能与肾密切相关。后阴即肛门，肛门对大便的排泄功能不仅与大肠有关，而且与肾有一定关系。婴幼儿和老年人控制二便的问题往往与肾虚有关。

The kidneys open into the ears, pudendum, urethra and anus Kidney essence is closely related to ear hearing. And hearing loss in the elderly is a manifestation of kidney essence deficiency. The reproductive and urination functions of pudendum and urethra are closely related to kidney. The function of defecating of anus is not only related to the large intestine, but also to the kidneys. The failure of controlling defecation in infants and the elderly is often related to kidney deficiency.

4. 肾在液为唾 肾经上挟舌根，舌下所出的津液为唾，唾为肾精所化。养生家们常以舌头轻抵上腭，待唾液满口腔后，缓缓咽之以存肾精。

The fluid of the kidneys is thick saliva The kidney meridian connects back of the tongue, and the fluid generated under the tongue is thick saliva which is transformed by kidney essence. Experts in health preservation often make their tongues lightly come to the upper palates and wait for saliva to fill the mouth cavity, and then they will slowly swallow the saliva to preserve kidney essence.

5. 肾在志为恐 过度惊恐可致肾气的固摄功能失常，导致二便失禁、滑精或滑胎等症。

The emotion of the kidneys is fear Excessive fear can lead to abnormal securing function of kidney qi, resulting in symptoms such as incontinence of urination and defecation, night emission, habitual abortion, etc.

6. 肾应冬 冬季为一年中气候最寒冷的季节，万物静谧闭藏。肾五行属水，为阴中之太阴，与冬气相通应，有封藏的特性。

The season of the kidneys is winter Winter is the coldest season of the year, with everything quiet and hidden. The kidneys belong to water in terms of five elements and yin within yin (taiyin), which correspond to winter and have the characteristic of sealing and storing.

第二节 六 腑
Section 2 Six Fu Viscera

一、胃
1 Stomach

胃位于左上腹部，上与食管相接，下与小肠相通。

The stomach is located in the upper left abdomen, connecting with esophagus on the upper end and small intestine on the lower end.

（一）胃的主要功能
1.1 The main functions of the stomach

胃主受纳、腐熟水谷 胃具有容纳食物，并将其加工成食糜的功能。

The stomach governs receiving and holding as well as decomposition The stomach has the function of receiving and holding the water and food as well as primarily digesting them and forming chyme.

（二）胃的生理特性
1.2 The physiological characteristics of the stomach

1. 胃主通降 胃的生理功能特点是以畅通下降为主。如果食物停滞于胃，可致胃胀痛、嗳气、吞酸、口臭等症。

The stomach dominating dredging and descending The physiological function of stomach is flowing downward without obstruction. If food stagnates in the stomach, it can cause distending pain in the stomach, belching, acid regurgitation, halitosis and other symptoms.

2. 胃喜润恶燥 胃腐熟食物有赖于胃津的濡润，如果胃内津液不足而干燥，饮食物就难以消化腐熟和下行。

The stomach likes moisturizing and hates dryness The decomposition of water and food depends on the moistening of stomach fluid. If the fluid in the stomach is insufficient and dryness occurs, it will be difficult for the water and food to digest, decompose and go down.

二、小肠

2 The small intestine

小肠位于腹中，上与胃相通，下与大肠连通。小肠的主要功能如下。

The small intestine is located in the abdomen, with the upper end connecting with the stomach and the lower end connecting with the large intestine. The main functions of the small intestine are as follows.

1. 小肠主受盛化物 小肠接受胃下传的食糜，将食糜进一步消化，吸收精微。在中医藏象学说中，常将消化功能归于脾的运化范畴，对于小肠的消化异常多从脾论治。

The small intestine governs receiving and holding as well as transforming The small intestine receives chyme transmitted from the stomach, and further digests it and absorbs the food essence. In the theory of visceral manifestations in TCM, the digestive function is often attributed to the transportation and transformation function of spleen, and the digestive abnormalities of the small intestine are mainly diagnosed and treated from the spleen.

2. 小肠主泌别清浊 指小肠对食糜作进一步消化，并将其分为清浊两部分：清者为精微部分，可重吸收回人体；浊者即食物残渣和水液。

The small intestine separates the clear from the turbid This function means that the small intestine further digests the chyme and divides it into two parts: the clear part is the food essence, which can be reabsorbed back to the human body; and the turbid part is food residues and fluid.

3. 小肠主液 指小肠在吸收谷精的同时，吸收大量津液的生理功能。

The small intestine govern fluid This physiological function means that small intestine absorbs a large amount of fluid while absorbing cereal essence.

三、胆

3 The gallbladder

胆位于右胁，依附于肝。胆的主要功能如下。

The gallbladder is located in the right hypochondrium and attached to the liver. The main functions of gallbladder are as follows.

1. 胆贮藏和排泄胆汁 胆汁由肝分泌而贮藏于胆，由胆排泄于小肠，有助于饮食物的消化。

The gallbladder stores and excretes bile Bile which is helpful for digestion is secreted by the liver and stored in the gallbladder, and excreted to the small intestine from the gallbladder.

2. 胆主决断 《素问·灵兰秘典论》载:“胆者,中正之官,决断出焉。”是指人对事物的决定和判断能力与胆气有关。如果胆气虚弱,遇事易怯懦而犹豫不决。

The gallbladder governs decision-making *Suwen Ling Lan Mi Dian Lun* (素问·灵兰秘典论) records: “The gallbladder is the viscus similar to the official of justice and is responsible for decision.” It means that people’s ability to decide and judge things is related to gallbladder qi. If gallbladder qi is weak, the person is easy to be timid and hesitant.

四、大肠

4 The large intestine

大肠位居腹中,上与小肠相接,其下端为肛门。大肠的主要功能如下。

The large intestine is located in the abdomen, connecting with the small intestine on the upper end, and the anus on the lower end. The main functions of the large intestine are as follows.

1. 大肠排泄糟粕 大肠接受小肠传递来的食物残渣,吸收一定水分后排出体外。

The large intestine conducts discharges faeces The large intestine receives food residues transmitted from the small intestine, absorbs some water and excretes residues out of the body.

2. 大肠主津 大肠具有接受食物残渣,吸收水分的功能。

The large intestine governs the thin fluid The large intestine has the function of receiving food residues and absorbing water.

五、膀胱

5 The bladder

膀胱位于小腹部,与肾相联通。膀胱的主要功能为贮尿和排尿,该功能与肾的气化、推动和固摄功能密切相关,因此多从肾治疗膀胱的遗尿、尿少等病变。

The bladder is located in the small abdomen and connected with the kidneys. The main function of it is to store urine and urinate, which is closely related to the qi transformation, promotion and securing functions of the kidneys. Therefore, diseases such as enuresis and oliguria of the bladder are treated from the kidneys.

六、三焦

6 Sanjiao

对三焦的认识主要有两种:一是认为三焦为六腑之一;二是将三焦作为划分内脏分布的区域,即膈以上的部位为上焦,膈与脐之间的部位为中焦,脐以下的部位为下焦。

There are two main understandings of sanjiao: one is that sanjiao is one of the six fu viscera; the other regards sanjiao as the distribution areas of viscera, that is, the part above diaphragm is the upper jiao, the part between diaphragm and umbilicus is the middle jiao, and the part below umbilicus is the lower jiao.

（一）三焦的主要功能

6.1 The main functions of sanjiao

1. 通行元气　元气由肾精所化生而根源于肾，通过三焦散布于各脏腑。

Circulating the primordial qi　The primordial qi is generated by kidney essence and originates from kidney, and it is distributed to zang–fu viscera through sanjiao.

2. 运行水液　三焦是水液散布运行的大通道。

Running fluid　Sanjiao is a big channel for fluid dispersion and circulation.

（二）上、中、下三焦的部位划分以及功能特点

6.2 The location division and functions of the upper, middle and lower jiao

1. 上焦　是指头至横膈之间，主要包括心肺。“上焦如雾”，是对位于上焦的肺宣发津液功能的形象概括。

Upper jiao　Upper jiao refers to the area between head and diaphragm, mainly including heart and lungs. The saying that “Upper jiao resembles mist” is a vivid comparison of the diffusion function of the lungs in the upper jiao.

2. 中焦　是指横膈与脐之间，主要包括脾胃。“中焦如沤”，是对胃腐熟消化水谷作用的形象概括。

Middle jiao　It refers to the area between diaphragm and umbilicus mainly including spleen and stomach. “Middle jiao resembles foam” is a vivid comparison of the decomposition function of the stomach in the middle jiao.

3. 下焦　是指脐以下至耻骨之间，主要包括小肠、大肠、肾和膀胱等。“下焦如渎”，是指膀胱和大肠像沟渠一样排泄二便。

Lower jiao　It refers to the area between the umbilicus and pubis, mainly including small intestine, large intestine, kidneys and bladder. “Lower jiao resembles a sluice” compares the function of discharging urine and faeces of the bladder and large intestine to that of an unobstructed ditch.

第三节　奇恒之腑

Section 3　Extraordinary fu–viscera

奇恒之腑是脑、髓、骨、脉、胆与女子胞的合称。它们在形态上多似腑而中空有腔，在功能上似脏而贮藏精气，故称为奇恒之腑。其中，胆又属于六腑。以下主要简单

介绍中医学对脑和女子胞的认识。

The term extraordinary fu–viscera is the collective name for brain, marrow, bone, vessels, gallbladder and uterus. Their shapes are more similar to the six fu viscera with hollow cavities, but they have the function of storing essence and qi, which means they are similar to the five zang viscera in functions. That's why they are named extraordinary fu–viscera. Among them, gallbladder also belongs to six fu viscera. The following is a brief introduction to the brain and uterus.

一、脑
1 The brain

脑位于颅内，与脊髓相通，由髓汇集而成。

The brain is located in the skull, connecting with the spinal cord, and is formed by the marrow.

（一）脑的主要功能
1.1 The main functions of the brain

脑具有主宰生命活动、主管精神活动和感觉活动（视听言动）的功能。

The brain has the function of dominating physiological activities and governing mental activities and sensory activities (vision, hearing, speech and movement).

（二）脑与五脏的关系
1.2 The relationship between the brain and the five zang viscera

在整体观念的影响下，中医学将人的精神活动分别归属于五脏。从意识思维而言，心藏神，肺藏魄，肝藏魂，脾藏意，肾藏志；从情感活动而言，心在志为喜，肝在志为怒，脾在志为思，肺在志为悲，肾在志为恐。所以，脑的病变多从五脏的精、气、血的失常来分析和治疗。

According to the holism concept, people's mental activities are assigned to the five zang viscera respectively. In terms of conscious thinking, the heart stores spirit, with the lungs storing inferior spirit, the liver storing soul, the spleen storing idea, and the kidney storing will; As for emotions, the emotion of the heart is joy, the liver is angry, the spleen is pensiveness, the lungs are sorrow, and the kidneys are fear. Therefore, brain lesions are mostly analyzed and treated from the abnormalities of essence, qi and blood in the five zang viscera.

二、女子胞
2 The uterus

女子胞位于小腹部，在膀胱后，直肠之前，下口与阴道相连。

The uterus is located in the lower abdomen, behind the bladder, before the rectum, and the lower opening is connected with the vagina.

（一）女子胞的主要功能

2.1 The main functions of the uterus

女子胞具有产生月经和孕育胎儿的功能。

The uterus has the functions of menstruating and gestating fetus.

（二）女子胞与脏腑的关系

2.2 The relationship between the uterus and zang-fu viscera

女性的月经及孕育胎儿与心、肾、肝、脾等有密切关系，中医治疗妇科病常以调理相关脏腑，作为影响女子胞的重要途径。

Women's menstruation and gestation of fetus are closely related to heart, kidneys, liver and spleen. TCM often regulates related zang–fu viscera as an important way to treat diseases in uterus.

1. 心主神明、心主血脉的作用 心神内守是女子按时来潮和适时排卵以成胎孕的重要条件。心主血脉，血脉充盈对女子胞的功能具有重要的资助和促进作用。

The heart governs the spirit, and the heart governs the blood and vessels Keeping the spirit in interior is an important condition for women's menstruation to come on time and ovulate at the right time to become pregnant. The heart governs the blood and vessels, and sufficient blood plays an important role in supporting and promoting the functions of the uterus.

2. 肾中精气的作用 女性在14岁左右，随着肾中精气的逐渐充盈，产生了“天癸”，这类物质能促进女子胞的发育成熟，女性月经来潮，从而具备生殖能力。在老年时期，肾中精气渐衰，天癸竭，女子胞的功能亦衰退。

The function of kidney essence At the age of about 14 years old, with the kidney essence becoming gradually sufficient, “tian gui” is produced. This kind of substance can promote the development and maturity of the uterus, so that women have menstruation, thus having reproductive capacity. When people enter the old age, the kidney essence is gradually reduced, with tian gui exhausted, and the reproductive function is also declined.

3. 肝藏血的作用 月经的来潮，胎儿的孕育，均依赖于血液，而肝藏血，能调节血量，疏泄血到子宫中去。

The liver stores blood Menstruation and gestation of fetus both depend on blood, and the liver's function of storing blood can regulate blood volume and drain blood into uterus.

4. 脾统血的作用 脾既是气血生化之源，也能统血，防止子宫出血过多。

The spleen contains blood In addition to being the source of qi and blood, spleen also contains blood and prevents excessive uterine bleeding.

第四节 经 络
Section 4 Meridians

经络学说是中国古人在长期的医疗实践中创造的一种理论，它对于指导针灸、推拿和气功都有重要意义。经络不同于神经或血管系统，但“经络的实质是什么”这一问题尚待进一步研究。

Meridian theory is a theory created by ancient Chinese in their long-term medical practice, which is of great significance for guiding acupuncture, massage and qigong. Meridians are different from nervous or vascular systems, but the problem of “what on earth meridians are” needs further study.

一、经络的概念
1 The concept of meridians

经络是经脉和络脉的总称。经络是运行气血，联络内脏与肢体，沟通上下内外，调节人体功能的通道系统。

Meridians include meridians and collaterals. Meridians are channels that circulate qi and blood, connect viscera and limbs, link the upper, lower, inside and outside parts, and regulates human body functions.

经络系统主要包括十二经脉、奇经八脉、络脉、经别。

The meridian system mainly includes twelve regular meridians, eight extra meridians, collaterals and divergent meridians.

二、十二经脉
2 The twelve regular meridians

十二经脉归属于不同的脏腑，从气血流注的次序而言，有手太阴肺经、手阳明大肠经、足阳明胃经、足太阴脾经、手少阴心经、手太阳小肠经、足太阳膀胱经、足少阴肾经、手厥阴心包经、手少阳三焦经、足少阳胆经、足厥阴肝经。它们的具体循行路线详见《针灸学》。

Twelve regular meridians belong to different zang-fu viscera. The list in order by the ebb-flow of qi and blood is: taiyin lung meridian of hand, yangming large intestine meridian of hand, yangming stomach meridian of foot, taiyin spleen meridian of foot, shaoyin heart meridian of hand, taiyang small intestine meridian of hand, taiyang bladder meridian of foot, shaoyin kidney meridian of foot, jueyin pericardium meridian of hand, shaoyang sanjiao meridian of hand, shaoyang gallbladder meridian of foot and jueyin liver meridian of foot.

Their specific running routes are shown in the book *Science of Acupuncture and Moxibustion* (针灸学).

三、奇经八脉

3 The eight extra meridians

奇经八脉是指走行路线奇特、不归属于脏腑的经脉，包括督脉、任脉、冲脉、带脉、阴跷脉、阳跷脉、阴维脉、阳维脉。督脉能联系十二经脉中的所有阳经，任脉能联系十二经脉中的所有阴经。冲脉能联通十二经脉。奇经八脉与十二经脉交织，起着调节十二经脉气血的作用。

The eight extra meridians refer to meridians with peculiar running routes and not belonging to zang–fu viscera They are governor meridian, conception meridian, thoroughfare meridian, belt meridian, yin heel meridian, yang heel meridian, yin link meridian and yang link meridian. The governor meridian can be linked to all yang meridians among the twelve regular meridians, and the conception meridian can be linked to all yin meridians among the twelve regular meridians. The thoroughfare meridian can be connected with all of the twelve regular meridians. The eight extra meridians are intertwined with the twelve regular meridians, playing a role in regulating their qi and blood.

第五章 常见病因
Chapter 5 Common Etiological Factors

病因是指能破坏人体相对平衡状态而导致疾病的原因，主要包括外感病因、内伤病因、继发病因。

Etiological factors refer to the factors that can destroy the relative balance of human body and lead to diseases, mainly including exogenous etiological factors, endogenous etiological factors, and secondary etiological factors.

第一节 外感病因
Section 1 Exogenous Etiological Factors

外感病因，是指由外而入，侵袭机体，引起外感疾病的致病因素。外感病因主要包括六淫、疫气。

Exogenous etiological factors refer to the factors that attack the body from the outside and cause exogenous diseases, mainly including six climatic exopathogens and pestilent qi.

一、六淫
1 Six climatic exopathogens

（一）六淫的概念
1.1 The concept of six climatic exopathogens

六淫是风、寒、暑、湿、燥、热（火）六种外感病邪的统称。六淫致病多由肌表、口鼻而入，具有季节性、地域性、相兼性，并可在一定条件下相互转化。

Six climatic exopathogens are the general name of six exogenous etiological factors, namely, wind, cold, summer heat, dampness, dryness and heat (fire). They mostly enter from skin, nose and mouth, which are seasonal, regional and compatible, and can be transformed into each other under certain conditions.

（二）六淫的性质和致病特点

1.2 The nature and etiological characteristics of the six climatic exopathogens

1. 风邪 Wind pathogen

（1）风为阳邪，其性开泄，易袭阳位　风性轻扬升散，具有升发、向上、向外的特性，故风邪致病，易伤人体属阳的部位，如头面、咽喉、肌表等。

Wind is a yang pathogen, characterized by opening and dispersing, and tending to impair yang parts　Wind floats and ascends, and has the characteristics of rising, dispersing, and moving upward and outward. Therefore, wind pathogen easily impairs yang parts of human body, such as head, throat, skin, etc.

（2）风性主动，善行而数变　风邪具有善动不居、游走不定、变化无常的性质，故其致病有病位游移、动摇不定和发病急骤的特性。

Wind causes movement, and it moves and changes swiftly　Wind is characterized by swift changes. So diseases caused by wind pathogen are marked by a sudden onset of symptoms in moving locations.

（3）风为百病之长　风邪是外感病因的先导，寒、湿、燥、热等邪气多依附于风而侵袭人体，如风与寒合为风寒，与热合为风热等。

Wind is the primary pathogen　Wind pathogen is the spearhead of exogenous etiological factors and liable to associate itself with cold, dampness, dryness and heat to attack human body. For example, wind is combined with cold to form wind-cold and combined with heat to form wind-heat.

2. 寒邪 Cold pathogen

（1）寒为阴邪，易伤阳气　寒邪侵袭，损伤阳气，阳失温煦，全身或局部可出现明显的寒象。

Cold is a yin pathogen and tends to impair yang qi　When cold pathogen invades, it will impair yang qi. That yang fails to warm the body can cause obvious cold in the whole body or locally.

（2）寒性收引　寒邪侵袭人体，可使气机收敛，腠理闭塞，经脉收缩而挛急。

Cold causes contraction　Cold pathogen can constrict qi movement, block interstices, and cause meridians to contract and convulse.

（3）寒性凝滞、主痛　寒邪侵袭人体，可使气血凝结，阻滞不通，不通则痛，故寒邪伤人多见疼痛症状。

Cold congeals and stagnates　Cold pathogen can also congeal qi and blood and cause stagnation which can lead to pain. Therefore, pain is common when cold pathogen impairs human body.

3. 暑邪 Summer heat pathogen

（1）暑为阳邪，其性炎热　暑为火热之气，具有炎热之性，故暑邪伤人多表现出一派阳热之象，出现壮热、心烦、面赤、烦躁、脉象洪大等症状。

Summer heat is a yang pathogen and causes flaming heat Summer heat is hot qi and is characterized by extreme hotness. So summer heat pathogen often causes hyperactive yang heat, with symptoms such as high fever, vexation, red facial complexion, dysphoria, surging and large pulse, etc.

（2）暑性升散，扰神伤津耗气 暑邪易于发散，使腠理开泄而大汗出，临床可见口渴喜饮、尿赤短少、气短乏力等伤津耗气症状。暑邪易上扰心神，而致心烦、头昏、面赤等症状。

Summer heat is characterized by ascending and dispersing, which disturbs the spirit, damages fluid and consumes qi Summer heat pathogen tends to disperse, making the interstices open and profuse sweat out. Symptoms such as thirst, scarce and dark urine, shortness of breath and fatigue can be seen in the clinic. Summer heat pathogen tends to disturb the heart spirit, causing vexation, vertigo, red facial complexion and other symptoms.

（3）暑多夹湿 暑邪为病，多合湿邪而弥漫机体，常见暑湿夹杂证候。临床除发热、烦渴等暑热表现外，常兼见四肢困倦、胸闷呕恶、大便溏泄不爽等湿阻症状。

Summer heat often combines with dampness Summer heat pathogen is often liable to mix itself with dampness pathogen to diffuse into the body, usually leading to combined summer heat and dampness syndrome. In addition to fever, polydipsia and other summer heat manifestations, symptoms of dampness and obstruction such as fatigue of limbs, oppression in chest, vomiting, loose stools and so forth are also seen clinically.

4. 湿邪 Dampness pathogen

（1）湿为阴邪，易阻气机，损伤阳气 湿为阴邪，易阻滞气机，使气机升降失常，出现胸闷、腹胀等症。湿邪侵袭人体，必困于脾，使脾阳不振，发为泄泻、水肿、小便短少等症。

Dampness is a yin pathogen and obstructs qi movement and impairs yang qi Dampness is a yin pathogen and tends to obstruct qi movement, resulting in abnormal ascending and descending of qi movement, which leads to symptoms such as oppression in chest, abdominal distension, etc. When damp pathogen invades the human body, it will be trapped in the spleen, which will lead to diarrhea, edema, scarce urine and other diseases.

（2）湿邪易袭阴位 湿邪有趋下之性，易伤人体下部，如水肿多以下肢较为明显。

Dampness pathogen tends to impair yang parts Dampness pathogen tends to move downward and affects the lower parts of the body. For example, edema is more obvious in lower limbs.

（3）湿性黏滞重浊 湿为重浊有质之邪，且湿性黏腻，故致病多见头身困重、分泌物黏浊、病程缠绵等特点。

Dampness is characterized by stickiness, stagnation, heaviness and turbidity Dampness pathogen is heavy and turbid as well as sticky and stagnant, so the disease is characterized by heavy head and body, sticky secretion and lingering course of disease.

5. 燥邪 Dryness pathogen

（1）燥性干涩，易伤津液　燥性干涩枯涸，易伤人体津液，出现各种干燥症状。

Dryness tends to desiccate and impair fluid　Dryness is dry and puckery, consuming fluid and causing various symptoms related with dryness.

（2）燥易伤肺　燥为秋令主气，与肺相应，故燥邪最易伤肺，可见干咳少痰，或痰黏难咯等症。

Dryness is likely to injure the lungs　Dryness is the major qi in autumn, which corresponds to the lungs. Therefore, dryness pathogen is most likely to injure the lungs, and causes symptoms such as dry cough with little phlegm, or makes phlegm too sticky to be coughed up.

6. 热（火）邪 Heat (fire) pathogen

（1）热（火）为阳邪，其性炎上　火为阳邪，其性升腾向上，具有明显的炎上特性，其致病主要表现在人体上部，可见咽喉红肿疼痛、耳鸣等。

Heat (fire) is a yang pathogen, and flames upward　Heat (fire) pathogen is a yang pathogen and is characterized by flaring up. It often affects the upper part of the body, causing symptoms such as red, swollen and painful throat, tinnitus and so on.

（2）易伤津耗气　热（火）邪侵犯人体，消灼煎熬阴津，耗伤气津，其致病表现为大汗出、口渴喜饮、倦怠乏力、少气懒言等气津两伤症状。

It consumes fluid and qi　When heat (fire) invades human body, it scorches yin fluid and consumes qi, causing deficiency of both qi and thin fluid, including symptoms such as profuse sweating, thirst, burnout, fatigue, panting, no desire to speak, etc.

（3）易致生风动血　火邪易于引起肝风内动和血液妄行，临床可出现四肢抽搐、两目上视、角弓反张或各种出血的病证。

It tends to generate wind and cause bleeding　Heat (fire) pathogen tends to stir endogenous wind and cause the blood to move recklessly. Clinically, it may cause limb convulsion, upward vision of eyes, opisthotonus or various bleeding symptoms.

（4）易扰心神　火热与心相通应，故火热之邪易扰心神，轻者心神不宁而心烦失眠，重者可扰乱心神，出现狂躁不安、神昏谵语等症。

It tends to disturb the heart spirit　Heat (fire) corresponds to the heart, so heat (fire) pathogen is easy to disturb the heart spirit The mild pathogen can cause disquieted heart spirit and insomnia, while the severe ones can disturb the mind spirit, resulting in mania, unconsciousness and delirium.

（5）易致疮痈　火热之邪入于血分，可聚于局部，腐蚀血肉，形成疮疡痈肿。其临床表现以疮疡局部红肿热痛为主要特征。

It tends to cause sores/carbuncles　Heat (fire) pathogen enters xuefen, which can gather locally, corrode flesh and blood, and form sores and carbuncles. Its clinical manifestations mainly include redness, swelling, heat and pain in the affected area.

二、疫气
2 Pestilent qi

（一）疫气的基本概念
2.1 The basic concept of pestilent qi

疫气是一类具有强烈致病性和传染性的病邪，是自然界一种毒疠之气。疫气的发生可由气候反常、环境污染、饮食不洁、预防隔离工作不严格、社会因素等引起，通过空气和接触传播，经过口鼻等途径，由外入内，侵袭人体，属于外感病因。

Pestilent qi is a kind of poisonous qi in nature, which causes epidemic pestilence. It is a kind of pathogen with strong pathogenicity and infectivity. The occurrence of pestilent qi can be caused by abnormal climate, environmental pollution, unclean diet, lax prevention and isolation, social factors, etc. It is an exogenous etiological factors which spreads through air and contact and invades human body from outside to inside through nose and mouth.

（二）疫气的性质及致病特点
2.2 The nature and etiological characteristics of pestilent qi

1. 传染性强，易于流行 疫气具有强烈的传染性和流行性，可通过口鼻等多种途径传播。处在疫气流行地区的人群，无论男女老少，体质强弱，只要接触疫气，都可能发生疫病。

It is highly contagious and easy to spread The pestilent qi is highly contagious and epidemic, and can be transmitted through various ways such as nose and mouth. People in epidemic areas who are exposed to pestilent qi are all susceptible to the epidemic diseases, regardless of their sex, age or constitution.

2. 一气一病，症状相似 一种疫气只能导致一种疫病发生，且每一种疫气所致疫病均有相似的临床特征和传变规律。如痄腮，一般都表现为耳下腮部肿胀。

One pestilent qi causes one disease with similar symptoms One pestilent qi can only lead to one epidemic disease with similar clinical characteristics and transmission rules. For example, mumps generally manifests as swelling of cheeks under the ears.

3. 发病急骤，病情危笃 疫气多属热毒之邪，其性疾速，致病具有发病急骤、来势凶猛、变化多端、病情险恶的特点，因而常出现热盛、伤津、扰神、动血、生风等临床表现。

The epidemic pestilence is characterized by rapid onset and dangerous conditions The pestilent qi is mostly heat toxin pathogen, so the epidemic pestilence caused by it is characterized by rapid and fierce onset and varied and sinister conditions. Therefore, clinical manifestations such as exuberant heat, consumed fluid, disturbance to mind, stirring blood and endogenous wind generation often occur.

第二节 内伤病因
Section 2 Endogenous Etiological Factors

内伤病因是指自内而生的邪气，多因人体情志、饮食、劳倦、安逸等不循常度，导致气血津液失调、脏腑组织异常而产生。内因包括七情内伤、饮食失宜、劳逸失度。

Endogenous etiological factors refer to the etiological qi born from within, which are mostly caused by the irregularity of human emotions, diet, work, rest, etc. These factors lead to imbalance of qi, blood and fluid and abnormal zang-fu viscera and tissues. They include seven emotions causing internal damage, improper diet and unbalanced work and rest.

一、七情内伤
1 Seven emotions causing internal damage

七情，即喜、怒、忧、思、悲、恐、惊七种正常的情志活动。七情内伤是七情的异常变化，是引起脏腑气机失调而导致疾病发生的常见致病因素。七情内伤的致病特点如下。

Seven emotions are seven normal emotional activities: joy, anger, worry, pensiveness, sorrow fear and fright. But seven emotions causing internal damage is an abnormal change of seven emotions, and it is a common etiological factor that causes the imbalance of qi movement of zang-fu viscera and leads to diseases. The etiological characteristics of seven emotions causing internal damage are as follows.

1. 直接伤及内脏 七情过激可直接影响脏腑活动而产生病理变化。不同的情志刺激可伤及不同的脏腑，产生不同的病理变化，如怒伤肝、喜伤心、思伤脾、悲忧伤肺，惊恐伤肾。

Injuring viscera directly Excessive seven emotions can affect zang-fu viscera activities directly and produce pathological changes. Different emotions can impair different viscera and cause different pathological changes, such as anger impairing liver, joy impairing heart, pensiveness impairing spleen, sorrow and worry impairing lungs and fright and fear impairing kidneys.

2. 影响气机 七情致病，可使脏腑气机紊乱，阴阳失调。不同的情志变化，其气机逆乱的表现也不尽相同，如怒则气上，喜则气缓，悲则气消，思则气结，恐则气下，惊则气乱。

Affecting qi movement Excessive seven emotions can cause disorders of the qi movement of zang-fu viscera and imbalanced yin and yang. Different emotions cause different manifestations of qi movement disorders, such as anger leading to qi ascending, joy leading to qi loose, sorrow leading to qi consumption, pensiveness leading to qi knotting, fear leading to qi sinking, and fright leading to qi turbulence.

二、饮食失宜

2 Improper diet

饮食失宜主要影响脾胃运化功能，引起消化功能障碍，还易生热、生痰、生湿，产生多种病变，成为疾病发生的一个重要原因。

Improper diet mainly affects the transportation and transformation function of spleen and stomach, causing digestive dysfunction, and also tends to generate heat, phlegm and dampness, resulting in a variety of pathological changes, making it a big cause of diseases.

1. 饮食不节 是指饮食质量或时间没有节制，没有规律。包括食量过少、食量过多或不能按照固定时间有规律地进食，可损伤脾胃，导致脾胃病变。

Irregular diet It means that the quantity of diet is uncontrolled or the time is irregular, including excessive hunger, binge eating or not eating at a regular time. They can all lead to spleen and stomach diseases.

2. 饮食不洁 是指饮食不清洁，或进食腐败变质有毒食物，或误食毒物。饮食不洁净会导致多种胃肠道疾病或引起寄生虫病。

Unclean diet It refers to eating unclean, spoiled or poisonous food, or even poisons by mistake. It can lead to many gastrointestinal diseases or parasitic diseases.

3. 饮食偏嗜 是指饮食偏于个人嗜好，膳食结构失宜，或饮食过寒过热，或饮食五味有所偏嗜，或某些营养缺乏而发生疾病。

Dietary predilection It refers to excessive indulgence in specific food, which results in inappropriate dietary structure. It includes eating cold or hot food, habitual preference for a particular flavour or taste or lack of certain nutrition.

三、劳逸失度

3 Unbalanced work and rest

劳逸失度，是指长时间过度劳累或过度安逸，导致脏腑经络及精、气、血、津液、神的失常而引发疾病。主要包括过劳与过逸两方面。

Unbalanced work and rest refers to long-term overwork or excessive leisure, which leads to disorders of zang-fu viscera, meridians, essence, qi, blood, fluid and spirit and causes diseases. It mainly includes overwork and excessive leisure.

1. 过劳 指过度劳累，包括劳力过度、劳神过度和房劳过度三个方面。劳力过度主要伤气，劳神过度主要损伤心脾，房劳过度主要耗伤肾中精气。

Overwork It includes excessive physical labor, excessive mental labor and excessive sexual intercourse. Excessive physical labor mainly impairs qi. Excessive mental labor mainly damages heart and spleen. And excessive sexual intercourse mainly consumes essence and qi in kidneys.

2. 过逸 指因病或生活过于安闲，不从事各种劳动和运动锻炼。长期形体少动，气血运行不畅继则脏腑功能减退，导致疾病。

Excessive leisure It means not engaging in all kinds of labor or exercise due to illness or too much leisure. Long-term physical inactivity will cause poor circulation of qi and blood, followed by hypofunction of zang-fu viscera, leading to diseases.

第三节 继发病因
Section 3 Secondary Etiological Factors

病理产物性病因是指在疾病发生和发展过程中所形成的病理产物，滞留体内而不去，成为新的致病因素，因其常继发于其他病理过程而产生，故又称“继发病因”，如痰饮、瘀血、结石等。

Pathological product etiology refers to the pathological product formed in the process of disease occurrence and development, which is trapped in the body and becomes a new etiological factor. Because it is often secondary to other pathological processes, it is also called “secondary etiological factor”, such as phlegm and fluid retention, static blood, concretion and so on.

一、瘀血
1 Static blood

瘀血是血液运行障碍，血液停滞所形成的病理产物，包括体内瘀积的离经之血，或因血液运行不畅，停滞于经脉或脏腑的血液。瘀血的致病特点如下。

Static blood is the pathological product formed by blood circulation disorder and blood stagnation, including blood stasis away from meridians in the body, and static blood in meridians or zang-fu viscera due to unsmooth blood circulation. The etiological characteristics of static blood are as follows.

1. 阻滞气机 瘀血停滞脏腑经络，或血行不畅，易于阻滞气机，导致气的升降出入失常。

Blocking qi movement Blood stagnation in zang-fu viscera and meridians or unsmooth blood circulation is easy to block qi movement, resulting in abnormal ascending, descending, entering and exiting movements of qi.

2. 影响血脉运行 瘀血阻于经脉之中，可致血运不畅，或血行停蓄，血液不能正常运行。

Affecting blood circulation Static blood blocked in meridians may cause unsmooth blood circulation, or stop blood circulation.

3. 影响新血形成 瘀血阻滞体内，影响气血运行，导致脏腑失于濡养，功能失常，影响新血生成。

Affecting the formation of new blood Static blood affects the circulation of qi and blood, leading to the loss of nourishment and dysfunction of zang–fu viscera, thus affecting the formation of new blood.

4. 病位固定，病证繁多 瘀血停滞，多难及时消散，故其致病病位相对固定。又因瘀血停滞部位不同，临床表现也不同，故病证繁多。

Fixed disease locations and various syndromes Most static blood is difficult to dissipate in time, so the disease location hardly changes. Static blood can also occur in different parts, and the clinical manifestations are also different, so there are various diseases and syndromes.

二、痰饮
2 Phlegm and fluid retention

痰饮是机体水液代谢障碍所形成的病理产物，又是致病因素。痰饮的致病特点如下。

Phlegm and fluid retention is not only a pathological product formed by the disorder of fluid metabolism, but also an etiological factor. The etiological characteristics of phlegm and fluid retention are as follows.

1. 易于阻滞气机 痰饮多为有形的病理产物，易于阻滞气机，使脏腑气机升降出入异常。如痰饮在肺，肺失宣降，出现咳嗽喘息、胸部满闷，甚则不能平卧等症。

Tending to block qi movement Phlegm and fluid retention is mostly a tangible pathological product, which is easy to block qi movement and causes abnormal ascending, descending, entering and exiting movements of qi. Phlegm and fluid retention in the lungs causes the lungs to fail to govern upward and outward diffusion as well as descent and purification, resulting in symptoms such as cough, gasping, chest tightness, and even inability to lie on the back.

2. 易于内扰心神 痰浊内扰，影响及心，扰乱神明，可见一系列神志异常的病证。如痰浊上蒙清窍，可见头昏目眩、精神不振等症状。

Tending to disturb the heart spirit Phlegm affects the heart and disturbs the spirit, causing a series of syndromes and symptoms related with abnormal consciousness. If it covers clear orifices, then dizziness, listlessness and other symptoms can be seen.

3. 症状复杂，变化多端 痰之为病，其病理变化多种多样，在不同的部位表现出不同的症状，可归纳为咳、喘、悸、眩、呕、满、肿、痛八大症。

Complex and varied symptoms Phlegm's pathological changes are varied, showing different symptoms in different parts, which can be summarized into eight major symptoms: cough, panting, palpitation, dizziness, vomiting, fullness, swelling and pain.

4. 影响水液代谢 痰饮形成后，影响肺、脾、肾、三焦等脏腑的功能活动，如痰湿困脾、痰饮阻肺、痰饮停滞下焦等，进而影响水液代谢。

Affecting fluid metabolism Phlegm and fluid retention affects the functions of zang-fu viscera such as lungs, spleen, kidneys and sanjiao. For example, phlegm dampness trapping spleen, phlegm retention blocking lungs and phlegm retention stagnating lower jiao all affect fluid metabolism.

三、结石

3 Concretion

结石是指体内某些部位形成并停滞为病的砂石样病理产物。结石的致病特点如下。

Concretion refers to a sandstone-like pathological product which is formed and stagnates in some parts of the body. The etiological characteristics of concretion are as follows.

1. 多发于胆、胃、肝、肾、膀胱等脏腑 结石为病，以肝胆结石、肾膀胱结石最常见。

More common in gallbladder, stomach, liver, kidneys and bladder Gall-stone, liver-stone, kidney-stone and bladder-stone are the most common concretions.

2. 病程较长，轻重不一 结石的大小不等，停留部位不一，其临床表现各异。

Long course of disease with different severity Concretions have different sizes, staying positions and clinical manifestations.

3. 阻滞气机，损伤脉络 结石为有形实邪，阻滞气机，可引起局部胀痛、水液停聚等。结石嵌滞局部，损伤脉络，可引起出血。

Blocking qi movement and damaging vessels Concretion is a kind of tangible pathogen, which blocks qi movement and causes local distending pain, fluid retention, etc. If embedded locally, it may damage the vessels and cause bleeding.

第六章 基本病机
Chapter 6 Basic Pathogenesis

病机，即疾病发生、发展变化及转归的机理，其着重研究疾病发生和人体产生病理反应的全过程及其规律。

Pathogenesis is the mechanism of the occurrence, progress, change and prognosis of the disease, focusing on the whole process and laws of disease occurrence and pathological reaction of human body.

第一节 发病原理
Section 1 Pathological Principles

一、发病的基本原理
1 Basic pathological principles

（一）正气不足是疾病发生的内在根据
1.1 Deficiency of vital qi is the internal basis for the occurrence of diseases

正气的强弱是决定发病与否的关键因素和内在依据，对发病起主导作用，如正虚感邪而发病，正虚生邪而发病，当正气不足，脏腑功能减退，多表现为虚证或虚实夹杂证。

The strength of vital qi is the key factor and internal basis to determine whether the disease occurs or not, and plays a leading role in the disease, such as the disease caused by deficient vital qi affected by exogenous or endogenous etiological factors, and the disease caused by deficiency of vital qi causing hypofunction of zang-fu viscera, which are mostly manifested as deficiency syndrome or syndrome of intermingled deficiency and excess.

（二）邪气是疾病发生的重要条件
1.2 Pathogenic qi is an important condition for the occurrence of diseases

邪气是发病的原因，影响发病的性质、类型、特点，病情和病位。在某些情况下，如邪气的毒力和致病力特别强，超过人体正气抗御能力，会导致疾病的发生。如疠气、高压、虫兽伤等。

Pathogenic qi is the cause of the disease, which affects the nature, type, characteristic, condition and location of the disease. If the virulence and pathogenicity of the pathogenic qi are too strong for vital qi to resist, diseases will occur. Pathogenic qi includes pestilent qi, high pressure, injury by animal and insect, etc.

（三）正邪斗争的胜负决定发病与否

1.3 The outcome of the struggle between vital qi and pathogenic qi determines whether the disease occurs or not

在邪正相争过程中，正气与病邪斗争的胜负，决定疾病的发生与否和发病的轻重缓急。

Vital qi and pathogenic qi struggle with each other, and the outcome determines the occurrence and priority of diseases.

二、影响发病的因素

2 The factors affecting the onset of the disease

影响发病的因素包括气候变化、地域特点、生活条件，以及体质特点、精神状态等。如气候的异常变化、气候及水土差异会引起季节病、地区多发病；久居阴暗潮湿之处，易受寒湿邪气所伤，出现关节疼痛；体质较弱或情绪异常波动可导致气血失调、脏腑功能失常而发病。

These factors include climate change, regional characteristics, living conditions, constitutions, mental states and so on. For instance, abnormal climate changes and climate, water and soil differences will cause seasonal and regional diseases; People living in a dark and humid place for a long time are vulnerable to cold and dampness, and feel pains in their joints; Weak constitution or abnormal mood swings can lead to imbalance of qi and blood and dysfunction of zang–fu viscera.

三、发病途径

3 The pathways of disease

（一）外感病邪

3.1 Exogenous etiological factors

病邪主要通过皮毛和口鼻，由表入里，侵犯脏腑。

They mainly enter from the outside to the inside through skin, nose and mouth, and invade zang–fu viscera.

（二）内伤病因

3.2 Endogenous etiological factors

以邪伤为主者，多因脏腑、气血功能失调及脏器组织结构损伤而发病。

In this case, patients are mainly affected by endogenous etiological factors causing dysfunction of zang-fu viscera, qi and blood and damage of organ structure.

（三）其他病因致病的发病途径

3.3 Pathological types

1. 感而即发 指机体感邪后随即发病的发病类型。

Immediate onset after contraction It refers to the pathological type of immediate onset after the body is contracted.

2. 伏而后发 指邪伏藏而后发病的发病类型。

Onset after incubation It refers to the pathological type of pathogenic qi hidden and then diseases occurring.

3. 徐发 指徐缓而病的发病类型。

Gradual onset This type means gradual onset of diseases after being in contact with pathogens.

4. 继发 指在原有疾病的基础上继发新的病变。

Secondary onset It means the secondary new lesions occur on the basis of the original diseases.

5. 复发 指原病再度发作或反复发作，复发大多与一定的诱发因素有关。

Recurrence It refers to the recurrence or relapse of the original disease, which is mostly related to certain inducing factors.

第二节 基本病机
Section 2 Basic Pathogenesis

基本病机，是指机体在致病因素作用下所产生的基本病理反应，是疾病发生后病变本质变化的一般规律。主要包括邪正盛衰、阴阳失调、气血津液失常，以及“内生五邪”。

Basic pathogenesis refers to the basic pathological reaction of the body to etiological factors, which is the general law of pathological changes after the occurrence of diseases. It mainly includes rising and falling of vital qi and pathogenic qi, yin-yang disharmony, abnormal qi, blood and fluid, and “five endogenous pathogenic qi”.

一、邪正盛衰

1 Rising and falling of vital qi and pathogenic qi

邪正盛衰，是指在疾病过程中，致病邪气与机体抗病能力之间相互斗争所发生的盛衰变化，关系到疾病的发展与转归，以及疾病的虚实病理变化。

The rising and falling of vital qi and pathogenic qi refers to the power changes in the struggle between pathogenic qi and disease resistance in the process of disease, including the development and prognosis of disease, as well as the pathological changes of deficiency and excess of disease.

（一）邪正盛衰与虚实变化

1.1 Rising and falling of vital qi and pathogenic qi and the change of deficiency and excess

1. 虚实病机 Deficiency and excess pathogenesis

（1）实性病机　主要是指邪气亢盛，正气未衰，以邪盛为主要矛盾的一类病理变化。多见于疾病的初期或中期，病程相对较短。

Excess pathogenesis　It mainly refers to a kind of pathological changes in which pathogenic qi is excessive, while vital qi is not declining, namely, excess pathogenic qi is the major cause of the disease. It is more common in the early or middle stage of the disease, and the course of the disease is relatively short.

（2）虚性病机　主要是指正气不足，邪不太盛，以正气亏虚为主要矛盾的一类病理变化。多由体质素虚，或疾病后期正气不足，大病久病之后，伤阴损阳，导致正气虚弱。

Deficiency pathogenesis　It mainly refers to a kind of pathological changes with deficiency of vital qi, while pathogenic qi is not so excess, namely, deficiency of vital qi is the main cause of the disease. It is due to usual deficiency of physical constitution, or deficiency of vital qi in the later stage of diseases, and after a serious illness, yin and yang are damaged, resulting in deficiency of vital qi.

2. 虚实夹杂 Intermingled deficiency and excess

（1）实中夹虚　以邪实为主，兼有正气不足者。如邪热炽盛，消灼津液而致实热伤津，而见高热、烦渴、尿少、齿舌干燥等为主要表现者。

Excess complicated with deficiency　In this case, pathogenic qi is excess, but also complicated with deficient vital qi. For example, excess etiological heat burns fluid and causes fluid deficiency, leading to symptoms such as high fever, polydipsia, oliguria, dry teeth and tongue.

（2）虚中夹实　以正虚为主，兼有实邪停留，或复感邪气者。如脾阳虚衰，水湿内生，以食少、神疲、水肿、痰多等为主要表现者。

Deficiency complicated with excess　In this case, vital qi is deficient, but also complicated with retained or regained excess pathogenic qi. For example, endogenous water dampness occurs due to spleen yang deficiency, resulting in symptoms such as poor appetite, mental fatigue, edema and excessive phlegm.

（二）邪正盛衰与疾病转归

1.2 Rising and falling of vital qi and pathogenic qi and change and prognosis of diseases

1. 正胜邪退　指疾病趋于好转和痊愈的一种转归。如风寒感冒，病邪表浅，正气亦能抗邪外出，若予以解表宣肺，则病邪驱除，正气修复。

Vital qi prevailing and pathogenic qi declining　It refers to a kind of prognosis that the disease tends to resolve and get better. In the case of common cold with wind–cold syndrome, the etiological factors are superficial, and vital qi can also resist them. If the patient is treated with reliving the exterior and dispersing the lungs, the etiological factors will be expelled and vital qi will be repaired.

2. 邪胜正衰　指在邪正消长盛衰变化过程中，疾病趋于恶化的一种转归。如外感热病过程出现正不敌邪，此时若能及时施治，也可避免恶化。

Pathogenic qi prevailing and vital qi declining　It refers to a kind of prognosis that the disease tends to deteriorate. For example, vital qi fails to resist pathogenic qi when exogenous fever occurs. But if it can be treated in time, deterioration can also be avoided.

3. 正虚邪恋　指疾病后期，正气已虚，邪气未尽，病势缠绵的一种转归。如外邪犯肺，若因正气素虚，或治疗不彻底，可致咳嗽日久不愈，甚至发展成为慢性咳喘病。

Vital qi being deficient with pathogenic qi lingering　It refers to a kind of prognosis in the late stage of the disease, in which vital qi is deficient, but pathogenic qi is not exhausted, and the disease is lingering. In the case of exogenous pathogen invading the lungs, deficiency of vital qi or incomplete treatment will cause cough not to be cured for a long time, and even develop into chronic cough and asthma.

4. 邪去正虚　指疾病后期，病邪已去，但正气耗伤的一种状态。多见于急、重病的后期。

Pathogenic qi declining and vital qi being deficient　It refers to a state in which the pathogenic qi has gone but the vital qi is consumed in the late stage of the disease. It is more common in the late stage of acute and serious illness.

二、阴阳失调

2 Yin-yang disharmony

阴阳失调是指在疾病的发生发展过程中，由于各种致病因素的影响，导致机体的阴阳双方失去相对的平衡协调而出现的阴阳偏盛、偏衰、互损、格拒、亡失等一系列病理变化。

Yin–yang disharmony refers to a series of pathological changes in the process of disease occurrence and development due to the influence of various etiological factors, including excess or deficiency of either yin or yang, mutual impairment between yin and yang, expulsion of yin and yang, collapse of yin or yang.

（一）阴阳偏胜

2.1 Excess of either yin or yang

1. 阳偏胜　指疾病过程中表现的一种功能亢奋、热量过剩的病理状态。如肝火上炎导致肝气疏泄太过，出现目赤头痛、急躁易怒、吐血等。

Yang excess　It refers to a pathological state of hyperactivity and excess heat in the process of disease. For example, liver fire flaring up leads to excessive flow of qi, causing red eyes, headache, irritability, hematemesis, etc.

2. 阴偏胜　指疾病过程中表现的一种阴寒性病理产物积聚的病理状态。如寒湿困阻脾脏阳气，出现腹胀腹泻、不思饮食等。

Yin excess　It refers to a pathological state in which a pathological product characterized by yin cold accumulates in the process of disease. For example, cold dampness blocks spleen yang, resulting in abdominal distension, diarrhea, poor appetite, etc.

（二）阴阳偏衰

2.2 Deficiency of either yin or yang

1. 阳偏衰　指疾病过程中，阳气虚损，功能活动减退或衰弱，温煦功能减退的一种病理状态。常见畏寒喜暖、四肢不温、喜静蜷卧等。

Yang deficiency　It refers to a pathological state in which yang qi is deficient, causing functional activities, including warm function, are decreased or weakened. It usually causes fear of cold, liking for warm, not warm limbs, liking for lying up quietly, etc.

2. 阴偏衰　指疾病过程中，阴液亏损，阴不制阳，导致阳气相对偏旺，功能活动虚性亢奋的一种病理状态。常见五心烦热、骨蒸潮热、盗汗、颧红等。

Yin deficiency　It refers to a pathological state in which yin fluid is deficient and yin fails to control yang, which leads to relatively excess yang qi and virtual hyperactivity of functional activities. It usually causes dysphoria with feverish sensation in chest, palms and soles, hectic fever, tidal fever, night sweating, hectic cheek and so on.

（三）阴阳互损

2.3 Mutual impairment between yin and yang

1. 阴损及阳　指由于阴液亏损，致使阳气的生化不足，或阳气无所依附而耗散，形成以阴虚为主的阴阳两虚病变。如肝阳上亢，病情进一步发展，亦可耗损肝肾阳气，而见畏寒肢冷、面白等。

Yin deficiency involving yang It refers to the deficiency of both yin and yang mainly due to yin deficiency. It is because the deficiency of yang qi generation, or the dissipation of yang qi without attachment due to the deficiency of yin fluid. For instance, if upper hyperactivity of liver yang develops further, it can also consume yang qi in liver and kidneys, causing fear of cold, cold limbs, white face, etc.

2. 阳损及阴 指由于阳气亏损，致使阴液的生成减少，形成以阳虚为主的阴阳两虚病变。如津液代谢障碍所致水肿，而见日益消瘦、烦躁不安等。

Yang deficiency involving yin It refers to the deficiency of both yin and yang state mainly due to yang deficiency. It is because the decrease of yin fluid generation due to the loss of yang qi. For instance, edema caused by fluid metabolism disorder can lead to increasing emaciation, dysphoria and so on.

三、精气血津液失常

3 Abnormal essence, qi, blood and fluid

（一）精的失常

3.1 Abnormal essence

1. 精亏 主要指肾精不足。如先天禀赋不足或房劳过度等，出现小儿生长发育异常，成年人体弱多病，男子精少不育等。

Essence deficiency It mainly refers to kidney essence deficiency. For example, insufficiency of natural endowment or excessive sexual intercourse can lead to abnormal growth and development of children, frailness of adults, oligospermia and infertility of men and so on.

2. 精瘀 指男子精滞精道，排精障碍。如房事不节可致精泄不畅而瘀滞。

Essence stasis It refers to men's sperm stagnating in the seminal tract, and difficult to be excreted. For example, excessive sexual intercourse can cause poor sperm discharge and stagnation.

（二）气的失常

3.2 Abnormal qi

1. 气虚 指气的生化不足或耗散太过，从而使脏腑组织功能活动减退的病理变化。如脾气虚，可见食少、消瘦、四肢无力等。

Qi deficiency It refers to the pathological changes of insufficiency of qi generation or excessive dissipation of qi, which leads to the decline of functional activities of zang–fu viscera and tissues. For example, deficiency of spleen qi can cause poor appetite, emaciation, weakness of limbs, etc.

2. 气机失调 指由于致病邪气的干扰，或脏腑功能失调，导致气的升降出入运动失常所引起的病理变化，包括气滞、气逆、气陷、气闭、气脱等。

Qi movement disorder It refers to the pathological changes of the abnormal ascending, descending, entering and exiting movements of qi due to etiological pathogens or the dysfunction of zang–fu viscera, including qi stagnation, qi reverse flow, qi sinking ,qi blockage, qi desertion, etc.

（三）血的失常

3.3 Abnormal blood

1. 血虚 指血液不足，濡养功能减退的一种病理变化。如面色、唇、甲淡白无华，健忘，神疲等。

Blood deficiency It refers to a pathological change of blood insufficiency and impaired moistening and nourishing function, including symptoms such as pale complexion, lips and nails, amnesia, spiritlessness, etc.

2. 血液运行失常 指由于某些致病邪气或脏腑功能失调，导致血液运行瘀滞不畅或运行加速的病理变化，包括血瘀和出血两种。

Abnormal blood circulation It refers to the pathological changes of blood stasis or accelerated blood circulation due to pathogenic qi or dysfunction of zang–fu viscera, including blood stasis and bleeding.

（四）津液代谢失常

3.4 Abnormal fluid metabolism

1. 津液不足 指津液亏少导致脏腑、组织官窍失其濡润滋养，产生干燥失润的病理变化。如夏季多汗尿少，或气候干燥而见口、鼻、皮肤干燥等。

Fluid deficiency It refers to the pathological change of dryness and loss of moisture and nourishment of zang–fu viscera, tissues and orifices caused by fluid insufficiency, such as hyperhidrosis and scanty urine in summer, or dry mouth, nose and skin due to dry climate.

2. 津液输布、排泄障碍 指津液不能正常转输和布散导致津液在体内环流迟缓，或者在某一局部发生滞留。如脾失健运、肺失宣降、肾阳不足，气化失职而见水肿、少尿等。

Disorder of fluid distribution and excretion It refers to the slow circulation of fluid in the body or its retention in a certain part due to abnormal transfer and distribution of fluid. Such as edema or short urine due to qi transformation disorder which may be caused by dysfunction of spleen in transportation, lungs failing to govern upward and outward diffusion as well as descent and purification or kidney yang deficiency.

第三节　内生五邪
Section 3　Five Endogenous Pathogenic Qi

“内生五邪”是指在疾病的发展过程中，由于脏腑阴阳失调，气、血、津液代谢异常所产生的类似风、寒、湿、燥、火五种外邪致病特征的病理变化。分别称为“内风”“内寒”“内湿”“内燥”“内火”。

“Five endogenous pathogenic qi” refer to the pathological changes similar to the etiological characteristics of five climatic exopathogens, namely, wind, cold, dampness, dryness and fire, which are caused by yin–yang disharmony of zang–fu viscera and abnormal metabolism of qi, blood and fluid in the development of diseases. They are called “endogenous wind”, “endogenous cold”, “endogenous dampness”, “endogenous dryness” and “endogenous fire”.

一、风气内动
1 Wind stirring internally

风气内动，即是“内风”。表现为眩晕、麻木、抽搐、震颤等“动摇”特征的一类病理变化。

Wind stirring internally produces the “endogenous wind”, causing a kind of pathological changes characterized by vertigo, numbness, convulsions and tremors.

1. 肝阳化风　多是情志所伤、操劳太过等耗伤肝肾之阴，筋脉失养所产生的病理变化。表现为肢体麻木、口眼㖞斜、半身不遂等。

Hyperactive liver yang causing wind　It is mostly caused by damaged by excess of seven emotions, overwork, etc., which consumes yin of liver and kidney and causes malnutrition of muscles and tendons. It is manifested as numbness of limbs, facial paralysis, hemiplegia, etc.

2. 热极生风　多见于热性病的热盛阶段。临床以四肢抽搐、目睛上吊、角弓反张等为主要表现，并伴有高热、神昏等。

Extreme heat causing wind　It is more common in the heat exuberance stage of febrile disease. Clinically, the main manifestations are limb convulsions, upward vision of eyes, opisthotonus, etc., accompanied by high fever and faintness.

3. 阴虚风动　机体阴液枯竭，无以濡养筋脉而产生的病理变化。常表现为筋惕肉瞤、手足蠕动等。

Stirring wind due to yin deficiency　It is caused by yin fluid deficiency leading to malnutrition of muscles and tendons. Common symptoms are muscular twitching and cramp, wriggling of limbs, etc.

4. 血虚生风 血液亏虚，血不荣经而产生的病理状态。多表现为肢体麻木、筋肉跳动等。

Blood deficiency causing wind It is caused by deficient blood failing to nourish meridians. Most of the symptoms are numbness of limbs, throbbing of muscles and so on.

二、寒从中生

2 Cold generated from within

寒从中生，是指机体阳气虚衰，温煦气化功能减退，阳不制阴，虚寒内生的病理变化。如阳气不足，温煦失职，出现畏寒肢冷等。

Cold generated from within refers to the pathological changes of endogenous deficiency-cold due to yang-qi deficiency which causes impaired warming and transformation functions and yang failing to control yin, including symptoms such as fear of cold and cold limbs due to impaired warming function of qi.

三、湿浊内生

3 Endogenous dampness-turbidity

湿浊内生，多因体内津液输布、排泄障碍，导致水湿痰饮内生的病理变化。如胸闷、大便不爽、身体困重等。

Endogenous dampness-turbidity refers to the pathological changes of water-dampness and phlegm retention due to fluid distribution and excretion disorders, such as chest tightness, unpleasant stool, heavy body, etc.

四、津伤化燥

4 Fluid deficiency causing dryness

津伤化燥，指体内津液不足，导致人体各组织器官失于濡润而出现干燥枯涩症状的病理变化。如肺燥宣降失司，常见干咳、咯血等。

Fluid deficiency causing dryness refers to the pathological change of dryness caused by insufficient fluid in the body, which leads to the loss of moisture and nourishment of various tissues and organs. For example, dryness in the lungs causes lungs to fail to govern upward and outward diffusion as well as descent and purification, and dry cough or hemoptysis often occurs.

五、火热内生

5 Endogenous fire

火热内生，指由于阳盛有余或阴虚阳亢而致的火热内扰，功能亢奋的病理变化。如阳气过盛或痰湿、瘀血、食积等，郁久化火，或阴虚火旺，引起骨蒸颧红、烦躁等。

Endogenous fire refers to the pathological changes of fire disturbing internally and hyperactivity of various functions caused by excessive yang or a relative hyperactivity of yang due to yin deficiency. For instance, excessive yang qi, long–term phlegm–dampness, blood stasis or dyspepsia transforming into fire, or yin deficiency leading to fire hyperactivity, can cause hectic fever, hectic cheek, dysphoria and so forth.

第七章　养生与防治原则
Chapter 7　Principles of Health Preservation and Prevention and Treatment

养生是指保养生命，以延长寿命，提高生命质量，减少疾病的发生。防治原则，是预防和治疗疾病时依据的基本法则。只有在治则的指导下，才能针对具体的病证制定有针对性的治疗方法，即治疗方法是对治疗原则的具体体现和实施。

Health preservation refers to maintaining life to prolong life span, improve quality of life and reduce the occurrence of diseases. The principles of prevention and treatment of diseases are the basic rules for preventing and treating diseases. Only under the guidance of treatment principles can we formulate targeted treatment methods for specific diseases and syndromes, that is, treatment methods are the concrete embodiment and implementation of treatment principles.

第一节　养生原则
Section 1　Principles of Health Preservation

养生的原则主要包括顺应自然、惜养肾精、慎重脾胃、形神兼顾。

The principles of health preservation mainly include conforming to nature, cherishing kidney essence, minding spleen and stomach, and taking into account both body and spirit.

一、顺应自然
1 Conforming to nature

中医学认为“人以天地之气生，四时之法成”，即人类是自然界的产物，只有不违背自然界的规律，才能减少疾病的发生。就四季而言，在春夏顺应外界阳气的渐增而多活动，在秋冬顺应外界的阴气渐增而适度休息。就一日而言，在白昼应活动，在夜晚宜休息。这些道理虽然简单，但很多现代人经常违背，导致阴阳颠倒，疾病丛生。

TCM holds that “human beings come to life through the qi of heaven and earth and matures in accordance with the laws of the four seasons”, that is, human beings are the products of nature, and only by not violating the laws of nature can we reduce the occurrence of diseases. As far as the four seasons are concerned, we should do more activities in spring and summer when yang qi increases in nature, and take moderate rest in autumn and winter when yin qi increases. As far as a day is concerned, we should be active during the day and rest at night. Although these principles are simple, many modern people often violate them, which leads to the reversal of yin and yang and numerous diseases.

二、惜养肾精

2 Cherishing the kidney essence

肾是“先天之本”，藏有大量的精，精是神的基础，是生命力的本源物质，可以促进人体的生长发育，尤其与人的生殖繁衍有关。养生家强调肾容易虚，精难以补，所以要爱惜肾精，成年人不可纵欲，过度纵欲会消耗肾精而导致早衰。

Kidneys are the “congenital origin”, which store a large amount of essence. Essence is the foundation of spirit and the original substance of life force, which can promote the growth and development of human body, especially promoting human reproduction and procreation. Experts in health preservation emphasize that the kidneys are easy to be deficient and essence is difficult to tonify, so we should cherish kidney essence, and adults should not give way to their carnal desires which will consume kidney essence and lead to senilism.

三、慎重脾胃

3 Minding the spleen and stomach

脾胃为气血生化之源，后天之本。如果脾胃虚弱，难以受纳和运化食物，不但气血生成不足，而且服药也难以吸收，严重影响治病的疗效。中国人讲“病从口入”，强调饮食要有节制、讲卫生，不可有五味偏嗜。此外，服药时也要避免伤及脾胃，常用健脾养胃药。

Spleen and stomach are the source of qi and blood and the acquired foundation. If the spleen and stomach are too weak to receive, transport or transform food, not only will the generation of qi and blood be insufficient, but also it will be difficult to absorb medicines, which will seriously affect the efficacy. Chinese people say that “diseases enter by the mouth”, emphasizing that diet should be moderate and hygienic, and that there should be no flavor predilection. In addition, we should avoid impair the spleen and stomach when taking medicine, and use medicines for strengthening the spleen and nourishing the stomach.

四、形神兼顾

4 Taking into account both body and spirit

健康的肉体是正常精神活动的物质基础，而精神可驾驭肉体。养生家强调养性调神，一方面通过适度的身体锻炼，如打太极拳、练习八段锦等促进气血流通，另一方面注意“恬惔虚无”“安神定志”，避免为物欲驱使，保持心神清明，控制好自己的身体和情绪。

A healthy body is the material basis of normal mental activities, and spirit can control the body. Experts in health preservation emphasize nourishing the mind. On the one hand, they promote the circulation of qi and blood through moderate physical exercises, such as doing taijiquan (shadow boxing) and baduanjin (eight trigrams boxing); on the other hand, they pay attention to "calmness and indifferent to fame or gain" and "tranquillization and settling minds", avoiding being driven by material desires, keeping their minds clear and controlling their bodies and emotions.

第二节　治未病
Section 2　Preventive Treatment of Diseases

"治未病"是指预防疾病，包括以下两个方面。

"Preventive treatment of diseases" refers to preventing diseases, including the following two aspects.

一、未病先防
1 Preventing diseases before onset

在疾病未发生之前，一方面应当注意增强人体正气，提高抗病能力；另一方面要注意避免各种邪气的侵害，防止环境、水源和食物的污染，注意生活与工作环境。

Before the disease occurs, on the one hand, attention should be paid to strengthening the vital qi of the human body and improving the disease resistance; on the other hand, we should avoid all kinds of pathogenic qi, prevent the pollution of environment, water and food, and pay attention to maintaining good living and working environment.

二、既病防变
2 Preventing deterioration after onset

在疾病发生的初始阶段，就应当争取早期诊断、早期治疗，防止病情进一步发展，以达到早期治愈疾病的目的。

In the initial stage of the disease, we should strive for early diagnosis and treatment to prevent the disease from deterioration, so as to cure the disease at an early stage.

第三节　治病求本
Section 3　Treatment Aiming at Its Root Causes

治病求本是治疗疾病的基本原则，是指必须寻求出病证的本质，针对其本质进行治疗。

Treatment aiming at its root causes is the basic principle of treating diseases, which means that we must seek out the root causes of diseases and syndromes and treat them accordingly.

一、标与本的概念

1 The concept of manifestation and root cause

标与本是相对的概念，一般而言，反映内在本质的病因病机为本，为一般治疗时的重点；外在的症状为标，在紧急情况下，治标比治本更为重要。

Manifestation and root cause are a pair of opposite concepts. Generally speaking, root cause refers to the etiology and pathogenesis reflecting the internal essence, and it is the focus of general treatment; while manifestation refers to external symptoms, and it is more important to treat the manifestations than the root causes in acute conditions.

（一）急则治标

1.1 Symptomatic treatment in acute condition

急则治标，是指症状危急时，先处理症状。例如大出血患者，若出血量大，无论什么病因病机，都应先紧急止血，待病情缓解后，再根据出血的病因病机以治本。

Symptomatic treatment in acute condition means that at emergency levels, symptoms should be treated first. For example, when treating patients with massive hemorrhage, doctors should stop bleeding urgently regardless of the etiology or pathogenesis. And after remission, they can treat the root causes of hemorrhage according to the etiology and pathogenesis.

（二）缓则治本

1.2 Radical treatment in chronic case

缓则治本，是在症状不急不重时所采用的一种治疗原则。治本可以消除病因病机，属于标的症状可以自消。

Radical treatment in chronic case is a treatment principle adopted when symptoms are not urgent or serious. Treating the root causes can eliminate the etiology and pathogenesis, and the symptoms can eliminate themselves accordingly.

（三）标本兼治

1.3 Treating both manifestation and root cause of diseases

标本兼治，是指病情复杂但不危急时采取的治疗原则。标本兼顾而同治，才能取得较好的治疗效果。例如阳盛伤阴的发热患者出现大便干结而腹痛，可同时采用清热与滋阴的方法。

Treating both manifestation and root cause of diseases refers to the treatment principle adopted when the condition is complicated but not critical. In this case, good therapeutic effect can be achieved only when both manifestations and root causes are taken into account and treated at the same time. For example, patients with fever caused by excessive yang damaging yin may have symptoms of dry stool and abdominal pain, and they can be treated with the methods of clearing heat and nourishing yin at the same time.

二、逆治

2 Orthodox treatment

逆治是指逆着病证的病机性质而治的常规治疗原则。逆治主要有以下四种治法。

Orthodox treatment refers to the routine treatment principle of treating against the pathogenesis of diseases and syndromes. There are four main methods of orthodox treatment.

1. 寒者热之 指寒性病证出现寒象，用温热药进行治疗。

Treating cold syndrome with heat methods It means treating cold syndromes with cold manifestations with warm or hot medicines or formulae.

2. 热者寒之 指热性病证出现热象，用寒凉药进行治疗。

Treating heat syndrome with cold methods It means treating heat syndromes with heat manifestations with cool or cold medicines or formulae.

3. 虚则补之 指虚性病证出现虚弱表现，用补益药进行治疗。

Treating deficiency syndrome with tonifying methods It means treating deficiency syndromes with deficiency manifestations with tonic medicines or formulae.

4. 实则泻之 指实性病证出现实性表现，用攻邪药进行治疗。

Treating excess syndrome with purgative methods It means treating excess syndromes with excess manifestations with purgative medicines or formulae.

三、从治

3 Retrograde treatment

从治是指顺从着病证的外在假象而治的一种治疗原则。这一治则适用于本质与现象不完全一致的病证。从治主要有以下四种治法。

Retrograde treatment refers to the treatment principle that obeys the external illusion of diseases and syndromes. This rule is applicable to diseases and syndromes whose manifestations and root causes are not completely consistent. There are mainly the following four treatment methods.

1. 热因热用 指用温热药治疗具有假热现象病证的治法，适用于真寒假热证。

Treating false-heat syndrome with heat methods It refers to the treatment of syndromes with false heat manifestations with warm or hot medicines or formulae, which is suitable for syndrome of true cold disease with false heat manifestation.

2. 寒因寒用 指用寒凉药治疗具有假寒现象病证的治法，适用于真热假寒证。

Treating false-cold syndrome with cold methods It refers to the treatment of syndromes with false cold manifestations with cool or cold medicines or formulae, which is suitable for syndrome of true heat disease with false cold manifestation.

3. 塞因塞用 指用补益药治疗具有闭塞症状的虚证，适用于真虚假实证。

Treating obstructive syndrome with tonifying methods It refers to the treatment of deficiency syndromes with obstructive manifestations with tonic medicines or formulae, which is suitable for syndrome of true deficiency disease with false excessive manifestation.

4. 通因通用 指用通利药治疗具有通泄症状的实证，适用于真实假虚证。

Treating incontinent syndrome with dredging methods It refers to the treatment of excess syndrome with incontinent manifestations with purgative medicines or formulae, which is suitable for syndrome of true excess disease with false deficient manifestation.

第四节 扶正祛邪
Section 4 Strengthening Vital Qi and Eliminating Pathogenic Qi

一、扶正与祛邪的原则
1 The principles of strengthening vital qi and eliminating pathogenic qi

扶正与祛邪，是针对虚证和实证所制定的两个基本治疗原则。

Strengthening vital qi and eliminating pathogenic qi are two basic treatment principles for deficiency syndrome and excess syndrome.

1. 扶正 指使用扶助正气的药物，或施行针灸、推拿、饮食等疗法，改善体质，提高人体的抗病能力。

Strengthening vital qi It refers to improving constitution and the disease resistance of human body through vital qi-strengthening medicines or formulae, acupuncture, massage, dietetic therapy and other therapies.

2. 祛邪 指使用祛除邪气的药物，或针灸、推拿、手术等疗法，以消除病理反应。

Eliminating pathogenic qi It refers to eliminating pathological reactions through pathogenic qi-eliminating medicines or formulae, acupuncture, massage, surgery and other therapies.

使用扶正与祛邪治则，首先要分清证候虚实，其次在用药上要注意轻重缓急。扶正时要避免扶助邪气；祛邪时要避免过度伤及正气，尤其是要注意保护脾胃。

To apply the principles of strengthening vital qi and eliminating pathogenic qi, we should first distinguish the deficiency and excess of syndromes, and then achieve rational medication.

When strengthening vital qi, we should avoid strengthening pathogenic qi; and when eliminating pathogenic qi, we should avoid excessive impairment to vital qi, especially paying attention to protecting spleen and stomach.

二、扶正与祛邪的应用

2 The application of strengthening vital qi and eliminating pathogenic qi

（一）单用

2.1 Single use

1. 扶正　用于以正气不足为主要矛盾，邪气轻微的虚证。常用补气法、养血法、滋阴法、温阳法等。

Strengthening vital qi　It is used for deficiency syndrome with deficiency of vital qi as the main cause of the disease and slight pathogenic qi. Commonly used methods include invigorating qi, nourishing blood, nourishing yin and warming yang.

2. 祛邪　用于邪气盛而正气尚不虚的实证。常用汗法、下法、清热解毒法、活血化瘀法、化痰法、消食法等。

Eliminating pathogenic qi　It is used for excess syndrome with exuberance of pathogenic qi and relatively normal vital qi. Commonly used methods include diaphoresis, purgative method, clearing heat and removing toxicity, promoting blood circulation and removing blood stasis, resolving phlegm and promoting digestion.

（二）兼用

2.2 Combined use

又称为攻补兼施，适用于虚实错杂证，根据邪正盛衰变化而决定两者的主次。

Also known as reinforcement and elimination in combination, it is suitable for the syndrome of combined deficiency and excess, and the priority of reinforcement and elimination is determined by the rising and falling of vital qi and pathogenic qi.

（三）先后使用

2.3 Successive use

1. 先祛邪后扶正　在虚实错杂证中，邪盛为主，如果扶正则易助邪，可先祛邪，邪被清除后再扶正。

Eliminating pathogenic qi first and then strengthening vital qi　In the syndrome of combined deficiency and excess, if exuberant pathogenic qi is the main cause, we can eliminate it first, and then strengthen vital qi, or pathogenic qi may also be strengthened.

2. 先扶正后祛邪　在虚实错杂证中，若正气太虚，难以承受攻邪药的副作用时，可先扶正，而后祛邪。

Strengthening vital qi first and then eliminating pathogenic qi In the syndrome of combined deficiency and excess, if vital qi is too deficient to bear the side effects of pathogenic qi–eliminating medicines or formulae, we can strengthen vital qi first and then eliminate pathogenic qi.

第五节 调整阴阳
Section 5 Coordinating Yin and Yang

根据阴阳学说，人体的基本病机是阴阳失调。调整阴阳的偏盛或偏衰，促进阴阳恢复动态平衡，可使疾病痊愈。

According to the yin–yang theory, the basic pathogenesis of human body is yin–yang disharmony. Thus, coordinating the excess or deficiency of either yin or yang and promoting the restoration of dynamic balance between yin and yang can help to cure diseases.

一、损其有余
1 Impairing the excess

损其有余是针对阴阳偏盛制定的治疗原则。阴邪或阳邪的亢盛都是“邪气盛则实”，阳邪偏盛导致实热证，应用“热者寒之”以散热；阴邪偏盛导致实寒证，应用“寒者热之”的方法散寒。

Impairing the excess is the treatment principle formulated for excess of yin or yang. The hyperactivity of yin pathogen or yang pathogen belongs to “exuberance of pathogenic qi causing excess syndrome”. And excess of yang pathogen leads to excessive heat syndrome, so we should “treat heat syndrome with cold methods” ; while excessive yin pathogen leads to excessive cold syndrome, so we should “treat cold syndrome with heat methods”.

二、补其不足
2 Tonifying deficiency

补其不足是针对阴阳偏衰制定的治疗原则。阴阳虚衰属于“精气夺则虚”，阳偏衰不能制阴而阴盛，出现虚寒证，当补阳以制阴；阴偏衰不能制阳而阳亢，出现虚热证，当补阴以制阳。

Tonifying deficiency is the treatment principle formulated for deficiency of yin or yang. Deficiency of yin or yang belongs to “lack of essence and qi causing deficiency syndrome”. And if deficient yang fails to control yin, which leads to relatively excess yin, namely, yang deficiency syndrome, we should tonify yang to control yin; if deficient yin fails to control yang, which leads to relatively excess yang, namely, yin deficiency syndrome, we should tonify yin to control yang.

第六节　三因制宜
Section 6　Full Consideration of Three Factors

三因制宜包括因时、因地和因人制宜，这是在整体观念和辨证论治指导下确立的治则。

Full consideration of three factors refers to considering climatic and seasonal conditions, the environment, and individual constitution, which is a treatment principle established under the guidance of the holism concept and treatment based on syndrome differentiation.

一、因时制宜
1 Full consideration of climatic and seasonal conditions

四时气候的变化，对人体生理和病理都会产生一定的影响，治疗疾病时必须考虑时间的特点，例如在夏季，气候较热，人体腠理疏松开泄，即使外感风寒致病，也不宜大量使用辛温药，以免汗液开泄太过；在冬季治疗热证时，应当慎用寒凉药，避免大量的寒凉药损伤了阳气。

The change of climate at four seasons will have a certain impact on human physiology and pathology, so we must consider the climatic and seasonal conditions when treating diseases. For example, in summer, the climate is hot, and the interstices of human body open and discharge. Even if exogenous wind–cold causes diseases, it is inappropriate to use a large number of pungent and warm herbs in case profuse sweating occurs; when treating heat syndrome in winter, we should use cold and cool herbs with caution to avoid damage of yang qi.

二、因地制宜
2 Full consideration of the environment

不同的地区气候差别大，而且居民的生活饮食习惯不同，所以人的体质不同，感受相同的病因后症状可能不同，需要辨证论治。例如气候寒冷的高原地区，治疗多用温热药；而气候温暖潮湿的地区，治疗常用清热或化湿药。

Different regions have different climates, and residents' living and eating habits are different, so people's constitutions and their symptoms after being affected by the same etiological factors are also different. Therefore, treatment should be based on syndrome differentiation. For example, in plateau areas with cold climate, warm and hot medicines and formulae are often used for treatment; in warm and humid areas, heat–clearing or dampness–eliminating medicines and formulae are commonly used.

三、因人制宜

3 Full consideration of individual constitution

在辨证论治时，应按患者的年龄、性别、体质的特点，来选用适宜的治法和方药。例如小儿患外感病后，病情变化较快，常有易寒易热、易虚易实的特点，用药量宜轻，要随病情变化及时调整治疗方案。老年人脏腑功能不同程度地衰弱，患病多为虚证或虚实夹杂证，治疗要注意扶正，如需攻邪，用药量应比青壮年轻，避免攻邪过度而损伤正气。

In treatment based on syndrome differentiation, appropriate treatment methods and prescriptions should be selected according to the characteristics of patients' age, sex and constitution. For example, after children suffer from exogenous diseases, their conditions change rapidly, which are often characterized by shift changes from cold to heat or deficiency to excess. So the dosage should be small, and the treatment plan should be adjusted in time according to the change of conditions.Another example is that the functions of zang–fu viscera of the elderly are weak to varying degrees, and most of the diseases are deficiency syndrome or syndrome of combined deficiency and excess. Thus, we should pay attention to strengthening vital qi in treatment, and if we need to eliminate pathogenic qi, the dosage should be smaller than that of young adults, so as to avoid damaging vital qi.

第八章　中医诊断疾病的方法
Chapter 8　Methods of Diagnosing Diseases in Traditional Chinese Medicine

中医诊断疾病的方法称为诊法，是中医诊察、收集病情资料的基本方法和手段，主要包括望、闻、问、切“四诊”。

The methods of diagnosing diseases in TCM are called diagnostic methods, which are the basic methods and means of diagnosing and collecting disease data in TCM, mainly including “four diagnostic methods” of inspection, listening and smelling, inquiry as well as palpation and pulse taking.

人体是一个以五脏为中心的有机整体，脏腑、形体、官窍间通过经络相互联系，维持着机体生理功能的协调平衡。体内的生理、病理变化，必然会反映于外，所以通过诊察疾病显现于外部的各种征象，可以分析疾病的原因、性质、病位和邪正关系，了解脏腑的变化，从而为辨证论治提供依据。

The human body is an organic whole centered on the five zang viscera, and the zang–fu viscera, body constituents and orifices are interrelated through meridians, maintaining the coordination and balance of the body’s physiological functions. Physiological and pathological changes in the body will inevitably be reflected in the outside. Therefore, by examining various manifestations of diseases, we can analyze the cause, nature, location and the relationship between vital qi and pathogenic qi of diseases and understand the changes of viscera, thus providing basis for syndrome differentiation and treatment.

望、闻、问、切四种诊法，分别从不同的角度诊察病情、认识疾病，对于中医辨证具有同等重要的意义。临床诊病时，应四诊合参，才能客观准确、全面系统地收集病情资料，作出正确的诊断。

The four diagnostic methods of inspection, listening and smelling, inquiry as well as palpation and pulse taking, which diagnose the conditions and understand the diseases from different perspectives, are of equal significance to TCM syndrome differentiation. In clinical diagnosis, the four diagnostic methods should be combined, so as to collect the disease data objectively, accurately, comprehensively and systematically and make correct diagnosis.

第一节　望　诊
Section 1　Inspection

望诊是医生运用视觉观察患者的神、色、形、态、舌象、头面、五官及排出物等，以了解健康状况，测知病情的诊察方法。

Inspection is a diagnostic method for doctors to observe patients' spirit, color, body statue, movement, tongue manifestation, head and face, five apertures, secretion and excretion by vision, so as to understand their health status and detect their illness.

一、望神色形态
1 Inspection of spirit, color,body statue and movement

（一）望神
1.1 Inspection of spirit

望神是通过观察神的得失有无，以分析病情、判断预后的诊察方法。临床上一般可将神分为得神、少神、失神、假神及神乱 5 类。

Inspection of spirit is a diagnostic method to analyze the condition and judge the prognosis by observing the gains and losses of spirit. Clinically, the conditions of spirit can be generally divided into five categories: presence of spirit, insufficiency of spirit , loss of spirit, false spirit and mental disorder.

1. 得神　是精气充足神旺的表现。可见神志清楚，思维敏捷，言语清晰，目光明亮灵活，精彩内含，面色荣润含蓄，表情自然，体态自如，动作灵活，反应灵敏。可见于正常人，也可见于病情轻浅之人，说明精气未衰，脏腑未伤，预后良好。

Presence of spirit　It means abundant essence,qi and spirit. Its manifestations include clear consciousness, nimble thought, clear speech, bright, beady and flexible eyeballs, a moist lustrous face, natural facial expressions, free postures, smooth body movements and quick responses. The presence of spirit can be seen in healthy people or people with illness of mild conditions and surface locations, which indicates that the essence and qi are not declining, and the zang–fu viscera are not impaired, and that the prognosis is good.

2. 少神　即精气不足的表现。可见精神不振，思维迟钝，少气懒言，两目乏神，肢体倦怠，动作迟缓。多见于轻病或恢复期患者，亦可见于体质虚弱者。

Insufficiency of spirit　It means lack of essence and qi. Its manifestations include lassitude, slow thinking, panting, no desire to speak, sluggish eyeballs, flabby muscle and slow body movements. It is more common in patients with mild illness or in convalescence, and can also be seen in those with weak constitution.

3. 失神　是精亏气败神衰的表现。可见两目晦暗，目无光彩，面色无华，精神萎靡，意识模糊，反应迟钝，手撒尿遗，骨枯肉脱，形体羸瘦。多见于久病重病之人，提示预后不良。

Loss of spirit　It indicates deficiency of essence, qi and spirit. It can be seen that dull eyes with sluggish eyeballs, a dark complexion lacking lustre, listlessness, vague consciousness, slow response, outstretched hands, enuresis, dry bones and withered flesh, and marked emaciation. It is more common in people with long-term and serious diseases, indicating poor prognosis.

4. 假神　指垂危患者出现精神暂时“好转”的虚假表现，常见于精气极度衰竭之人，为临终前的预兆。如原本目光晦滞，突然目似有光，但却浮光外露；本为面色晦暗，突然两颧泛红如妆；本已神昏或精神极度萎靡，突然神识失清，想见亲人，言语不休；本来毫无食欲，久不能食，突然思食、索食等。假神是脏腑精气极度衰竭，正气将脱，虚阳外越，阴阳即将离决所致。

False spirit　It refers to the false signs of temporary “improvement” in spirit of dying patients, which is common in people with extreme exhaustion of essence and qi, and is a omen before death. Its manifestations include: a sudden change from dull eyes with sluggish eyeballs to floating brightness in the eyes; a sudden change from a dark complexion to flushed cheeks; a sudden change from mental unconsciousness or listlessness to clear consciousness, willingness to see loved ones and talkative voice; a sudden change from no appetite and low food intake into increased appetite and hunger, etc. False spirit is caused by the extreme exhaustion of essence and qi in zang–fu viscera, collapse of vital qi, deficiency yang flying out, and divorce of yin and yang.

5. 神乱　指神志错乱失常。临床常表现为狂躁、淡漠、痴呆等，多见于狂、癫、痴、痫等患者。

Mental disorder　It refers to insanity. Clinical manifestations include mania, apathy, dementia, etc., which are more common in patients with madness, insanity, epilepsy and delusion.

（二）望色

1.2 Inspection of color

望色是通过观察面部与肌肤的颜色和光泽，以了解病情的诊察方法。

Inspection of color is a diagnostic method to detect the illnesses by observing the color and luster of face and skin.

1. 常色　即正常无病的面色。其特点是明润、含蓄。明润，即面部皮肤光明润泽。含蓄，即面部色泽隐藏于皮肤之内，而不特别显露，是精气内含而不外泄的表现。常色有主色、客色之分。

Normal complexion　It means normal and healthy complexion. It is characterized by lustre and implicature. Lustre means the complexion is moist and lustrous. Implicature means the complexion is hidden in the skin, and not exposed, which manifests that the essence is contained in the body but not leaked. Normal complexion can be divided into governing complexion and visiting complexion.

（1）主色　是与生俱来的面色，是个体一生基本不变的面色。

Governing complexion　It is the congenital complexion, and almost remains unchanged throughout an individual's life.

（2）客色　因外界因素的影响，而微有相应变化的面色，称为客色。如随四时之变，人之面色也有春稍青、夏稍赤、长夏稍黄、秋稍白、冬稍黑的变化，但均不离明润、含蓄之本色。

Visiting complexion　It refers to the complexion slightly changing with the influence of external factors. For example, with the change of four seasons, people's complexion also changes from slightly blue in spring, slightly red in summer, slightly yellow in late summer, slightly white in autumn to slightly black in winter, but they are all moist, lustrous and non-exposed.

2. 病色　即疾病状态下面部色泽的异常变化。其特征是色泽晦暗枯槁或显露。观察病色之关键在于辨别五色善恶及五色主病。

Sick complexion　It is the abnormal changes in both color and lustre of the face under a morbid state. It is characterized by dull, withered or exposed color. The key to observe the sick complexion lies in distinguishing the benign complexion and malignant complexion and understanding the diseases indicated by the five colors.

（1）五色善恶　凡五色光明润泽者为善色，说明虽病而脏腑精气未衰，预后良好；凡五色枯槁晦暗者为恶色，提示病情深重，脏腑精气衰败，多预后不佳。

Benign complexion and malignant complexion　The five colors that are relatively bright and moist belong to benign complexions, indicating that although under a morbid state, the essence and qi of zang-fu viscera remain sufficient and have a favourable prognosis; while those that are dark and withered are malignant complexions, indicating critical conditions, essence and qi failure of zang-fu viscera and an unfavourable prognosis.

（2）五色主病　五色即青、赤、黄、白、黑5种不同的面色，可反映不同脏腑的病变及病邪的性质。

Five colors indicating diseases　Five different complexions, namely, blue, red, yellow, white and black, can indicate the pathological changes of different zang-fu viscera and the nature of etiological factors.

①青色：主寒证、气滞、血瘀、疼痛、惊风。

Blue: It indicates cold syndrome, qi stagnation, blood stasis, pain and convulsion.

②赤色：主热证。满面通红者，属实热证；两颧潮红者，属阴虚证。

Red: It indicates heat syndrome. Patients whose faces are reddened allover have excessive heat syndromes; The flushed cheeks indicate yin deficiency syndrome.

③黄色：主脾虚、湿证。面目一身俱黄者，为黄疸。其中黄色鲜明如橘皮色者，属阳黄，乃湿热为患；黄色晦暗如烟熏色者，属阴黄，乃寒湿为患。

Yellow: It indicates spleen deficiency syndrome and dampness syndrome. Those with yellow faces, eyeballs and skin are jaundice. If the yellow is as bright as orange peel, it belongs to yang yellow and indicates damp heat; if the yellow is as dark as smoke, it belongs to yin yellow and indicates cold and dampness.

④白色：主气血亏虚、寒证、亡阳、脱血。

White: It indicates deficiency of qi and blood, cold syndrome, yang depletion and blood loss.

⑤黑色：主肾虚、寒证、水饮、血瘀、剧痛。

Black: It indicates kidney deficiency, cold syndrome, water retention, blood stasis and severe pain.

（三）望形态

1.3 Inspection of body statue and movements

望形态是通过观察患者形体胖瘦、强弱及动静姿态，以诊察疾病的方法。

Inspection of body statue and movements is a method to diagnose diseases by observing the patient's body shapes, physical strengths, and dynamic and static postures.

1. 望形体 体强指形体强壮，提示内脏坚实，气血充盛，即使患病预后也较好。体弱指形体虚弱，提示内脏虚弱，气血不足，或病重难于治疗，预后较差。体胖多属阳气不足，或多痰多湿。体瘦多为脾胃虚弱，或中焦有热，或阴虚火旺。

Inspection of body statue Strong body indicates solid internal organs, abundant qi and blood and good prognosis even if the disease occurs. Physical weakness indicates visceral weakness, deficiency of qi and blood, or serious diseases which are difficult to treat and has poor prognosis. Fat body is mostly due to deficiency of yang qi, or excessive phlegm and dampness. Thin body is mostly due to deficiency of spleen and stomach, heat in the middle jiao, or excessive fire due to yin deficiency.

2. 望姿态 主要观察患者的行、坐、卧、立时的动作与体态。若行走之际，突然停步不前，以手护心或脘腹者，多为真心痛或脘腹痛；以手护腰，弯腰曲背，行动艰难，多为腰腿病。坐而仰首，伴咳喘痰多，多见于哮病、肺胀等病证；但卧不能坐，坐则晕眩，不耐久坐，多为肝阳化风，或气血俱虚。若卧时面常向里，喜静懒动，身重不能转侧，多属阴证、寒证、虚证；卧时面常向外，躁动不安，身轻自能转侧，多属阳证、热证、实证；仰卧伸足，掀去衣被，多属实热证；蜷卧缩足，喜加衣被者，多属虚寒证。若站立不稳，伴眩晕者，多属肝风内动；不耐久站，站立时常欲依靠他物支撑，多属气血虚衰。

Inspection of movements It mainly observes the patient's walking, sitting, lying and standing movements and postures. If the person suddenly stops when walking and touches his heart or abdomen with hands, he may have real heart pain or abdominal pain; pinching waist with hands, bending back, and moving hard often indicate waist and leg diseases. Sitting and looking up, accompanied by cough, gasp and profuse phlegm, is more common in asthma, lung distension and other diseases; if the person can't sit for a long time but lie down, or he will be dizzy, he may have hyperactive liver yang causing wind or deficiency of both qi and blood. Lying down with face inward, liking for quiet, laziness, and body being too heavy to turn sideways indicate yin syndrome, cold syndrome and deficiency syndrome; while lying down with face outward, restlessness, and body being easy to turn sideways mostly belong to yang syndrome, heat syndrome and excess syndrome; lying on the back, stretching the feet, and stripping away off clothes and quilts indicate excessive heat syndrome; while curling up, shrinking the feet, and liking to add clothes and quilts indicate deficiency cold syndrome. Standing unsteadily, accompanied by dizziness mostly belongs to internal stirring of liver wind; having difficulties in standing for a long time and wanting to lean against other things when standing are mostly due to deficiency of qi and blood.

二、望头颈五官

2 Inspection of head, face, neck and five apertures

（一）望头面

2.1 Inspection of head and face

1. 望头部 Inspection of head

（1）形态　小儿头形过大，伴智力低下者，为先天不足，肾精亏损，水液停聚。头形过小，伴智力低下者，为先天不足，肾精亏损。

Shape　If the child's head is too large, accompanied by mental retardation, it is due to congenital deficiency, kidney essence loss, and fluid retention. If the head is too small, accompanied by mental retardation, it is due to congenital deficiency and kidney essence loss.

（2）头发　头发润泽而浓密，为精血充足。头发稀疏、色黄干枯者，为精血不足。青年白发，有家族史而无所苦者，一般不作病态论；若伴健忘、腰膝酸软者，属肾虚；伴心悸、失眠、健忘者，为劳神伤血。

Hair　Moist and thick hair indicates sufficient essence and blood. Sparse and dry hair with yellow color is due to deficiency of essence and blood. If young people with white hair have family history and no trouble because of it, it is not considered to be morbid; but if the white hair is accompanied by forgetfulness, soreness and weakness of waist and knees, it belongs to kidney deficiency; if accompanied by palpitation, insomnia, forgetfulness, it indicates excessive mental labor damaging blood.

2. 望面部　若眼睑浮肿，多为水肿病。若一侧或两侧腮部以耳垂为中心肿起，边缘不清，局部灼热疼痛，称为痄腮，为外感温毒所致。若患侧口角下垂或㖞斜，为口眼㖞斜。单纯口眼㖞斜者，为风邪中络；若有半身不遂者，则为中风之中经络；若有神志改变者，则为中风之中脏腑。

Inspection of face Swollen eyelids are, mostly caused by edema. If one or both cheeks are swollen with earlobe as the center, unclear edges and local burning pain, it is called mumps, which is caused by exogenous warm toxicity. If the affected corner of the mouth is drooping or oblique, it is wry eye and mouth. And simple facial paralysis is caused by wind pathogen attacking collaterals; if there is hemiplegia, it is attacking meridians in stroke; if there is a change of mind, it is attacking the zang-fu viscera in stroke.

（二）望颈项

2.2 Inspection of neck

1. 外形变化 颈前喉结处结块肿大，一侧或两侧，随吞咽移动，称为瘿瘤，多因肝郁气结痰凝所致，或与地方水土有关。颈侧颌下有肿块如豆，累累如串珠，称为瘰疬，多由肺肾阴虚，虚火炼津为痰，或感受风热时毒，结于颈项所致。

Changes in appearance If the laryngeal prominence in front of the neck is lumped and swollen, and one or both sides move with swallowing, it is called goiter, which is mostly caused by stagnation of liver qi and phlegm coagulation, or related to geographic factors. There are lumps like beans and beads under the jaw at the neck side, which are called scrofula. They are commonly caused by yin deficiency of lungs and kidneys engendering deficiency fire, which forms phlegm, or by wind-heat toxicity.

2. 动态变化 颈项软弱，抬头无力者，称为项软。若见于小儿者，多属先天不足；见于久病者，多属气血大伤；若重病项软，头倾视深，属肾精亏竭。后项强硬，俯仰不利，转动不便，称为项强。伴恶寒发热、脉浮者，多为风寒侵袭太阳经脉；伴高热神昏者，多为热极生风。若睡醒后觉项强不舒，肩背疼痛者，为落枕，多因睡姿不当所致。

Dynamic change Weak neck and weakness in head-up are called soft neck. If it is seen in children, it is mostly due to congenital deficiency; if found in people with chronic diseases, it is caused by serious damage of qi and blood;if the serious diseases have the symptoms of soft neck, inclined head and deep vision, it is kidney essence deficiency. Tough scruff with difficulties in moving and rotating is called stiff neck. If it is accompanied by aversion to cold, fever and floating pulse, it is caused by wind-cold invading taiyang meridians; if accompanied by high fever and faint, it is mostly extreme heat causing wind. Uncomfortable and stiff neck with pain in shoulder and back after waking up is called laozhen (stiff neck), which is mostly caused by improper sleeping position.

（三）望五官

2.3 Inspection of five apertures

望五官是通过观察目、耳、鼻、口等的异常变化，以诊察疾病的方法。

Inspection of five apertures is a method to diagnose diseases by observing abnormal changes in eyes, ears, nose and mouth.

1. 望目 目的各部与五脏是相对应的：瞳仁属肾，称水轮；黑睛属肝，称风轮；白睛属肺，称气轮；目眦及血络属心，称血轮；眼睑属脾，称肉轮。

Inspection of eyes Each part of the eye corresponds to the five zang viscera: the pupil belongs to the kidneys, and is called the water wheel; cornea belongs to the liver and is called wind wheel; white of the eye belongs to the lungs and is called qi wheel; canthus and blood collaterals belong to the heart and are called blood wheels; eyelid belongs to the spleen and is called flesh wheel.

（1）目色 全目赤肿为肝经风热，目眦色赤为心火，白睛色赤为肺热，眼睑红肿湿烂为脾有湿热，白睛发黄为黄疸，目眦淡白为血虚。

Color of the eyes Red and swollen eyes indicate wind–heat in liver meridian. Red canthi indicate heart fire. The white of the eye becoming slightly red indicate lung heat. Red and swollen eyelids indicate damp–heat in spleen. The white of the eye becoming yellow indicate jaundice. Pale canthi indicate blood deficiency.

（2）目形 眼突颈肿属瘿病。目窠微肿如新卧起之状，是水肿病初起。睑缘红肿起结节如麦粒，为针眼，为风热邪毒，或脾胃蕴热上攻于目所致。

Shape of the eyes Protuberant eyes and swollen neck indicate goiter. The eye socket is slightly swollen as if just waking up, indicating the beginning of edema. Nodules on red and swollen eyelid margin like kernels are hordeolum, which is caused by wind–heat pathogenic qi, or heat accumulated in spleen and stomach attacking the eyes.

（3）目态 瞳仁散大，多属肾精耗竭，为濒死危象，亦可见于中毒；瞳仁缩小，多属中毒所致。

State of the eyes Enlarged pupils are mostly caused by kidney essence exhaustion, which indicate a near–death crisis or poisoning; Pupil contraction is mostly caused by poisoning.

2. 望耳 耳轮淡白，主寒证或气血虚；耳轮干枯色黑，主肾精亏耗。耳薄小者，多为肾虚；耳轮甲错者，多属血瘀。

Inspection of ears Pale helix indicate cold syndrome or deficiency of qi and blood; dry and black helix indicate kidney essence depletion. Thin ears are mostly due to kidney deficiency. Squamous and dry helix indicate blood stasis.

3. 望鼻 Inspection of nose

（1）色泽 鼻头色青为虚寒或腹痛，色黄为里有湿热，色白为气虚或失血，色赤为脾肺二经有热，色黑为有水气。

Color of the nose　Blue nose indicates deficiency cold or abdominal pain, yellow dampness–heat inside, white qi deficiency or blood loss, red heat in spleen and lung meridians, and black fluid retention.

（2）形态　鼻头红肿，多属肺胃蕴热或血热；鼻头色赤有小丘疹，称酒渣鼻，多为肺胃热壅；鼻翼扇动，多为邪热壅肺。

Shape of the nose　Red and swollen nose is mostly due to heat accumulation in lungs and stomach or blood heat; Red nose with small papules, called rosacea, is mostly caused by heat congestion in lungs and stomach; If the nostrils flare, it is due to pathogenic heat congesting the lungs.

（3）鼻内分泌物　鼻流清涕者，多属外感风寒；鼻流浊涕者，多为外感风热；涕黄质黏量少，或伴有血丝，多为燥邪所致；若久流浊涕且腥臭者，为鼻渊，属湿热蕴蒸；阵发性清涕量多，伴喷嚏频作者，为鼻鼽，多属肺虚兼风寒外袭；鼻腔出血，为鼻衄，多因燥热灼伤鼻络。

Nasal secretions　Clear nasal discharge is mostly due to exogenous wind–cold; Turbid nasal discharge is mostly due to exogenous wind–heat; Small amount of yellow and sticky nasal discharge, or accompanied by a little blood is mostly caused by dryness pathogen; Turbid and fishy nasal discharge for a long time is sinusitis, which is due to dampness–heat amassing and steaming; Paroxysmal clear nasal discharge with large amount and accompanied by frequent sneezing is allergic rhinitis, which is mostly caused by lung deficiency and external assault by wind–cold wind–cold; Nasal hemorrhage is epistaxis, which is mostly caused by dryness and heat burning nasal collaterals.

4. 望口唇　唇色淡白者，主血虚；鲜红者，为阴虚火旺；深红者，主实热；红绛而干者，是热盛津伤；青紫者，为瘀血内停。口疮多因心脾积热上蒸所致。口角流涎者，多属脾虚湿盛，或中风口㖞。

Inspection of mouth and lips　Pale lips indicate blood deficiency; Bright red lips indicate hyperactivity of fire due to yin deficiency; Crimson lips are due to excessive heat; Crimson and dry lips indicate consumption of fluid due to intense heat; Blue and purple lips are caused by internal stagnation of blood. Oral ulcers are mostly caused by heat amassing in heart and spleen and steaming upward. Thin saliva mostly indicates dampness excessiveness due to spleen deficiency and dampness, or wry mouth due to stroke.

三、望排出物

3 Inspection of Secretion and Excretion

望排出物是观察患者分泌物、排泄物的形、色、质、量的变化，以诊断病情的方法。其变化总的规律是色白、质稀者多属虚证、寒证，色黄、质稠者多属实证、热证。

Inspection of excretion is a method to observe the changes of the shape, color, quality and quantity of patients' secretions and excretions to diagnose their illnesses. The general rule is that those with white color and thin quality belong to deficiency syndrome and cold syndrome, while those with yellow color and thick quality belong to excess syndrome and heat syndrome.

（一）望痰

3.1 Inspection of Phlegm

痰色白而清稀，为寒痰；痰色白、滑、量多而易咳者，为湿痰；痰少而黏，难咳出者，属燥痰；痰色黄而黏稠，为热痰；咳吐腥臭脓血痰者，为肺痈。

White and thin phlegm is cold phlegm; White, slippery, substantial phlegm which is easy to cough up is wet phlegm; Small amount of sticky phlegm which is difficult to cough up belongs to dry phlegm; Yellow and sticky phlegm is hot sputum; Fishy pus and phlegm with a little blood is caused by lung abscess.

（二）望呕吐物

3.2 Inspection of Vomitus

呕吐物清稀无臭，多为寒呕；秽浊酸臭，多为热呕；酸腐，夹有未消化食物，多属伤食；呕吐清水痰涎，伴胃脘振水声者，为痰饮中阻；呕吐黄绿苦水，多属肝胆湿热，肝气犯胃所致。

Clear and odorless vomitus is mostly cold vomitus; Dirty and sour vomitus is mostly hot vomitus; Acid and rotten vomitus with undigested food is mostly caused by food damage; Vomiting clear water, phlegm and thin saliva, accompanied by the sound of water in the stomach, is due to phlegm retention obstructing middle-jiao; Vomiting yellow-green bitter water is mostly caused by dampness-heat of liver and gallbladder and liver qi invading stomach.

四、望舌

4 Inspection of Tongue

望舌，又称舌诊，是观察舌象以了解病情的诊察方法。

Inspection of tongue, also known as tongue diagnosis, is a diagnostic method to observe the tongue manifestations to understand the illnesses.

（一）舌的形体结构

4.1 The structure of the tongue

诊舌的部位主要是舌体，舌体又称舌质。舌体的前端称为舌尖，舌体的中部称为舌中，舌体的后部、人字形界沟之前称为舌根，舌体两侧称为舌边。

The main part of tongue diagnosis is tongue body, which is also called tongue quality.

It is divided into the tip which refers to the front end of the tongue body, the middle part of the tongue, the root which refers to the back part of the tongue body and the front of the herringbone sulci terminal, and the edges of the tongue.

（二）舌诊原理

4.2 The principle of tongue diagnosis

1. 舌与脏腑的联系 结构上，五脏六腑都直接或间接地通过经络、经筋与舌相联系。功能上，舌质的形质和颜色与气血的盛衰和运行状态有关，舌苔和舌质的润燥与津液的盈亏有关。

The connection between tongue and zang–fu viscera In terms of structure, the zang–fu viscera are directly or indirectly connected with tongue through meridians and meridian tendons. In terms of function, the shape and color of tongue body are related to the rising and falling as well as the circulation of qi and blood, and the moisture of tongue coating and tongue body is related to fluid.

2. 脏腑在舌面上的分部 舌尖属心肺，舌边属肝胆，舌中属脾胃，舌根属肾。

The distribution of zang–fu viscera on the tongue The tip belongs to heart and lungs; the edges belong to liver and gallbladder; the middle part belongs to spleen and stomach; the root belongs to kidneys.

（三）舌诊的方法和注意事项

4.3 Methods and precautions for tongue diagnosis

1. 舌诊方法 望舌时，患者可采取坐位或仰卧位，面向自然光线，头略扬起，自然将舌伸出口外，舌体放松，舌面平展，舌尖略向下，尽量张口使舌体充分暴露。望舌的顺序：先望舌质，再望舌苔。望舌质时，则按照舌尖、舌中、舌边、舌根的顺序依次观察。

Methods When observing the tongue, practitioners can let the patient can take a sitting or supine position, face the natural light, raise his head slightly, naturally extend the tongue out of the mouth, relax the tongue body, spread the tongue surface flat, with tongue tip slightly downward, and try to open his mouth to fully expose the tongue body. The order of inspection of the tongue is: first look at the tongue body, and then look at the tongue coating. When looking at the tongue body, observe it in the order of tip, middle part, edges and root of tongue.

2. 注意事项 ①光线充足；②伸舌自然，使舌面平坦舒展；③察舌苔时应注意排除染苔，如某些食物或饮料可使苔色失真。

Precautions ① Adequate light; ② Extend the tongue naturally, so that the tongue surface is flat and stretched; ③ When examining tongue coating, attention should be paid to eliminating stained coating. For example, some foods or drinks can change the coating color.

（四）正常舌象

4.4 Normal tongue manifestation

望舌主要观察舌质和舌苔两方面的变化。望舌质主要包括舌质的神、色、形、态，以候脏腑虚实、气血盛衰；望舌苔主要诊察苔质和苔色，以辨病邪深浅、邪正消长。

Inspection of the tongue mainly observes the changes of tongue body and tongue coating. Inspection of tongue body mainly includes observing its spirit, color, shape and state, so as to diagnose the deficiency and excess of zang–fu viscera and the rise and fall of qi and blood; Inspection of tongue coating mainly includes observing coating quality and coating color, so as to distinguish the depth of etiological factors and the waning and waxing of etiological factors.

正常舌象的特征　舌质淡红、鲜明、滋润，舌体大小适中，柔软灵活；舌苔均匀、薄白而湿润，简称为“淡红舌，薄白苔”。正常舌象受年龄、性别、体质、禀赋等影响，可以产生生理性变异。

The characteristics of normal tongue manifestations　These characteristics include: pink, bright, moist, soft and flexible tongue body with moderate size as well as uniform, thin, white and moist tongue coating, which can be concluded as “pink tongue with thin and white coating”. But normal tongue manifestation can also be influenced by age, sex, constitution, endowment, etc., and appear physiological variation.

（五）望舌质

4.5 Inspection of tongue body

1. 望舌神　即观察舌质的荣枯以辨有神、无神，可推断疾病预后。

Inspection of tongue spirit　It means observing the lustrous and withered states of tongue body to distinguish between presence and loss of spirit, and infer the prognosis of diseases.

（1）荣舌　舌质滋润，红活鲜明，舌体灵动自如，为有神，为脏腑气血充盛，虽病亦属善候。

Lustrous tongue　The tongue body is moist, pink, vivid and flexible. It indicates presence of spirit, sufficient qi and blood in zang–fu viscera. And even the patient is ill, it also has a good prognosis.

（2）枯舌　舌质干枯，色泽晦暗，活动不灵，为无神，为脏腑气血衰败，病势危重，预后不良。

Withered tongue　The tongue body is dry in quality, dull in color and ineffective in activity, indicating loss of spirit, declining of qi and blood in zang–fu viscera, critical diseases and poor prognosis.

2. 望舌色　即通过观察舌质颜色的变化，以了解疾病的有关情况。

Inspection of tongue color It means observing the changes of tongue color to understand the relevant situation of diseases.

（1）淡红舌　即舌色淡红润泽，为脏腑功能正常、气血和调的表现。见于健康人，或病情轻浅者。

Pink tongue　It means that the tongue is light pink and moist, which is the manifestation of normal function of zang-fu viscera and harmony of qi and blood. It can be seen in healthy people or those with mild illness.

（2）淡白舌　比正常舌色浅淡，主阳虚证，或气血两虚证。

Pale tongue　The color is lighter than the normal tongue, which indicates yang deficiency syndrome or syndrome of deficiency of both qi and blood.

（3）红舌　较正常舌色红，甚至呈鲜红色，主实热或阴虚。

Red tongue　Its color is redder than the normal tongue, even bright red, which is mainly due to excess heat or yin deficiency.

（4）绛舌　较红舌颜色更深，或略带暗红色，主里热亢盛或阴虚火旺。

Crimson tongue　It is darker than the red tongue, or slightly kermesinus, indicating exuberance of interior heat or hyperactivity of fire due to yin deficiency.

（5）青紫舌　指全舌呈现紫色，或局部现青紫斑点，主血行瘀滞。

Purple tongue　It means the whole tongue is purple, or has local blue and purple spots, which are mainly caused by blood stasis.

3. 望舌形　舌形指舌质的形状。

Inspection of tongue shape　It means observing the shape of the tongue.

（1）老嫩舌　舌质坚敛苍老，纹理粗糙或皱缩者为老舌，多见于实证；舌质娇嫩，纹理细腻者为嫩舌，多见于虚证。

Tough tongue and tender tongue　Solid and old tongue with rough or shriveled texture is called tough tongue, which is more common in excess syndrome; Delicate tongue with fine texture is tender tongue, which is more common in deficiency syndrome.

（2）胖瘦舌　舌体比正常人大而厚，伸舌满口，为胖大舌，主水湿内停或痰湿热毒上泛。舌体比正常舌瘦小而薄，为瘦薄舌，主气血两虚或阴虚火旺。

Bulgy tongue and thin tongue　Bulgy tongue is larger and thicker than the normal one, and is full of mouth when stuck out, and indicates dampness retention or phlegm dampness and heat toxin flowing upward. Thin tongue is smaller and thinner than normal tongue, and indicates deficiency of both qi and blood or hyperactivity of fire due to yin deficiency.

（3）点刺舌　点指突起于舌面的红色或紫红色星点；刺指舌乳头突起如刺，摸之棘手。点刺舌主脏腑热盛或血分热盛。

Tongue with spots and pricks　Spots refer to red or purplish spots protruding from the tongue surface; Pricks refer to the tongue papilla protruding like pricks, which is difficult to touch. Tongue with spots and pricks indicates heat exuberance in zang-fu viscera or heat exuberance in xuefen.

（4）裂纹舌 舌面上出现各种形状的裂纹、裂沟，主邪热炽盛、阴液亏虚、血虚不润、脾虚湿盛。

Fissured tongue It means cracks and furrows of various shapes appear on the tongue surface, indicating exuberance of heat pathogen, deficiency of yin fluid, blood deficiency failing to moisten and dampness exuberance due to spleen deficiency.

（5）齿痕舌 舌体边缘有牙齿压迫的痕迹，主脾虚、水湿内盛。

Teeth–printed tongue It means there are traces of teeth compression on the edge of the tongue body, and indicates spleen deficiency and dampness exuberance.

4. 望舌态 舌态指舌体的动态。强硬舌多见于热入心包，或高热伤津，或风痰阻络；痿软舌主气血两虚或阴虚；歪斜舌多见于中风或中风先兆；震颤舌多为肝风内动；短缩舌多因寒凝筋脉、热极动风、气血亏虚、肝风夹痰所致。

Inspection of tongue state Tongue state refers to the dynamics of the tongue body. Stiff tongue is more common in heat entering pericardium, or high fever impairing fluid, or wind–phlegm obstructing collaterals; Flaccid tongue indicates deficiency of both qi and blood or yin deficiency; Skewed tongue is more common in stroke or is stroke precursor; Trembling tongue is mostly caused by internal stirring of liver wind; Shortened and contracted tongue is mostly caused by cold coagulation of tendons and vessels, extreme heat stirring wind, deficiency of qi and blood, and liver wind with phlegm.

5. 望舌下络脉 将舌尖翘起，舌系带两侧可见青紫色脉络，即为舌下络脉。正常人络脉不扩张，也无分支或瘀点。若舌下络脉青紫迂曲，或粗胀，主血瘀气滞，或痰热内阻，或寒凝血瘀。

Inspection of sublingual vessels Blue–purple veins seen on both sides of the lingual frenum when tilting the tip of the tongue are the sublingual vessels. In normal people, these vessels do not expand, and there are no branches or petechiae. If the sublingual vessels turn blue and tortuous, or coarse and swollen, it is mainly due to blood stasis and qi stagnation, or phlegm–heat obstructing internally, or cold coagulation and blood stasis.

（六）望舌苔

4.6 Inspection of tongue coating

1. 望苔质 苔质即舌苔的质地。

Inspection of the character of tongue coating.

（1）薄厚苔 透过舌苔能隐隐见到舌质者，为薄苔；不能透过舌苔见到舌质者，为厚苔。薄苔主表证，亦见于正常人；厚苔主里证，见于痰湿、食积。

Thin coating and thick coating If tongue quality can be seen through tongue coating, it is thin coating; If tongue quality cannot be seen through tongue coating, it is thick coating. Thin coating indicates superficies syndrome, and can also be seen in normal people; Thick coating indicates interior syndrome, such as phlegm-dampness and dyspepsia.

（2）润燥苔　舌苔润泽有津，干湿适中，为润苔；舌面水分过多，扪之湿滑，为滑苔；舌苔干燥，扪之无津，甚则舌苔干裂，为燥苔。润苔主津液未伤；滑苔主水湿内聚；燥苔主热盛津伤，或阳虚气不化津。

Moist coating and dry coating　Moist coating means the tongue coating is moist, neither too dry or too soggy; Slippery coating means the tongue surface is too soggy and slippery when touching; Dry coating means the tongue coating is dry with no fluid, and cracked. Moist coating indicates that fluid is not impaired; Slippery coating indicates fluid retention; Dry coating indicates injury of fluid due to exuberant heat, or failure of qi transforming fluid caused by yang deficiency.

（3）腐腻苔　苔质疏松，颗粒粗大，如豆腐渣堆积舌面，揩之易去，称为腐苔；质致密，颗粒细小，如涂有油腻之状，揩之不去，称为腻苔。多由湿浊、痰饮、食积所致。

Curdy coating and greasy coating　Curdy coating means the coating character is loose and coarse, and on the tongue surface there are granules like tofu dregs which are easy to wipe away. Greasy coating means the coating character is dense and greasy with fine granules which are difficult to wipe away. They are mostly caused by dampness-turbidity, phlegm retention and dyspepsia.

（4）剥落苔　舌苔全部或部分脱落，脱落处可见舌底光滑无苔，称为剥落苔。多主胃气匮乏，胃阴大伤，或气血两虚。

Crumbling coating　Crumbling coating means all or part of the tongue coating falls off, and the tongue surface is slippery without coating. It indicates lack of stomach qi, severe impairment of stomach yin, or deficiency of both qi and blood.

2. 望苔色　苔色的变化主要有白苔、黄苔、灰黑苔三类。

Inspection of the color of tongue coating　The color of tongue coating mainly includes white, yellow and gray black.

（1）白苔　指舌面上所附着的苔呈现白色。多主寒证，亦可见于正常人。

White coating　It refers to the white coating attached to the tongue surface. It mainly indicates cold syndrome, and can also be seen in normal people.

（2）黄苔　指舌苔呈现黄色。多主热证，苔色越黄，提示邪热越甚。

Yellow coating　It means that the tongue coating is yellow. It mainly indicates heat syndrome, and the yellower the coating color, the more serious the heat pathogen is.

（3）灰黑苔　苔色浅黑，为灰苔；苔色深灰，为黑苔。多主阴寒内盛或里热炽盛。

Gray black coating　If the color is light gray, it is gray coating; If the color is dark gray, it is black coating. They mainly indicate internal cold or heat exuberance.

第二节 闻 诊
Section 2 Listening and Smelling

闻诊是医生通过听声音和嗅气味，以诊察疾病的方法。

The method of listening and smelling is a way for doctors to detect diseases by listening to sounds and sniffing smells.

一、听声音
1 Listening to the sound

听声音是通过听辨患者所发出的语言、呼吸、咳嗽、呕吐、呃逆、嗳气、太息等声响，以判断病变寒热虚实等性质的诊病方法。

Listening to the sound is a diagnostic method to judge the nature of cold, heat, deficiency and excess of pathological changes by listening to the sounds of language, breathing, cough, vomiting, hiccup, belching and sighing made by patients.

（一）正常声音
1.1 Normal sound

正常人生理状态下的声音称为常声，具有发声自然、声调和畅、柔和圆润、语言流畅、应答自如、言与意符等特点，表示人体气血充盈，发声器官和脏腑功能正常。

Normal people's physiological voice is called normal voice, which has the characteristics of natural vocalization, smooth tone, soft and mellow sound, fluent language, free response, relevant answers, etc., indicating that the human body is full of qi and blood, and the vocal organs and zang–fu viscera function normally.

（二）病变声音
1.2 Sound after pathological changes

1. 发声 语声高亢，洪亮有力，声音连续者，多属阳证、实证、热证；语声低微细弱，懒言而沉静，声音断续者，多属阴证、虚证、寒证。新病音哑或失音者，多属实证，多因外感风寒或风热袭肺，或痰湿壅肺所致，即所谓“金实不鸣”。久病音哑或失音者，多属虚证，多为肺肾阴虚，肺失滋润所致，即所谓“金破不鸣”。若患者自觉胸中憋闷不畅，时时发出长吁或短叹声，称为太息，多为肝郁气滞所致。

Sound High, loud, powerful and continuous voice mostly indicates yang syndrome, excess syndrome and heat syndrome; Low, weak and intermittent voice, with no desire to speak and liking for quietness, mostly indicates yin syndrome, deficiency syndrome and cold syndrome. New diseases with dumb voice or aphonia are mostly excess syndrome, and caused by exogenous wind-cold or wind-heat attacking the lungs, or phlegm-dampness obstructing the lungs, that is, the so-called "muffled metal failing to sound". Long-term diseases with dumb voice or aphonia mostly belong to deficiency syndrome, which is caused by yin deficiency of lungs and kidneys and loss of moisture of lungs, that is, the so-called "broken metal failing to sound". If the patient feels oppressed and unsmooth in his chest, and always gives out a long sigh or a short sigh, it is called sighing, which is mostly caused by stagnation of liver and qi.

2. 语言 语言的异常主要是心神的病变。

Language The abnormality of language is mainly caused by the pathological changes of mind.

（1）谵语 指神志不清，语无伦次，声高有力。多属热扰心神之实证。

Delirium It refers to unconsciousness, incoherence of language with high and powerful voice. It mostly indicates excess syndrome of heat disturbing the mind.

（2）郑声 指神志不清，语言重复，时断时续，声音低弱。属于心气大伤，精神散乱之虚证。

Fading murmuring It refers to unconscious murmuring haltingly with frequent repetitions and a low, faint voice. It often indicates deficiency syndrome of great damage to heart qi causing mental disorder.

（3）狂言 指精神错乱，声嘶力竭，语无伦次，骂詈不休，喧扰妄动。多见于狂病，因痰火扰心所致。

Raving It refers to deranged mind, wild and illogical talk, scolding endlessly, and making noises. It is more common in manic psychosis, which is caused by phlegm and fire disturbing the heart.

（4）言謇 指说话不流利，含糊不清，缓慢涩滞，语不达意。见于中风先兆或中风后遗症。

Slurred speech It refers to unclear and slow speech, tongue stiffness, and words failing to express the patients' clear mental consciousness. It can be seen as stroke precursor or be one sequela of stroke.

3. 呼吸 Breath

（1）喘 即气喘，指呼吸困难，短促急迫，甚则张口抬肩，鼻翼扇动，难以平卧的表现。发作急骤，呼吸深长，息粗声高，唯以呼出为快者，为实喘；多因风寒袭肺，或痰浊、痰热壅肺所致。病势缓慢，呼吸短浅，急促难续，息微声低，唯以深吸为快，动则喘甚者，为虚喘；多因肺肾亏虚，气失摄纳所致。

Panting It refers to dyspnea, rapid breathing, and even breathing with mouth open, shoulders raised and alaenasi flaring and inability to lie on the back. Rapid attack, deep and long breathing with high sound of breathing, and ability to only exhale quickly belong to panting of excess type; it is mainly caused by wind-cold attacking the lungs, or phlegm turbidity and phlegm heat obstructing the lungs. Slow onset, short breath with difficulty to continue and low and faint sound of breathing, and ability to only inhale quickly belong to panting of deficiency type; it is mainly caused by deficiency of lungs and kidneys which cannot control qi.

（2）哮　指呼吸困难，急促似喘，喉间有哮鸣音的表现。多因痰饮内伏，复感外邪所致。

Wheezing　It refers to dyspnea, shortness of breath like panting, and wheezing sound in throat. It is mainly caused by phlegm retention attacked by exopathogens.

喘以气息急迫、呼吸困难为主，哮以喉间哮鸣声为特征。喘不兼哮，但哮必兼喘。临床上哮与喘常同时出现，所以常并称为哮喘。

Panting is mainly characterized by urgent breath and dyspnea, while wheezing is characterized by throat wheezing. Panting is not necessarily accompanied by wheezing, but wheezing is sure to be accompanied by panting. Clinically, they often appear at the same time, so these two together are often called asthma.

（3）短气　指自觉呼吸短促而不相接续，气短不足以息的轻度呼吸困难。虚证短气，兼有形瘦神疲、声低息微等，多因体质衰弱或元气虚损所致；实证短气，常兼有呼吸声粗，或胸部窒闷，或胸腹胀满等，多因痰饮、胃肠积滞等所致。

Shortness of breath　It refers to mild dyspnea of conscious shortness of breath without continuity. Shortness of breath of deficiency type accompanied by tangible thinness and fatigue, low sound of breathing, etc., is mostly caused by physical weakness or deficiency of primordial qi; Shortness of breath of excess type, often accompanied by rough breathing sounds, chest tightness, chest and abdomen distension, etc., is mostly caused by phlegm retention, gastrointestinal stagnation, etc.

4. 咳嗽　咳声重浊，咳痰清稀色白，多属外感风寒，肺失宣肃所致；咳声不扬，痰稠色黄，不易咳出，兼咽喉疼痛者，多因热邪壅肺，肺失宣肃所致；咳有痰声，色白量多，易于咳出，多因脾失健运，聚湿生痰，痰湿阻肺所致；干咳无痰，或痰少黏稠，伴咽喉、皮肤干燥，多属燥邪犯肺，或肺阴亏虚；咳声低微、气怯，多属肺气亏虚。

Cough　If the cough sound is heavy and turbid, and the expectoration is clear and thin, it is mostly caused by exogenous wind–cold and the lungs failing to govern upward and outward diffusion as well as descent and purification; If the cough sound is not loud, the expectoration is thick and yellow which is not easy to cough up, and accompanied by throat pain, it is mostly caused by heat pathogen obstructing the lungs and the lungs failing to govern upward and outward diffusion as well as descent and purification; If the cough has sound of phlegm, the expectoration is white and profuse and easy cough up, it is mostly caused by dysfunction of spleen in transportation, aggregation of dampness forming phlegm, and phlegm dampness blocking lungs; Dry cough without phlegm or little viscous phlegm, accompanied by dry throat and skin, is mostly due to dryness invading the lung, or lung yin deficiency; If the cough sound is low and qi is weak, it mostly belongs to lung qi deficiency.

5. 呕吐、呃逆、嗳气 呕吐指胃内容物从口中吐出的症状；呃逆指从咽喉发出的不由自主的冲击声，为声短而频、呃呃作响的症状；嗳气指胃中气体上出咽喉所发出的一种声长而缓的症状。三者皆由胃气上逆所致。

Vomiting, hiccup, and belching Vomiting refers to the symptom of stomach contents spit out from the mouth; Hiccup refers to the involuntary impact sound from the throat, which is short, frequent and uh–uh–rattling; Belching refers to long and slow release of gas from the stomach through the mouth. All three are caused by adverse rising of stomach qi.

二、嗅气味

2 Smelling

嗅气味是根据患者体内所散发的各种气味，以及分泌物、排泄物和病室的气味，以判断病证。气味酸腐臭秽者，多属实热；气味偏淡或微有腥臭者，多属虚寒。

Smelling is to judge the disease and syndrome according to various odors emitted by patients, as well as the odors of secretions, excretions and wards. Sour, rancid and filthy odors mostly indicate excess heat; Light or slight fishy odors mostly indicate deficiency cold.

（一）病体之气

2.1 The qi of the sick body

1. 口气 口出酸臭之气，属内有宿食；口出臭秽之气，属胃热。

Breath Sour and smelly breath indicates undigested food within the body; Stinky breath indicates stomach heat.

2. 鼻臭 鼻出臭气，常流浊涕，为“鼻渊”，多因肺热或脾胃湿热所致。

Nose Smelly nose with turbid nasal discharge is sinusitis, which is mostly caused by lung heat or damp heat of spleen and stomach.

3. 排泄物之气味 咳吐浊痰脓血，有腥臭气，为肺痈；大便酸臭，多为宿食停滞；小便黄赤浊臭，多属湿热。

The smell of the excretions Coughing or vomiting turbid phlegm, pus and blood with fishy smell is lung abscess; Sour and smelly stool mostly indicates undigested food stagnation; Yellow, red, turbid and smelly urine mostly is due to dampness–heat.

（二）病室之气

2.2 Qi in the ward

病室有血腥味，多属失血证；病室有尸臭气味，多为脏腑衰败；病室有尿臊气（氨气味），多见于水肿病晚期；病室有烂苹果样气味（酮体气味），多见于消渴病晚期。

If there is blood smell in the ward, it is mainly caused by blood loss syndrome; Odor of corpse in the ward mostly indicates the decline of zang–fu viscera; The urine smell (ammonia smell) in the ward is more common in the late stage of edema; The rotten apple–like smell (ketone body smell) is more common in the late stage of consumptive thirst.

第三节　问　诊
Section 3　Inquiry

问诊是医生通过对患者或陪诊者进行有目的的询问，以了解疾病的发生、发展、诊治经过、现在症状和其他有关情况，从而诊察病情的一种方法。

Inquiry is a diagnostic method for doctors to know the occurrence, development, diagnosis and treatment process, current symptoms and other related conditions by asking patients or medical chaperon purposefully.

一、问诊的方法与注意事项
1 The methods and precautions of inquiry

问诊时，要善于抓住主症、确定主诉，并围绕主诉有目的地进行深入、细致的询问，同时要边问边辨，问辨结合。

When inquiring, doctors should be good at grasping the main symptoms, determining the chief complaint, and making in–depth and meticulous inquiries around the chief complaint purposefully. At the same time, they should combine asking and distinguishing.

问诊时，应在安静适宜的环境下进行。对于某些病情不便当众表述的患者，更应单独询问。语言要通俗易懂，切忌使用患者听不懂的医学术语。

The inquiry should be conducted in a quiet and suitable environment. For some patients whose illness is inconvenient to express in public, they should be asked separately. The language should be easy to understand, and medical terms that patients can’t understand should be avoided.

二、问诊的内容
2 The content of the inquiry

（一）问一般情况
2.1 Inquiring about the general information

一般情况包括姓名、性别、年龄、婚否、发病节气、职业、籍贯、现住址等。

General information includes name, gender, age, marriage, solar term when the disease occurs, occupation, native place, current address, etc.

（二）问主诉

2.2 Inquiring about the chief complaint

主诉是患者就诊时最感痛苦的症状、体征及持续时间。

The chief complaint is the the patient's most painful symptom, sign and duration at the current time.

（三）问病史

2.3 Inquiring about medical history

问现病史包括发病情况、病变过程、诊治经过、现在症状四部分。问既往史包括患者既往健康状况及既往患病情况。问个人生活史包括生活经历、精神情志、生活起居、婚姻生育等。问家族史是指询问与患者有血缘关系的亲属的健康和患病情况。

Inquiring about the history of present illness includes four parts: incidence, pathological changes, diagnosis and treatment process, and present symptoms. Inquiring about the past history includes the patient's past health status and previous illness. Inquiring about personal life history including life experience, spirit and emotion, daily life, marriage and childbirth, etc. Inquiring about family history refers to asking about the health and illness of the blood relatives of patients.

三、问现在症状

3 Inquiring about the current symptoms

问现在症状是指对患者就诊时所感到的痛苦和不适，以及与其病情相关的全身情况进行详细询问。

Inquiring about present symptoms refers to asking patients about the pain and discomfort they feel as well as the general conditions related to their illness at the time of seeing a doctor.

清代陈修园在《医学实在易》中记载了“十问歌”，即“一问寒热二问汗，三问头身四问便，五问饮食六问胸，七聋八渴俱当辨，九问旧病十问因，再兼服药参机变，妇人尤必问经期，迟速闭崩皆可见，再添片语告儿科，天花麻疹全占验”。“十问歌”内容言简意赅，目前仍有指导意义。

In Qing Dynasty, Chen Xiuyuan recorded “the Song of Ten Inquiries” in *Yixueshizaiyi* (医学实在易), that is, “Firstly inquire for cold and heat and secondly inquire for the sweating; Thirdly for the head and body and fourthly for the excretion; Fifthly for the diet and sixthly for the chest; Seventhly the deafness and eighthly the polydipsia should to be identified; Ninthly for the chronic illness and tenthly for the cause of disease; Then take medicine and waiting for further chance variation. Inquire the menstrual period for women in particular and the late menses, early menses, amenorrhea and metrorrhagia will be clear. Lastly inquire about the pediatrics, and the smallpox and measles will be diagnosed." "The Song of Ten Inquiries" is concise and still has guiding significance.

（一）问寒热

3.1 Inquiring about cold and heat

问寒热指询问患者有无怕冷或发热的感觉。

It refers to asking patients if they have an aversion to cold or have a fever.

寒即怕冷，是患者的主观感觉，临床有恶风、恶寒、畏寒之别。恶风是指患者遇风觉冷，避之可缓的症状，较恶寒轻。恶寒是指患者自觉怕冷，多加衣被或近火取暖而寒冷不缓解者。畏寒是指患者身寒怕冷，加衣覆被，或近火取暖而寒冷能缓解者。

Cold means having an aversion to cold, which is the subjective feeling of patients. It is divided into aversion to wind, aversion to cold and fear of cold in clinic. Aversion to wind refers to the symptoms that patients feel cold when encountering wind and can feel better when avoiding it, which is lighter than aversion to cold. Aversion to cold refers to the symptoms that patients are afraid of cold, and even they add more clothes or warm near fire, the cold is not relieved. Fear of cold refers to patients who are afraid of cold, add clothes and cover or keep warm near fire, and the cold can be relieved.

热即发热，除指体温高于正常外，还包括体温正常而自觉全身或某一局部发热。

Heat refers to having a fever, which means that the body temperature is higher than normal, and it also includes normal body temperature with feeling of fever in the whole body or local areas.

临床常见的类型包括：

Common clinical types include:

1. 恶寒发热 指恶寒与发热同时并现，多见于外感病初期。

Aversion to cold with fever It refers to the simultaneous occurrence of aversion to cold and fever, which is more common in the early stage of exogenous diseases.

2. 但寒不热 指只感怕冷而不觉发热的症状。多属阴盛或阳虚所致的里寒证。

Chill without fever It refers to the symptoms of being afraid of cold without feeling fever. It belongs to interior cold syndrome caused by yin excess or yang deficiency.

3. 但热不寒 指只发热不觉寒冷，或反恶热的症状。多属阳盛或阴虚所致的里热证。

Fever without chill It refers to the symptoms of fever without feeling cold, or aversion to heat instead. It mostly indicates interior heat syndrome caused by yang excess or yin deficiency.

4. 寒热往来 指恶寒与发热交替发作，为半表半里证的特征，可见于少阳病和疟疾。

Alternate attacks of chill and fever It refers to the alternate attack of aversion to cold and fever, which is a characteristic of neither exterior nor interior syndrome, and can be seen in Shaoyang disease and malaria.

（二）问汗

3.2 Inquiring about sweating

问汗指询问患者有无汗出异常的情况。

It refers to inquiring the patient if there is abnormal sweating.

1. 无汗 指当汗出而不出汗。表证无汗多见于表实寒证；里证无汗多为阴寒内盛，或阳气虚衰，或津血亏虚。

Anhidrosis It means not sweating when sweating is needed. superficies syndrome without sweat is more common in exterior excess cold syndrome; Interior syndrome without sweat is mostly caused by yin–cold excess, yang–qi deficiency, or deficiency of fluid and blood.

2. 有汗 指不当汗出而汗出，或汗出较多。表证有汗多见于伤风表证和风热表证。里证有汗常表现为以下几种情况：

Sweating It refers to sweating when sweating is not needed, or profuse sweating. superficies syndrome with sweating is more common in exterior wind syndrome and exterior wind–heat syndrome. Sweating in interior syndromes is often manifested in the following types:

（1）自汗 指不因外界环境因素的影响，经常日间汗出不止，活动后尤甚。常见于气虚、阳虚证。

Spontaneous sweating It means sweating during the day, especially after activities, without the influence of external environmental factors. It is common in qi deficiency and yang deficiency syndromes.

（2）盗汗 指不因外界环境因素的影响，入睡时汗出，醒则汗止。多见于阴虚证。

Night sweating It refers to sweating when falling asleep and stopping sweating after waking up without the influence of external environmental factors. It is more common in yin deficiency syndrome.

（3）战汗 指先见全身寒冷战抖，而后汗出。多见于外感热病中，提示邪正剧争，常为病情变化的转折点。

Sweating following shiver It refers to a cycle of sudden coldness followed by shivering and sweating in externally contracted febrile conditions, seeing the whole body trembling with cold and then sweating. It is often seen in exogenous febrile disease, suggesting fierce struggle between vital qi and pathogenic qi, which is often the turning point of disease change.

（三）问疼痛

3.3 Inquiring about pain

疼痛有虚实之分。因气机闭塞，气血运行不畅，为“不通则痛”，属因实致痛；因气血不足，或阴阳亏损，脏腑经络失养，为“不荣则痛”，属因虚致痛。

Pain can be divided into deficiency and excess. Pain caused by the occlusion of qi movement and the poor circulation of qi and blood, namely, “pain caused by obstruction”, indicates excess syndromes; Pain caused by deficiency of qi and blood, or loss of yin and yang and malnutrition of zang–fu viscera and meridians, namely, “pain caused by lacking nourishment”, indicates deficiency syndromes.

1. 问疼痛的性质 Inquiring about the nature of pain

（1）胀痛　指疼痛伴有胀满的感觉，多与气滞有关。

Distending pain　It refers to pain with a sensation of fullness and distension. It is most commonly caused by qi stagnation.

（2）刺痛　指疼痛如针刺之状，是瘀血的特征。

Stabbing pain　It refers to pain as if pricked by a needle. It is one characteristic of static blood.

（3）走窜痛　指痛处游走不定，或走窜攻痛。发生于胸胁、脘腹者，多因气滞所致；发生于肢体关节者，多见于风邪偏盛之痹病。

Migratory pain　It refers to pain that migrates from one area to another area. Migratory pain in the rib area, stomach and abdomen is often associated with liver qi stagnation; whereas migratory joint pain is often associated with bi disease caused by excess wind pathogen.

（4）固定痛　指痛处固定不移。痛在胸胁、脘腹等处，多属血瘀所致；痛在肢体关节，多见于寒或湿偏盛所致之痹病。

Fixed pain　It means that the pain is fixed. Pain in chest and abdomen, is mostly caused by blood stasis; pain in joints, is more common in bi disease caused by excess cold or dampness.

（5）冷痛　指疼痛伴有冷感而喜暖，属寒证。

Cold pain　It refers to pain with a cold sensation that alleviates with warmth. It indicates cold syndrome.

（6）灼痛　指疼痛伴有灼热感，喜凉恶热，属热证。

Burning pain　It refers to pain with a burning sensation that alleviates with cold and has an aversion to heat. It indicates heat syndrome.

（7）绞痛　指疼痛剧烈如刀绞，多为有形实邪或寒邪凝滞所致。

Colicky pain　It refers to sharp pain as if lacerated by a knife. It is most commonly caused by tangible pathogens or cold pathogen stagnation.

（8）隐痛　指疼痛不甚剧烈，尚可忍耐，但绵绵不休，多属虚证。

Dull pain　It means that the pain is tolerable and less pronounced, but persistent. It most indicates deficiency syndrome.

（9）空痛　指疼痛伴有空虚感觉，多属气血精髓亏虚。

Empty pain　It refers to pain with an empty sensation. It is most commonly caused by deficiency of qi and blood and essence.

（10）重痛　指疼痛伴有沉重感觉，多因湿邪困阻气机所致。

Heavy pain　It refers to pain with a sensation of heaviness. It is most commonly caused by dampness obstructing qi movement.

（11）酸痛　指疼痛伴有酸软感。多因湿邪侵袭，或肾虚所致。

Aching pain　It refers to pain accompanied by a feeling of soreness and weakness. It often occurs as a result of dampness attacking the body or kidney deficiency.

（12）闷痛　指疼痛带有满闷、憋闷的感觉。多因痰浊内阻所致。

Stuffy pain　It refers to pain accompanied by feeling of oppression. It is mainly caused by internal obstruction of phlegm turbidity.

（13）掣痛　指痛由一处而连及他处，抽掣牵扯作痛，多因经脉阻滞不通，或经脉失养所致。

Dragging pain　It refers to the pain that occurs in one part of the body but perceives in some other parts of the body. It is mostly caused by the blockage of meridians or the loss of nourishment of meridians.

一般而言，新病疼痛，痛势剧烈，持续不解，或痛而拒按者，多属实证；久病疼痛，痛势较轻，时痛时止，或痛而喜按者，多属虚证。冷痛喜温，遇寒痛剧，得温痛减者，属寒证；灼痛喜凉，痛处发热，遇寒觉舒者，属热证。

Generally speaking, if new illness causes pain which is severe and persistent, or is amplified when being pressed, it is mostly excess syndrome; if long-term disease causes mild and intermittent pain which will be relieved when being pressed, it mostly belongs to deficiency syndrome. Cold pain which likes warmth, and will be amplified when encountering cold and be relieved when getting warm indicates cold syndrome; burning pain which likes cold and is hot, and can be relieved when encountering cold indicates heat syndrome.

2. 问疼痛的部位 Inquiring about the spot of pain

（1）头痛　指头的某一部位或整个头部疼痛的症状。如头痛连项者，属太阳经；两侧头痛者，属少阳经；前额连眉棱骨痛者，属阳明经；颠顶痛者，属厥阴经等。

Headache　It refers to a symptom of pain in one part of the head or the whole head. Headache that radiates to the occipital region is Taiyang headache; Headache that is located in the temples on both sides is Shaoyang headache; Frontal headache that radiates to the supraorbital bone is Yangming headache; Headache that is located in the parietal region is Jueyin headache.

（2）胸痛　指胸部正中或偏侧疼痛，多为心肺病变。如虚里部位作痛，或痛彻臂内者，病位在心；胸膺部位作痛，常兼咳喘者，病位在肺。

Chest pain　It refers to the pain in the middle or two sides of the chest, which is mostly due to cardiopulmonary disease. Pain which locates in the xuli part, or perceives in the arm indicates the disease is in the heart; Pain in the chest, and often accompanied by cough and panting, indicates the disease is in the lungs.

（3）胁痛　指胁的一侧或两侧疼痛。多与肝胆病变有关。

Hypochondriac pain　It refers to pain on one or both sides of hypochondrium. It is mainly due to hepatobiliary diseases.

（4）脘痛　指上腹部、剑突下疼痛。因寒、热、气滞、瘀血、食积所致者，属实证；因胃阴虚或胃阳不足所致者，属虚证。

Epigastric pain　It refers to the pain under the upper abdomen and xiphoid process. Epigastric pain caused by cold, heat, qi stagnation, blood stasis and dyspepsia belongs to excess syndrome; epigastric pain caused by deficiency of stomach yin or deficiency of stomach yang belongs to deficiency syndrome.

（5）腹痛　指胃脘以下、耻骨毛际以上的部位发生疼痛。因寒凝、热结、气滞、血瘀、食积、虫积等所致者，属实证；由气虚、血虚、阳虚等所致者，属虚证。

Abdominal pain　It refers to the pain below the epigastric region and above the pubic hair. Abdominal pain caused by cold coagulation, heat stagnation, qi stagnation, blood stasis, dyspepsia, insect accumulation, etc., belongs to excess syndrome; abdominal pain caused by qi deficiency, blood deficiency and yang deficiency belongs to deficiency syndrome.

（6）腰痛　指腰脊正中或腰部两侧疼痛。多因肾虚失养、寒湿侵袭、瘀血或结石阻滞等导致。

Low back pain　It refers to pain in the middle of the lumbar spine or on both sides of the waist. It is mainly caused by kidney deficiency, cold and dampness invasion, blood stasis or concretion blocking.

（7）四肢痛　指四肢、肌肉、筋脉、关节等部位疼痛。常见于痹病。疼痛游走不定者为行痹，以感受风邪为主；疼痛剧烈，遇寒尤甚，得热痛缓者为痛痹，以感受寒邪为主；重着而痛，阴雨天加重者，为着痹，以感受湿邪为主；四肢关节灼热肿胀而痛者，为热痹，因感受湿热之邪所致。

Limb pain　It refers to pain in limbs, muscles, tendons and joints and is common in bi disease. Limb pain that migrates from one area to another area indicates migratory bi which is mainly caused by wind pathogen; If the pain is severe and will be amplified when encountering cold and be relieved when getting warm, it belongs to painful bi which is mainly caused by cold pathogen; Limb pain which is heavy and painful and aggravated in rainy days belongs to stationary bi which is mainly caused by dampness pathogen; If the joints of limbs are burning, swelling and painful, it indicates heat bi, which is caused by dampness and heat pathogens.

（8）周身疼痛　指头身、腰背、四肢等部位均觉疼痛。一般新病周身疼痛，多属实证，常因感受风寒湿邪而致；若久病卧床不起而周身作痛，则属虚证，乃气血亏虚，失其荣养所致。

Pain in the whole body　It refers to pain in head, waist, back, limbs and other parts of the entire body. Generally, new disease suffers from pain all over the body mostly belongs to excess syndrome which is mainly caused by wind, cold and dampness pathogens; If the patient is bedridden for a long time and suffers from pain all over the body, it belongs to deficiency syndrome, which is caused by deficiency of qi and blood and lacking nourishment.

（四）问饮食口味

3.4 Inquiring about food and taste

问饮食口味指询问患者口渴与饮水、食欲与进食量及口中味觉等情况。

Inquiring about food and taste refers to asking patients about thirst and water drinking, appetite and food intake, and taste in the mouth.

1. 口渴与饮水　口不渴饮提示津液未伤，多见于寒证、湿证；口渴欲饮提示津液损伤，多见于燥证、热证；渴不多饮常见于湿热证、痰饮内停、瘀血内停及温病营分证。

Thirst and water drinking　If the patient is not thirsty and has no desire to drink, it indicates that fluid is not impaired, which is more common in cold syndrome and dampness syndrome; If the patient is thirsty and desires to drink, it indicates fluid impairment, which is more common in dryness syndrome and heat syndrome; If the patient is thirsty but lacks drinking, it is common in dampness-heat syndrome, phlegm retention, blood stasis stagnation and yingfen syndrome of epidemic febrile disease.

2. 食欲与食量　食欲指对进食的要求和进食的欣快感觉，食量即实际的进食量。

Appetite and food intake dose　Appetite refers to the desire and the euphoric feeling of eating, and food intake dose is the actual amount of eating.

（1）食欲减退　指进食的欲望减退，或食之无味，食量减少，甚至不想进食的症状。虚者多因脾胃虚弱，实者多因饮食积滞或湿邪内阻等所致。

Anorexia　It refers to the symptoms of decreased desire to eat, tastelessness, reduced food intake or even no desire to eat. Deficiency syndrome is mostly caused by deficiency of spleen and stomach, while excess syndrome is mostly caused by dyspepsia or internal blocking of dampness pathogen.

（2）消谷善饥　指食欲亢进，进食量多，但食后不久即感饥饿的症状。多因胃火炽盛所致。多见于消渴病，或瘿病。

Rapid digestion of food and polyorexia　It refers to the symptoms of excessive appetite and excessive food intake, but hunger soon after eating. It is mainly caused by excessive stomach fire and is common in diabetes or goiter.

（3）饥不欲食　指有饥饿感，但不想进食，或进食不多。多因胃阴不足，虚火内扰所致。

Hunger but with no desire to eat It means the patient feels hungry, but does not want to eat, or does not eat much. It is mainly caused by deficiency of stomach yin leading to deficiency fire disturbing internally.

3. 口味 指口中异常味觉或气味。口淡多见于脾胃虚弱、寒湿中阻及寒邪犯胃。口苦多见于肝胆火旺，或肝胆湿热。口酸多因肝胃郁热或伤食所致。口甜多见于脾胃湿热或脾虚之证。口咸多与肾虚及寒水上泛有关。口黏腻多由湿热、痰热，或痰湿、寒湿中阻所致。

Taste It refers to abnormal taste or smell in the mouth. Tastelessness is more common in syndromes of deficiency of spleen and stomach, cold and dampness blocking middle jiao and cold pathogen invading stomach. Bitter taste in mouth is more common in syndromes of hyperactivity of liver and gallbladder fire or dampness–heat of liver and gallbladder. Sour taste is mostly caused by heat stagnation in liver and stomach or food damage. Sweet taste is more common in syndromes of dampness–heat of spleen and stomach or spleen deficiency. Salty taste is mostly related to kidney deficiency and cold–water flooding upward. Sticky and greasy taste is mostly caused by dampness–heat, phlegm–heat, phlegm–dampness or cold–dampness blocking middle jiao.

（五）问睡眠

3.5 Inquiring about sleep

问睡眠主要询问睡眠时间的长短、入睡的难易、有无多梦等情况。

Inquiring about sleep mainly asks about the length of sleep, the difficulty of falling asleep, and whether dreaminess occurs.

1. 失眠 指经常不易入睡，或睡而易醒、难以复睡，或睡而不酣、时易惊醒，甚至彻夜不眠的症状。由阴血亏虚，或心虚胆怯，或阴虚火旺所致者，属虚证；由邪气内扰而致者，属实证。

Insomnia It refers to the symptoms that it is often difficult to fall asleep, sleep but wake up easily and difficult to sleep again, light sleep and wake up easily, or even stay up all night. Insomnia caused by deficiency of yin and blood, timidity due to deficiency of heart qi, or hyperactivity of fire due to yin deficiency belongs to deficiency syndrome; Insomnia caused by pathogenic qi disturbing internally belongs to excess syndrome.

2. 嗜睡 指神疲困倦，睡意很浓，经常不自主入睡的症状。多因阳虚阴盛，或痰湿内盛所致。

Hypersomnia It refers to the symptoms of exhaustion, sleepiness and frequent involuntary sleep. It is mostly caused by yang deficiency and yin excess, or phlegm–dampness excess.

（六）问二便

3.6 Inquiring about urine and faeces

应注意询问二便的性状、次数、便量、排便感等内容。

Attention should be paid to inquiring about the characteristics, frequency, volume and defecation feeling.

1. 大便 健康成人一般每日或隔日大便一次，为黄色成形软便，排便顺畅，便内无脓血、黏液及未消化的食物。

Faeces Healthy adults generally defecate once a day or every other day, and the faeces is yellow and soft, with smooth defecation and no pus, blood, mucus and undigested food.

（1）便次异常 Abnormal faeces frequency

①便秘：指大便秘结不通，排便时间延长，或欲便而艰涩不畅的症状。多因热结肠道，或津液亏少，或阴血不足所致。亦有因气机郁滞，或气虚传送无力，或阳虚寒凝而致者。

Constipation: It refers to the symptoms of hard stools and difficult, prolonged defecation time, or difficulty in defecation. It is mostly caused by heat accumulating in the intestines, deficiency of fluid, or deficiency of yin blood. It can also be caused by stagnation of qi movement, qi being too deficient to transmit stools, or cold coagulation due to yang deficiency.

②泄泻：指便次增多，便质稀薄，甚至便稀如水样的症状。外感风寒、湿热、疫毒之邪，或内伤饮食，或脾胃虚弱，或命门火衰，或情志失调等，均可导致泄泻。

Diarrhea: It refers to the symptoms of increased faeces times, loose faeces quality and even watery stools. Diarrhea can be caused by exogenous wind-cold, dampness-heat or epidemic toxin, food damage, deficiency of spleen and stomach, decline of vital gate fire, or emotional disorder.

（2）便质异常 Abnormal faeces quality

①完谷不化：指大便中含有较多未消化的食物残渣。新起者多为食滞胃肠，病久多属脾胃虚寒、肾虚命门火衰。

Diarrhea with undigested food: It means that the stool contains more undigested food residues. New disease is caused by retention of food in stomach and intestines, and long-term disease is caused by deficiency cold of spleen and stomach, kidney deficiency and decline of vital gate fire.

②溏结不调：若大便时干时稀，多因肝郁脾虚所致；若大便先干后稀，多属脾胃虚弱。

Irregular stool: If stool is characterized by alternating loose and dry stool, it is mostly caused by liver depression and spleen deficiency; If the stool is dry first and then loose, it is mostly due to deficiency of spleen and stomach.

③脓血便：指大便中夹有脓血、黏液。多见于痢疾或肠癌。

Stool with pus and blood: It refers to stool with pus, blood and mucus. It is more common in dysentery or intestinal cancer.

④便血：指血自肛门排出，包括血随便出，或便黑如柏油状，或单纯下血的症状。多因脾胃虚弱，气不摄血，或胃肠积热，湿热蕴结等所致。便血有远血与近血之分。若血色暗红或紫黑，或便黑如柏油状者，为远血，多见于胃脘等部位出血。若便血鲜红，血附在大便表面或于排便前后滴出者，为近血，多见于内痔、肛裂等病变。

Hematochezia: It refers to the passage of fresh blood through the anus, including the symptoms of blood with stools, black “tarry” faeces or expulsion of fresh bright red blood without stools. It is mainly caused by deficiency of spleen and stomach which leads to qi failing to control blood, or heat accumulation in stomach and intestine and accumulation of dampness–heat. Hematochezia can be divided into distant anal bleeding and nearby anal bleeding. If the blood color is dark red or purple black, or black “tarry”, it indicates distant anal bleeding, which is more common in epigastric bleeding. If the blood in the stool is bright red, and is attached to the stool surface or drips before and after defecation, it is nearby anal bleeding, which is more common in internal hemorrhoid, anal fissure and other lesions.

（3）排便感异常　肛门灼热常见于湿热泄泻或湿热痢疾。里急后重指腹痛窘迫，时时欲便，肛门重坠，便出不爽的症状，常见于湿热痢疾。排便不爽多因湿热蕴结或肝气犯脾或食滞胃肠所致。大便失禁多因脾肾虚衰、肛门失约所致。肛门气坠多属脾虚中气下陷。

Abnormal defecation feeling　A burning sensation of the anus is common in dampness–heat diarrhea or dampness–heat dysentery. Tenesmus is characterized by abdominal pain, a feeling of constantly needing to pass stools, weight–bearing sensation of the anus and a sense of incomplete evacuation after defecation, and it is common in dampness–heat dysentery. Defecation with sensation of incomplete defecation is mostly caused by dampness–heat accumulation, liver–qi invading spleen or retention of food in stomach and intestines. Fecal incontinence is mostly caused by spleen and kidney deficiency and anus failing to control stools. Sinking anus belongs to spleen deficiency causing spleen qi sinking.

2. 小便　健康成人日间排尿 3 ～ 5 次，夜间 0 ～ 1 次。

Urine　Healthy adults urinate 3–5 times during the day and 0–1 time at night.

（1）尿量异常　尿量增多常见于虚寒证。多尿兼多饮、多食、消瘦等症者，为消渴病。尿量减少多因津液损伤或水液停聚所致，常见于各种热病和水肿、癃闭、鼓胀等疾病。

Abnormal urine volume　Increased urine volume is common in deficiency cold syndrome. Diabetes occurs in patients with polyuria and polydipsia, polyphagia and emaciation. The decrease of urine volume is mostly caused by fluid impairment or fluid retention, which is common in various diseases such as febrile disease, edema, dribbling and retention of urine and swelling.

（2）尿次异常　小便频数多因膀胱湿热，或肾气不固所致。癃闭指以排尿困难，尿量减少，甚至小便闭塞不通为主症的病证。主要由肾与膀胱气化失司所致。

Abnormal urination frequency　It is mostly caused by dampness-heat of bladder or non-consolidation of kidney qi. Dribbling and retention of urine refers to the syndrome characterized by symptoms of dysuria, decreased urine volume and even obstruction of urine. It is mainly caused by the loss of control of qi transformation of kidneys and bladder.

（3）排尿感异常 Abnormal urination feeling

①小便涩痛：指排尿时自觉小便涩滞不畅、尿道灼热疼痛的症状。多因湿热蕴结，膀胱气化不利所致，多见于淋证。

Difficulty and pain in micturition: It refers to the symptoms of unsmooth urination and burning pain of urethra when urinating. It is mostly caused by dampness-heat accumulation and dysfunction of qi transformation of bladder, which is more common in stranguria.

②余沥不尽：指小便后点滴不尽的症状。多因肾气不固，膀胱失约所致。

Inexhaustible drip: It refers to the symptoms of inexhaustible drip after urinating, which is mainly caused by non-consolidation of kidney qi and malfunction of bladder.

③小便失禁：指小便不能随意控制而自遗的症状。多属肾气不固或下焦虚寒所致。

Incontinence of urine: It refers to the symptoms that urine cannot be controlled at will. It is mostly caused by non-consolidation of kidney qi or deficiency cold of lower jiao.

④遗尿：指成人或 3 周岁以上小儿，在睡眠中经常不自主地排尿的症状。多因禀赋不足，肾气亏虚，膀胱失约所致。

Enuresis: It refers to the symptoms that adults or children over 3 years old often urinate involuntarily during sleep. It is mainly caused by insufficiency of natural endowment, deficiency of kidney qi and malfunction of bladder.

第四节　切　诊
Section 4　Palpation and Pulse Taking

切诊是医生用手对患者体表某些部位进行触、摸、按、压，以获得病情资料的一种诊察方法。切诊包括脉诊和按诊两部分。

Palpation and pulse taking diagnosis is a diagnostic method in which doctors palpate, touch, push and press some parts of patients' body surface with their hands to obtain disease data. This method includes pulse taking and palpation.

一、脉诊
1 Pulse taking

脉诊，又称切脉，是医生用手指切按患者的脉搏，根据脉动应指的形象以了解病情、判断病证的一种诊察方法。

Pulse taking is a diagnostic method in which doctors understand the condition of illness and judge the syndrome by feeling patients' pulse and perceiving the sensations under the fingers.

脉象的形成，不仅与心脏的搏动、脉道的通利和气血的盈亏直接相关，而且与全身其他脏腑的功能活动关系密切。人体的血脉贯通全身，内连脏腑，外达肌表，运行气血，周流不休，所以脉象能反映全身脏腑和气血的状况。

The formation of pulse manifestation is not only directly related to the beating of the heart, the circulation of pulse channels and the amount of qi and blood, but also closely related to the functions of other zang–fu viscera of the whole body. The blood vessels run through the whole body, connecting the zang–fu viscera inside, reaching the muscle and skin outside, circulating qi and blood, and flowing around endlessly, and that's why the pulse manifestation can reflect the status of the zang–fu viscera and qi and blood of the whole body.

（一）诊脉的部位

1.1 The position of pulse taking

诊脉根据部位不同有遍诊法、三部诊法和寸口诊法，目前临床常用寸口诊法。

According to different positions of pulse taking, there are overall pulse diagnosis, three arteries pulse diagnosis and cunkou pulse diagnosis. At present, cunkou diagnosis is commonly used in clinic.

1. 遍诊法 指《素问·三部九候论》所提出的三部九候诊法。诊脉的部位分头、手、足三部，每部又各分天、地、人三候，故称三部九候诊法。

Overall pulse diagnosis It refers to the diagnosis method using the three positions and nine indicators proposed in *Su Wen* (素 问). It is pulse examination on three regions of the body: the head, hands and feet. Each region is sub–divided into upper, middle and lower sections. Altogether they form nine pulse–taking positions.

2. 三部诊法 指诊人迎、寸口、趺阳三脉，见于《伤寒杂病论》。

Three arteries pulse diagnosis It refers to the diagnosis of three arteries: renying, cunkou and fuyang, which is recorded in *Shanghan Zabing Lun* (*Treatise on Cold pathogenic and Miscellaneous Diseases*) (伤寒杂病论).

3. 寸口诊法 诊脉部位为腕后桡动脉搏动处。

Cunkou pulse diagnosis It is to feel the medial aspect of the styloid process where the radial artery pulsates.

（1）寸口脉分部 寸口脉分寸、关、尺三部，以腕后高骨（桡骨茎突）内侧为关部，关前为寸部，关后为尺部，两手共六部脉。

The division of the cunkou area The cunkou area is divided into cun, guan and chi positions. The inner side of the posterior high bone of wrist (styloid process of radius) is guan position, cun position is before guan position and chi position is after guan position. Altogether there are six positions in both hands.

（2）寸口分部候脏腑　左手寸部候心，关部候肝，尺部候肾；右手寸部候肺，关部候脾胃，尺部候肾（命门）。

Different divisions indicating zang–fu viscera　The cun position of the left hand indicates heart, with guan position indicating liver, and chi position indicating kidney; The cun position of the right hand indicates lungs, with guan position indicating the spleen and stomach, and chi position indicating kidney (vital gate).

（二）诊脉的方法和注意事项

1.2 Methods and precautions of pulse taking

1. 时间　清晨诊脉最好，也可在机体内外环境安静的条件下随时诊脉。每次诊脉每手应不少于 1 分钟，两手以 3 分钟左右为宜。

Time　It is best to take pulse in the early morning, and doctors can also take pulse at any time under the quiet environment inside and outside the body. The duration of pulse taking should be no less than 1 minute for each hand, and about 3 minutes for both hands is advisable.

2. 体位　患者取坐位或仰卧位，手臂平展，与心脏处于同一水平，手心向上，并在腕关节背部垫上脉枕，以便于切脉。

Posture　Patients take sitting or supine position, with flat arms at the same level as the heart and palms up, and put a pulse pillow on the back of wrist joint for pulse taking.

3. 平息　指诊脉时医生要保持呼吸自然均匀，用自己一呼一吸的时间去计算患者脉搏的至数。医生诊脉时必须虚心冷静，全神贯注。

Breathing evenly　It means that doctors should breathe naturally and evenly when taking pulse, and count the pulse rate of patients' pulse in one breath (a breathing cycle) of doctors. Therefore, doctors must be modest, calm and absorbed when taking a pulse.

4. 指法　可概括为布指、运指等。

Finger positioning method　It includes finger positioning method and finger movement method.

（1）布指　指医生用左手或右手的食指、中指与无名指诊脉。三指指端平齐，自然弯曲成弓形，并以中指确定关脉部位，食指按于关前的寸脉，无名指按于关后的尺脉，指目（指端隆起螺纹处）紧贴于脉动部位。患者身高臂长者，布指宜疏，反之宜密。

Finger positioning　It refers to doctors take pulse with the index finger, middle finger and ring finger of his left or right hand. The tips of the three fingers are flush, naturally bent and arched. The middle finger is used to to feel the guan position, with the index finger pressing on the cun position, and the ring finger on the chi position, and the finger eyes (the threaded part of the finger tip) should be closely attached to the pulse area. If patients are tall and have long arms, fingers should be positioned sparsely, and vice versa.

（2）运指 指运用指力的轻重、挪移及布指变化以体察脉象，包括举、按、寻、总按和单按等。轻指力触及皮肤者为举，又叫浮取；重指力按在肌肉与筋骨之间者为按，又叫沉取；手指用力适中，按至肌肉者，称为中取。指力从轻到重，从重到轻，左右前后推寻，以寻找脉动最明显的特征，称为寻。三指用同样的指力切三部脉，称总按；仅一指用力，重点辨某部脉，称单按。

Finger movement It refers to a method of moving and exerting different finger pressures on positions for pulse examination, including lifting, pressing, searching, general pressing and single pressing, etc. Touching the skin with light finger force belongs to lifting, which is also called floating; Pressing between muscles and tendons with heavy finger force is pressing, which is also called sinking; If the finger exerts moderate force and presses to the muscle, it is called taking pulse moderately. If finger force changes from light to heavy, then from heavy to light, pushing back and forth to find the most distinct part of pulsation, it is called searching. General pressing refers to exerting even finger pressures to take pulse of three arteries; Single pressing means using one finger to take pulse of only one artery.

（三）正常脉象

1.3 Normal pulse manifestation

正常人的脉象又称平脉。

The pulse manifestation of normal people is also called normal pulse.

1. 正常脉象的形态 寸关尺三部有脉，一息四五至，不浮不沉，不大不小，从容和缓，柔和有力，节律一致，尺脉沉取有一定力量，并随生理活动和气候环境的不同而有相应的正常变化。

The form of normal pulse A normal pulse can be felt in all of the cun, guan and chi positions, with a frequency of 4 to 5 beats in one breath. It is neither superficial nor deep. It is relaxed, smooth, soft, forceful and rhythmic. Pressing the chi position by sinking method, doctors can still feel the pulse. And a normal pulse also has corresponding normal changes with different physiological activities and climate environment.

2. 正常脉象的特点 平脉有胃、神、根三个特点。脉有胃气，指脉象从容和缓，不疾不徐；脉有神，指脉象柔和有力，节律整齐；脉有根，指沉取应指有力，尺部尤显。

The characteristics of normal pulse It is marked by the three essential elements: stomach qi, spirit and root. The pulse has stomach qi, which means that the pulse manifestation is calm and smooth, neither fast nor slow; The pulse has spirit, which means that the pulse manifestation is soft, forceful and the rhythmic; The pulse has root, which means the pulse is forceful when pressing with relatively large force, especially on the chi position.

3. 正常脉象的变异因素 不同季节，脉象会有一定变化，如春稍弦、夏稍洪、秋稍浮、冬稍沉。年龄越小脉搏越快，如 3 岁以内婴幼儿一息七八至为平脉，5 ～ 6 岁幼儿一息六至为平脉。瘦者肌肉薄则脉常浮，胖者皮下脂肪厚故脉常沉。

Factors causing variation of normal pulse manifestation A normal pulse varies in different seasons, for example, it becomes slightly stringy in spring, slightly surging in summer, slightly floating in autumn and slightly deep in winter. The younger the age, the faster the pulse. For example, the pulse rate of infants under 3 years old 7 to 8 beats in one breath of seven or eight, and that of infants aged 5 to 6 is 6 beats in one breath. They are all normal pulses. Thin people have thin muscles, which leads to relatively floating pulse, while plump people have thick subcutaneous fat, so they often have deep pulse.

（四）病理脉象

1.4 Pathological pulse manifestation

脉象的辨别是通过位、数、形、势四个方面来体察的。其中位是指脉动部位的浅深。数是指脉动频率的快慢和脉动节律的整齐与否。形是指脉动的形态，具体是指脉形的粗细、长短，脉管的紧张度及脉搏往来的流利度。脉势是指脉搏应指的强弱，与脉的紧张度和流利度也相关。

The pulse manifestation is examined from four aspects: position, frequency, shape and potential. Position refers to the depth of the pulse spot. Frequency refers to the speed and rhythm of pulse. Shape refers to the form of pulse, specifically refers to the thickness and length of pulse shape, the tension of pulse vessels and the fluency of pulsation. Pulse potential refers to the strength of pulse, which is also related to the tension and fluency of pulse.

1. 按脉位分类 Classification by pulse position

（1）浮脉 Floating pulse

脉象特征：轻取即得，重按稍减而不空。

Pulse characteristics: It can be easily felt with gentle touch. And it becomes a bit weaker when pressing down, but with no feeling of hollowness.

临床意义：表证，或久病虚证。生理性浮脉可见于夏秋季或形体偏瘦者。

Clinical indications: It indicates superficies syndrome, or deficiency syndrome of chronic disease. Physiological floating pulse can be seen in summer and autumn or those with thin body.

（2）沉脉 Deep pulse

脉象特征：轻取不应，重按始得。

Pulse characteristics: It is difficult to feel with light or moderate pressure but can be felt on heavy pressure.

临床意义：里证。有力为里实，无力为里虚。生理性沉脉可见于冬季或肥胖者。

Clinical indications: It indicates interior syndrome. Forceful one indicates interior excess, and weak pulse indicates interior deficiency. Physiological deep pulse can be seen in winter or obese people.

2. 按脉率分类 Classification by pulse frequency

（1）迟脉 Slow pulse

脉象特征：脉来迟慢，一息不足四至。

Pulse characteristics: It is late and slowly, with less than 4 beats in one breath.

临床意义：寒证。有力为实寒，无力为虚寒。若邪热结聚，也可见迟脉。生理性迟脉可见于久经锻炼之人。

Clinical indications: It indicates cold syndrome. Forceful pulse indicates interior excess cold, and weak pulse indicates deficiency cold. If etiological heat accumulates, slow pulse can also occurs. Physiological slow pulse can be seen in people who have been exercising for a long time.

（2）缓脉 Moderate pulse

脉象特征：一息四至，来去怠缓。

Pulse characteristics: It is a pulse with about 4 beats in one breath. The beats come and go slowly.

临床意义：湿病、脾胃气虚。

Clinical indications: It indicates dampness disease and spleen and stomach qi deficiency.

（3）数脉 Rapid pulse

脉象特征：脉来快数，一息五六至。

Pulse characteristics: It comes quickly, with more than 5 beats in one breath.

临床意义：热证。有力为实热，无力为虚热。生理性数脉可见于儿童和婴儿，以及正常人在运动和情绪激动时。

Clinical indications: It indicates heat syndrome. Forceful pulse indicates excess heat, and weak pulse indicates deficiency heat. Physiological rapid pulse can be seen in children and infants, as well as normal people during exercise and emotional excitement.

（4）结脉 Irregularly intermittent pulse

脉象特征：脉来缓慢，时有一止，止无定数。

Pulse characteristics: It arrives unhurriedly and stops at irregular intervals.

临床意义：结而有力主寒、痰、瘀血、癥瘕积聚；结而无力主气血虚弱。

Clinical indications: Forceful pulse indicates cold, phlegm, blood stasis and abdominal masses; Weak pulse indicates qi and blood deficiency.

（5）代脉 Regularly intermittent pulse

脉象特征：时有一止，止有定数，良久方来。

Pulse characteristics: It stops regularly for a relatively longer period of time.

临床意义：脏气衰微，或跌打损伤、痛证、惊恐。

Clinical indications: It indicates zang viscera qi decline, traumatic injury, pain syndrome or panic.

（6）促脉 Irregular–rapid pulse

脉象特征：脉来急速，时有一止，止无定数。

Pulse characteristics: It arrives urgently but irregularly interrupted.

临床意义：促而有力主阳热亢盛、气血壅滞、痰食停滞等实证；促而无力多为脏腑虚衰。

Clinical indications: Forceful pulse indicates excess syndromes such as exuberance of yang–heat, stagnation and jamming of qi and blood, stagnation of phlegm and food, etc.; and weak pulse indicates deficiency of zang–fu viscera.

3. 按脉形分类 Classification by pulse shape

（1）滑脉 Slippery pulse

脉象特征：往来流利，如珠走盘，应指圆滑。

Pulse characteristics: Its beats come and go fluently and smoothly like pearls rolling on a dish, feeling slick to the fingers.

临床意义：痰饮、食积、实热。青年人和妇女妊娠也常见滑脉，均属生理现象。

Clinical indications: It indicates phlegm retention, dyspepsia and excess heat. Slippery pulse is also common in young people and women during pregnancy, which is a physiological phenomenon.

（2）涩脉 Hesitant pulse

脉象特征：往来不畅，应指艰涩，如轻刀刮竹。

Pulse characteristics: Its beats come and go unsmoothly, feeling stagnant and obstructive to the fingers, like a knife scraping bamboo.

临床意义：涩而无力主精伤、血少；涩而有力主气滞、血瘀。

Clinical indications: Weak pulse indicates energy impairment and blood deficiency; and forceful pulse indicates qi stagnation and blood stasis.

（3）洪脉 Surging pulse

脉象特征：脉体宽大，充实有力，如波涛汹涌，来盛去衰。

Pulse characteristics: It is broad, large and forceful like roaring waves that crash onto the shore powerfully and slowly fade away.

临床意义：热盛。

Clinical indications: It indicates heat exuberance.

（4）细脉 Thready pulse

脉象特征：脉细如线，但应指明显。

Pulse characteristics: It feels thin and soft, like a silken thread, but it is distinct to the fingers.

临床意义：气血两虚、湿病。

Clinical indications: It indicates deficiency of both qi and blood and dampness disease.

（5）弦脉 Stringy pulse

脉象特征：端直以长，如按琴弦。

Pulse characteristics: It feels straight, long and tense, like the feeling of pressing a tight string of a musical instrument.

临床意义：肝胆病、痛证、痰饮。

Clinical indications: It indicates liver or gallbladder disease, pain syndrome and phlegm retention.

（6）紧脉 Tight pulse

脉象特征：绷急弹指，状如牵绳转索。

Pulse characteristics: It is tight and quick, feeling like pulling a twisted rope.

临床意义：实寒、痛证、食积。

Clinical indications: It indicates excess cold, pain syndrome and dyspepsia.

4. 按脉势分类 Classification by pulse potential

（1）虚脉 Feeble pulse

脉象特征：三部脉举之无力，按之空虚。

Pulse characteristics: It is weak at all three regions, with emptiness feeling when pressed with force.

临床意义：虚证。

Clinical indications: It indicates deficiency syndrome.

（2）实脉 Excess pulse

脉象特征：三部脉举按皆有力。

Pulse characteristics: It is forceful at all three regions using different pressure.

临床意义：实证。

Clinical indications: It indicates excess syndrome.

（3）濡脉 Soft pulse

脉象特征：浮细而软。

Pulse characteristics: It is superficial, thready and soft.

临床意义：虚证、湿证。

Clinical indications: It indicates deficiency syndrome and dampness syndrome.

（4）弱脉 Weak pulse

脉象特征：极软而沉细。

Pulse characteristics: It is extremely soft, and deep and weak

临床意义：气血不足。

Clinical indications: It indicates deficiency of qi and blood.

二、按诊
2 Palpation

按诊是医生用手直接触摸或按压患者的某些部位，以了解局部冷热、润燥、软硬、压痛、肿块或其他异常变化，从而推断出疾病部位、性质和病情轻重等情况的一种诊察方法。

Palpation is a diagnosis method in which doctors directly touch or press some parts of patients with their hands to detect local temperature, moistness, softness, tenderness, lumps or other abnormal changes, so as to determine the location, nature and severity of diseases.

（一）按诊的方法和体位
2.1 Methods and postures of palpation

按诊的手法主要有触、摸、按、叩四法。触法指以手指或手掌轻轻接触患者局部皮肤。摸法指以手指稍用力寻抚局部。按法指以重手按压或推寻局部。叩法是指医生用手叩击患者身体某部。按诊时患者可取坐位或仰卧位。

There are four methods of palpation: palpating, touching, pressing and knocking. The method of palpating means gently touching the local skin of the patient with fingers or palms. Touching refers to touching the local area with a little force with fingers. Pressing refers to pressing or pushing local parts relatively forcefully. Knocking refers to tapping a certain part of patients' body with hands. Patients can sit or lie on their backs when receiving palpation.

（二）按诊的内容
2.2 The content of palpation

1. 按肌肤 是指医生用手触摸某些部位的肌肤。

Pressing skin It means that doctors touch certain parts of patients' skin with their hands.

（1）诊寒热 肌肤寒冷，多为寒证；肌肤灼热，为阳热炽盛。

Diagnosis of temperature Cold skin indicates cold syndrome; Scorching skin is mostly due to exuberance of yang-heat.

（2）诊润燥、滑涩 皮肤干瘪者，为津液不足；肌肤润滑者，为津血充盛；肌肤枯涩者，为气血不足；肌肤甲错者，多为瘀血或血虚失荣所致。

Diagnosis of moistness Dry skin indicates insufficient fluid; Lubricated skin indicates sufficient fluid and blood; Dull and unsmooth skin is mainly due to deficiency of qi and blood; Squamous and dry skin armor is mostly caused by static blood or blood deficiency.

（3）诊疼痛 局部肌肤柔软，按之痛减者，为虚证；肌肤硬痛拒按，按之痛甚者，为实证。

Diagnosis of pain If the skin in the pain area is soft and the pain is relieved when being presses, it is deficiency syndrome; If the skin is hard and painful and is amplified when being pressed, it is excess syndrome.

（4）诊肿胀 用手按压肌肤肿胀部位，以辨别水肿和气肿。如按之凹陷，举手不能即起者，为水肿；按之凹陷，举手即起者，为气肿。

Diagnosis of swelling Pressing the swollen part of skin with hands helps to distinguish edema and qi swelling. If the swollen part pits after being pressed by hands and can't recover immediately when the hands are lifted up, it indicates edema; and if it can recover immediately, it indicates qi swelling.

2. 按手足 手足俱冷者，是阳虚寒盛；手足俱热者，多为阳盛热炽。

Pressing hands and feet Cold hands and feet are due to yang deficiency and cold excess; Hot hands and feet indicate yang excess and heat exuberance.

3. 按胸胁 包括按虚里、按脘部、按腹部。

Pressing the chest and hypochondrium It includes the examination of xuli, the epigastric part and the abdomen.

（1）按虚里 虚里位于左乳下第 4、第 5 肋间，为心尖搏动处。正常情况下，虚里搏动不显，仅按之应手，节律清晰；是心气充盛，宗气积于胸中，为平人无病的征象。虚里按之其动微弱者为不及，是宗气内虚之征，亦可因饮停心包所致；动而应衣太过，是宗气外泄之象。

Examining xuli Xuli is located at the apex of heart, between the 4th and 5th ribs below the left nipple. Under normal circumstances, the pulsation of xuli is rhythmic and not obvious, which can only be felt when being pressed; It indicates the heart qi is sufficient and that the pectoral qi gathers in the chest, and is a sign that people have no illness. If its pulsation is weak when being pressed, it indicates deficiency of pectoral qi or fluid retention in the pericardium; If the pulsation is too obvious, it indicates leakage of pectoral qi.

（2）按脘部 脘部痞满，按之较硬而疼痛者，属实证，多因实邪聚结胃脘所致；按之濡软而无痛者，属虚证，多因胃腑虚弱所致；脘部按之有形而胀痛，推之辘辘有声者，为胃中有水饮。

Examining the epigastric part If the epigastric part is full, and is hard and painful when being pressed, it indicates excess syndrome, which is mostly caused by the accumulation of excessive pathogen in the epigastric region; If it is full, and is soft and painless when being pressed, it belongs to deficiency syndrome, which is mostly caused by deficiency of stomach; If the epigastric part has distending pain when being pressed and a watery sound when being pushed, it is due to fluid retention in the stomach.

（3）按腹部 腹部按之凉而喜温者，属寒证；腹部按之热而喜凉者，属热证；腹痛喜按者，多属虚证；腹痛拒按者，多属实证。若腹部有肿块，肿块推之不移，痛有定处者，为癥积，病属血分；肿块推之可移，或痛无定处，聚散不定者，为瘕聚，病属气分。

Examining the abdomen If the abdomen is cold when being pressed and patients like warmth in the abdominal part, it indicates cold syndrome; If the abdomen is hot when being pressed and patients like cold in the abdominal part, it indicates heat syndrome; If it is relieved when being pressed, it indicates deficiency syndrome; and if it is amplified when being pressed, it is mostly excess syndrome. If there is a lump in the abdomen, and it does not move when being pushed, and the pain is fixed, it indicates abdominal masses accumulating which belongs to xuefen; If the lump can be moved, or the pain is migratory and changeable, it indicates abdominal masses gathering which belongs to qifen.

第九章　中医常用的辨证方法
Chapter 9　Syndrome Differentiation Methods Commonly Used in Traditional Chinese Medicine

辨证，就是在中医基础理论指导下，对患者的临床资料进行分析、综合，对照各种证的概念，从而对疾病的当前病理本质作出判断，并概括为具体证名的过程。常用的辨证方法有八纲辨证、气血津液辨证、脏腑辨证等。

Syndrome differentiation is a process of analyzing, synthesizing and comparing the concepts of various syndromes under the guidance of the basic theory of TCM, so as to judge the nature of diseases at a certain stage and summarize them into specific syndromes. Commonly used syndrome differentiation methods include syndrome differentiation of eight principles, syndrome differentiation of qi, blood and fluid, syndrome differentiation of zang-fu viscera and so on.

第一节　八纲辨证
Section 1　Syndrome Differentiation of Eight Principles

一、概念与意义
1 Concept and Significance

八纲是指阴、阳、表、里、寒、热、虚、实八类证候。

Eight principles refer to eight syndromes: yin, yang, superficies, interior, cold, heat, deficiency and excess.

八纲辨证就是根据望、闻、问、切四诊搜集和掌握的各种病情和资料，运用八纲进行分析综合，从而辨别病变部位的浅深、疾病性质的寒热虚实、邪正斗争的盛衰和疾病类别的阴阳。

Syndrome differentiation of eight principles refers to differentiate diseases into yin, yang, superficies, interior, cold, heat, deficiency and excess syndromes through analyzing the data collected by the four diagnostic methods, namely, inspection, listening and smelling, inquiry as well as palpation and pulse taking. The analysis focuses on the disease location, nature and strength between vital qi and pathogenic qi and the yin or yang of disease categories.

二、八纲的基本证候

2 Basic syndromes of eight principles

八纲的基本证候，即通过表里辨证、寒热辨证、虚实辨证、阴阳辨证四对纲领的辨证，区分出的表证与里证、寒证与热证、虚证与实证、阴证与阳证八个证候。

The basic syndromes of the eight principles are eight syndromes, namely, superficies syndrome, interior syndrome, cold syndrome, heat syndrome, deficiency syndrome, excess syndrome, yin syndrome and yang syndrome, which are distinguished through four pairs of syndrome differentiation: syndrome differentiation of superficies and interior, syndrome differentiation of cold and heat, syndrome differentiation of excess and deficiency, and syndrome differentiation of yin–yang.

（一）表里辨证

2.1 Syndrome differentiation of superficies and interior

表里辨证是辨别病变部位内外深浅、病情轻重和病变趋向的一对纲领。

It is to distinguish the location, severity and trend of diseases.

1. 表证 一般是指六淫、疫疠等邪气经皮毛、口鼻侵入时所表现的轻浅证候的概括。多见于外感病的初期阶段。

Superficies syndrome It generally refers to the summary of mild and shallow syndromes when pathogens such as six climatic exopathogens and epidemic pestilence affect skin, nose and mouth. It is more common in the initial stage of exogenous diseases.

临床表现：发热，恶寒（或恶风），头身疼痛，鼻塞流涕，喉痒咳嗽，舌苔薄白，脉浮等。

Clinical manifestations: fever, aversion to cold (or wind), head and body pain, nasal obstruction and runny nose, itchy throat and cough, thin and white tongue coating, floating pulse, etc.

2. 里证 泛指病位在内的一类证候。

Interior syndrome It generally refers to a class of syndromes in which diseases locate in the interior.

临床表现：里证的范围广泛，临床表现多种多样，凡非表证（及半表半里证）的特定证，一般都属里证的范畴。

Clinical manifestations: The scope of interior syndrome is wide, and the clinical manifestations are various. Any manifestations that do not belong to superficies syndrome (or neither superficies nor interior syndrome) generally belong to interior syndrome.

3. 半表半里证 外邪由表内传，尚未入里，邪正相搏于表里之间，称为半表半里证。

Neither superficies nor interior syndrome It occurs when exopathogens have not entered the interior and vital qi fights with pathogenic qi between the superficies and interior.

临床表现：寒热往来，胸胁苦满，心烦喜呕，默默不欲饮食，口苦，咽干，目眩，脉弦等。

Clinical manifestations: alternate attacks of chill and fever, fullness and discomfort in chest and hypochondrium, disquieted heart spirit and vomiting, poor appetite, bitter taste, dry throat, dizziness, stringy pulse, etc.

（二）寒热辨证

2.2 Syndrome differentiation of cold and heat

寒热，是辨别疾病性质的一对纲领。

Cold and heat are a pair of principles to distinguish the nature of diseases.

1. 寒证 是感受阴寒之邪，或自体阳虚所表现的证候。

Cold syndrome It is the syndrome resulting from excess of yin–cold attacking the interior or yang deficiency within the body.

临床表现：寒证的临床表现不一，常见：恶寒喜暖，面色皖白，肢冷蜷卧，口淡不渴，痰涎清稀，小便清长，大便稀溏，舌淡苔白滑，脉迟或紧等。

Clinical manifestations: The clinical manifestations of cold syndrome are various, and common symptoms include: aversion to cold and preference for warmth, pale complexion, cold limbs and curling up, tastelessness without thirst, clear phlegm and thin saliva, clear urine in large amounts, loose stool, pale tongue with white and slippery coating, slow or tight pulse, etc.

2. 热证 是感受阳热之邪，或自体阳盛阴虚所表现的证候。

Heat syndrome It is the syndrome resulting from excess of yang–heat pathogen attacking the interior or yin deficiency within the body.

临床表现：热证的临床表现不一，常见：恶热喜冷，口渴喜冷饮，面红目赤，烦躁不安，痰涕黄稠，吐血，衄血，小便短赤，大便干结，舌红苔黄而干燥，脉数等。

Clinical manifestations: The clinical manifestations of heat syndrome are also various, and common symptoms include: aversion to heat and preference for cold, thirst and preference for cold drinks, red face and eyes, dysphoria, yellow and thick phlegm and nasal discharge, hematemesis, bleeding from five aperture or subcutaneous tissue, deep–colored urine in small amounts, dry stool, red tongue with yellow and dry coating, rapid pulse, etc.

（三）虚实辨证

2.3 Syndrome differentiation of excess and deficiency

虚实辨证，是分析辨别邪正盛衰的一对纲领。虚指正气不足，实指邪气过盛。

Deficiency and excess are a pair of principles to analyze and distinguish the rising and falling of vital qi and pathogenic qi. Deficiency refers to deficiency of vital qi, while excess refers to excess of pathogenic qi.

1. 虚证 是指人体正气虚弱，生理功能表现不足或衰退的一类证候。

Deficiency syndrome It refers to a kind of syndrome with weak vital qi and insufficient or declining physiological functions.

临床表现：虚证可表现为多种证候，所以虚证的典型证候难以概括。

Clinical manifestations: Deficiency syndrome can be manifested as a variety of syndromes, so it is difficult to summarize the typical syndromes of deficiency syndrome.

2. 实证 是由于邪气亢盛，机体功能亢奋或代谢障碍，病理性产物停积而出现的一类证候。

Excess syndrome It is a kind of syndrome caused by excessive etiological qi, hyperactivity of body function or metabolic disturbance, and stagnation of pathological products.

临床表现：由于实邪的性质及部位不同，其临床表现亦不一致。

Clinical manifestations: Because of the different nature and location of excessive pathogens, excess syndromes' clinical manifestations are also inconsistent.

（四）阴阳辨证

2.4 Syndrome differentiation of yin-yang

阴阳是辨识疾病总的纲领，用以统括其余的六个方面，即表、热、实证属阳证，里、寒、虚证属阴证。

Yin and yang are the general principles to diagnose diseases, which means they are used to conclude the other six principles, namely, exterior, heat and excess syndromes belong to yang syndrome, and interior, cold and deficiency syndromes belong to yin syndrome.

1. 阴证和阳证 Yin syndrome and yang syndrome

（1）阴证 主要是指机体阳气虚衰，阴气偏盛所表现的病证。多属寒属虚，病位大多在里。临床表现多见精神萎靡，面色皖白，气短声低，舌淡苔白，脉沉迟细等。

Yin syndrome It mainly refers to the syndrome caused by deficiency of yang qi and excess of yin qi. It mainly indicates cold and deficiency, and the disease location is in the interior. Clinical manifestations include listlessness, pale complexion, shortness of breath and low voice, pale tongue with white coating, deep, slow and thready pulse, etc.

（2）阳证 主要是指邪热炽盛，机体阳气偏亢所表现的病证。多属热属实。临床表现多见精神兴奋，狂躁不安，面色红赤，气粗声高，壮热烦渴，小便黄赤，大便干结，舌红绛苔黄厚，脉洪数或滑数等。

Yang syndrome　It refers to the syndrome caused by excessive etiological heat and hyperactivity of yang qi. It mainly indicates heat and excess. Common clinical manifestations are mental excitement, mania, red complexion, thick breath and high voice, high fever and polydipsia, yellow red urine, dry stool, red or crimson tongue with thick yellow coating, surging and rapid or slippery and rapid pulse, etc.

2. 阴虚证与阳虚证　阴液不足为阴虚，阳气不足为阳虚。阴虚多有热象，阳虚多见寒象。

Yin deficiency syndrome and yang deficiency syndrome　Yin deficiency syndrome is caused by yin fluid deficiency and yang deficiency syndrome is caused by yang qi deficiency. And yin deficiency is often characterized by heat manifestations, while yang deficiency is often characterized by cold manifestations.

（1）阴虚证　形体消瘦，潮热盗汗，五心烦热，咽干口燥，舌红少苔或无苔，脉细数等。

Yin deficiency syndrome　Manifestations include emaciation, tidal fever and night sweating, dysphoria with feverish sensation in chest, palms and soles, dry throat and mouth, red tongue with little or no coating, thready and rapid pulse, etc.

（2）阳虚证　面色㿠白，肢冷畏寒，神疲乏力，气短自汗，阳痿早泄，尿频清长，便溏，舌苔白滑，脉沉迟等。

Yang deficiency syndrome　It manifests as pale complexion, cold limbs and fear of cold, fatigue, shortness of breath and spontaneous sweating, impotence and prospermia, clear urine in large amounts and frequent urination, loose stool, white and slippery tongue coating, deep and slow pulse, etc.

3. 亡阴证与亡阳证　阴液衰竭为亡阴，阳气衰竭为亡阳。亡阴证多见汗出黏腻，身热肢温，烦躁不安，甚则昏迷气粗，舌红而干，脉细数无力。亡阳证多见冷汗淋漓，面色苍白，手足厥冷，肌肤不温，精神淡漠，气息微弱，舌淡，脉微细欲绝。

Yin depletion syndrome and yang depletion syndrome　Yin fluid depletion causes yin depletion syndrome and yang qi depletion causes yang depletion syndrome. Yin depletion syndrome has symptoms of sticky and greasy sweat, warm body and limbs, dysphoria, and even coma and thick breath, red and dry tongue, and thready, rapid and weak pulse. Yang depletion syndrome manifests as cold sweat, pale complexion, deadly cold hands and feet, tepid skin, apathy, weak breath, pale tongue and faint and thready pulse.

三、八纲证候间的关系

3 Relationship between syndromes of eight principles

（一）证候相兼

3.1 Concurrent syndromes

证候相兼是指疾病在某一阶段出现证候相兼状况。其临床表现一般是相关纲领证候相加。

Concurrent syndromes refer to the coexistence of multiple syndromes (excluding those with opposite nature) in a certain stage of disease. The clinical manifestations are generally the sum of related syndromes.

（二）证候错杂

3.2 Intermingling syndromes

证候错杂是指疾病在某一阶段同时出现表与里、寒与热、虚与实等病位、病性相反的证候。主要有表里同病、寒热错杂、虚实夹杂等，其临床表现一般是相关纲领证候的症状、体征相加。

Intermingling syndromes refer to the coexistence of syndromes with opposite nature, such as superficies and interior, cold and heat, and deficiency and excess syndromes. It mainly includes simultaneous superficies and interior syndromes, intermingled cold and heat, intermingled deficiency and excess, etc. Their clinical manifestations are generally the sum of symptoms and signs of related syndromes.

（三）证候转化

3.3 Syndrome transformation

证候转化是指八纲中相互对立的证候之间在一定条件下可以发生相互转化。主要有表里出入、寒热转化、虚实转化等。

Syndrome transformation refers to the mutual transformation of syndromes with opposite nature under certain conditions. It mainly includes entering of superficies syndrome and exiting of interior syndrome, cold–heat transformation, deficiency–excess transformation and so on.

第二节 气血津液辨证
Section 2 Syndrome Differentiation of Qi, Blood and Fluid

一、概念与意义
1 Concept and significance

气血津液辨证是根据气血津液的相关理论，分析四诊所获得的临床资料，在八纲辨证的基础上判断是否存在气血津液病证的辨证方法。

Syndrome differentiation of qi, blood and fluid is a syndrome differentiation method to analyse clinical data obtained from four diagnostic methods and judge pathologies of qi, blood and fluid based on syndrome differentiation of eight principles according to the theory of qi, blood and fluid.

二、气血辨证
2 Syndrome differentiation of qi and blood

（一）气病辨证
2.1 Syndrome differentiation of qi disease

气病以气的生理功能减退、气机失调为基本病机。

The basic pathogenesis of qi disease includes impaired physiological functions of qi and qi movement disorder.

1. 气虚证 是指机体元气不足，以神疲乏力、少气懒言、脉虚等为主要表现的证候。

Syndrome of qi deficiency It refers to the syndrome of insufficient primordial qi, which is mainly manifested by fatigue, panting and no desire to speak, and feeble pulse.

临床表现：神疲乏力，少气懒言，头晕目眩，自汗，活动时诸症加剧，舌淡苔白，脉虚等。

Clinical manifestations: fatigue, panting and no desire to speak, dizziness, spontaneous sweating, aggravation of these symptoms during activities, pale tongue with white coating, feeble pulse, etc.

2. 气陷证 是指气虚无力升举而反下陷，以自觉气坠或内脏下垂为主要表现的证候。

Syndrome of qi sinking It refers to the syndrome of deficient qi failing to ascend and sinking instead, and it is mainly manifested by a feeling of qi sinking or visceroptosis.

临床表现：头晕目眩，少气倦怠，久痢久泄，腹部有坠胀感，脱肛或子宫脱垂等，舌淡苔白，脉弱等。

Clinical manifestations: dizziness, panting, burnout, chronic dysentery and diarrhea, abdominal swelling, prolapse of anus or uterus, pale tongue with white coating, weak pulse, etc.

3. 气滞证 是指气机阻滞，运行不畅，以胀闷、疼痛、脉弦为主要表现的证候。

Syndrome of qi stagnation It refers to the syndrome caused by stagnation of qi movement, with manifestations of distension, pain and stringy pulse.

临床表现：胸胁、乳房、脘腹等处胀闷或攻窜作痛，胀痛常随嗳气、矢气、叹息而减轻，或随忧思恼怒而加重，脉弦等。

Clinical manifestations: distension, tightness or migratory pain in chest, breast, abdomen, etc., which is often relieved with belching, flatus or sighing, or aggravated with anxiety or anger, and stringy pulse.

4. 气逆证 是指气机升降失常，逆而向上，以咳喘、呕恶、头痛眩晕等为主要表现的证候。

Syndrome of reversed flow of qi It refers to the syndrome of abnormal ascending and descending of qi movement and counterflow of qi, which is mainly manifested by cough and panting, vomiting, headache and dizziness.

临床表现：肺气上逆，可见咳嗽喘息；胃气上逆，见嗳气、呃逆、恶心、呕吐；肝气上逆，见眩晕、头痛、昏厥、呕血等。

Clinical manifestations: Adverse rising of lung qi causes cough and gasping; adverse rising of stomach qi causes belching, hiccup, nausea and vomiting; adverse rising of liver qi causes vertigo, headache, fainting, hematemesis and so on.

（二）血病辨证

2.2 Syndrome differentiation of blood disease

血病的主要病理变化为血液不足，或血行障碍。

The main pathological changes of blood are blood deficiency or blood circulation disorder.

1. 血虚证 是指血液亏虚，脏腑、经络和组织失养，以面、睑、唇、舌色淡白，脉细为主要表现的证候。

Syndrome of blood deficiency It refers to the syndrome of blood deficiency, malnutrition of zang–fu viscera, meridians and tissues, which is mainly manifested by pale face, eyelid, lips and tongue, and thready pulse.

临床表现：面白无华或萎黄，唇色淡白，头晕眼花，心悸失眠，手足发麻，爪甲苍白，妇女经量少色淡，经期错后，舌淡苔白，脉细无力等。

Clinical manifestations: pale or sallow complexion, pale lips, dizziness, palpitation and insomnia, numbness of hands and feet, pale nails, scanty menstruation with a pale menstrual colour, delayed period of menstruation, pale tongue with white coating, thready and weak pulse, etc.

2. 血瘀证 是指瘀血内阻，以疼痛、肿块、出血及瘀血、涩脉为主要表现的证候。

Syndrome of blood stasis It refers to the syndrome of internal obstruction of blood stasis, which is mainly characterized by pain, lump, bleeding, static blood and hesitant pulse.

临床表现：疼痛如针刺，痛有定处、拒按，入夜加剧；肿块在体表呈青紫色，在内部按之硬而不移。面色黧黑，肌肤甲错，口唇爪甲紫暗，或皮下紫斑，或腹部青筋外露，或下肢筋青胀痛，或大便色黑如柏油。妇女常见闭经。舌质紫暗，或见瘀点瘀斑，脉细涩等。

Clinical manifestations: pain is as if pricked by a needle, which is fixed and will be amplified when being pressed or at night; lump is blue–purple on the body surface, and it is hard and unmovable when being pushed. Other manifestations include: darkish complexion, squamous and dry skin, purple and dark lips and nails, subcutaneous purple spots, exposed abdominal veins, blue lower limb veins with distending pain, or black stool as tarry. Women may have amenorrhea. The tongue is purple and dark, or with petechiae and ecchymosis, and the pulse is thready and hesitant.

3. 血热证 是指脏腑火热炽盛，热迫血分，以出血和实热症状为主要表现的证候。

Syndrome of heat in blood It refers to the syndrome of exuberance heat in zang–fu viscera, which suppressing xuefen, causing symptoms of bleeding and excess heat.

临床表现：咳血，吐血，尿血，衄血，便血，月经先期、量多，心烦，口渴，舌红绛，脉滑数等。

Clinical manifestations: hemoptysis, hematemesis, hematuria, bleeding from five aperture or subcutaneous tissue, hematochezia, precocious menstruation with large amount, disquieted heart spirit, thirst, crimson tongue, slippery and rapid pulse, etc.

4. 血寒证 是指寒邪客于血脉，血行不畅，以拘急冷痛、形寒、肤色紫暗为主要表现的证候。

Syndrome of cold in blood It refers to the syndrome of cold pathogen in blood vessels, causing unsmooth blood circulation, and the main manifestations are spasm, cold pain, cold body and dark purple skin color.

临床表现：少腹冷痛，肤色紫暗，形寒肢冷，得温痛减，月经愆期，痛经，经色紫暗，夹有血块，舌紫暗苔白滑，脉沉迟涩等。

Clinical manifestations: lower abdominal cold pain, dark purple skin color, cold body and limbs, pain alleviates with warmth, delayed period with a dark purple menstrual colour and blood clots, dysmenorrhea, dark purple tongue with white and slippery coating, deep, slow and hesitant pulse, and so forth.

（三）气血同病辨证

2.3 Syndrome differentiation of simultaneous qi and blood disease

气为血之帅，血为气之母。在发病时，二者常相互影响，既见气病，又见血病，称为气血同病。

Qi is the commander of blood, and blood is the mother of qi. Qi disease and blood disease often exist and influence each other at the same time when disease occurs, which is called simultaneous qi and blood disease.

1. 气虚血瘀证 指气虚运血无力，而致血行瘀滞，以气虚和血瘀症状相兼为主要表现的证候。

Syndrome of blood stasis due to qi deficiency It refers to the syndrome of qi deficiency failing to circulate blood, which leads to blood stasis, and it is mainly manifested by concurrent qi deficiency and blood stasis symptoms.

临床表现：面色淡白或晦滞，身倦乏力，少气懒言，疼痛如刺，痛处不移、拒按，舌淡暗或有瘀斑，脉沉涩等。

Clinical manifestations: pale or dull complexion, tiredness and fatigue, panting and no desire to speak, pain as if pricked by a needle, fixed pain which will be amplified when being pressed, pale and dark tongue or with ecchymosis, deep and hesitant pulse, etc.

2. 气滞血瘀证 指气滞不行以致血运障碍，或血瘀导致气行阻滞，出现既有气滞又有血瘀的证候。

Syndrome of qi stagnation and blood stasis It refers to the disorder of blood circulation caused by qi stagnation, or the blockage of qi circulation caused by blood stasis, resulting in both qi stagnation and blood stasis.

临床表现：胸胁胀满、走窜疼痛，急躁易怒，面色紫暗，皮肤青筋暴露，兼见痞块刺痛拒按，妇女闭经或痛经、经色紫暗夹有血块，乳房胀痛等，舌质紫暗或有瘀斑，脉弦涩等。

Clinical manifestations: fullness of chest and hypochondrium, migratory pain, irritability, dark purple complexion, exposure of skin veins, mass with stabbing pain which will be amplified when being pressed, amenorrhea or dysmenorrhea of women, with a dark purple menstrual colour and blood clots, distending pain of breasts, dark purple tongue or with ecchymosis, stringy and hesitant pulse, etc.

3. 气血两虚证 指气血不能相互化生，以气虚与血虚症状共见为主要表现的证候。

Syndrome of deficiency of both qi and blood It refers to the syndrome in which qi and blood can not transform into each other, causing simultaneous presence of qi deficiency and blood deficiency symptoms.

临床表现：神疲乏力，少气懒言，自汗，面色淡白或萎黄，口唇、眼睑、爪甲颜色淡白，头晕目眩，心悸失眠，形体消瘦，肢体麻木，月经量少色淡、愆期，舌淡白，脉细弱等。

Clinical manifestations: fatigue, panting and no desire to speak, spontaneous sweating, pale or sallow complexion, pale lips, eyelids and nails, dizziness, palpitation and insomnia, emaciation, numbness of limbs, delayed period with a pale menstrual colour and scanty amount, pale tongue, thready and weak pulse, and so on.

4. 气不摄血证　指气虚不能统摄血液而致出血，以气虚与出血症状共见为主要表现的证候。

Syndrome of qi failing to control blood　It refers to the syndrome of qi failing to contain blood and allows the blood to flow out of the vessels, which is mainly manifested as simultaneous presence of qi deficiency and bleeding.

临床表现：吐血，便血，皮下瘀斑，崩漏，气短，倦怠乏力，面色白而无华，舌淡，脉细弱等。

Clinical manifestations: hematemesis, hematochezia, subcutaneous ecchymosis, metrorrhagia, shortness of breath, fatigue, pale complexion lacking lustre, pale tongue, thready and weak pulse, etc.

三、津液辨证

3 Syndrome differentiation of fluid disease

津液辨证是根据津液的生理和病理特点，对四诊所收集的各种病情资料进行分析、归纳，辨别疾病当前病理本质是否存在着津液病证的辨证方法。

Syndrome differentiation of fluid disease is a syndrome differentiation method that analyzes and induces all kinds of disease data collected by four diagnostic methods to distinguish whether there is fluid syndrome currently in accordance with the physiological and pathological characteristics of fluid.

（一）津液亏虚证

3.1 Syndrome of deficiency of fluid

津液亏虚证是由于体内津液亏少，形体、脏腑、官窍失其濡润滋养，以口渴欲饮、尿少便干、官窍及皮肤干燥等为主要表现的证候。

Syndrome of deficiency of fluid is the syndrome caused by deficient fluid failing to nourish body, zang-fu organs and orifices, and its main manifestations are thirst with desire to drink, short urine, dry stool, dry orifices and skin, and so forth.

临床表现：口渴咽干，唇燥而裂，皮肤枯瘪，眼球深陷，小便短黄而少，便干，舌红少津，脉细数无力等。

Clinical manifestations: thirst and dry throat, cheilosis, withered skin, deep sunken eyeballs, yellow-colored urine in small amounts urine, dry stool, red tongue with little fluid, thready, rapid and weak pulse, etc.

（二）痰证
3.2 Phlegm syndrome

痰证是指痰浊停聚或流窜于脏腑、经络及组织之间，临床以痰多、胸闷、呕恶、眩晕、体胖等为主要表现的证候。

Phlegm syndrome refers to the syndrome of phlegm stagnation or phlegm moving between zang–fu viscera, meridians and tissues, which is mainly manifested by excessive phlegm, chest distress, vomiting, dizziness and fatness.

临床表现：咳嗽咳痰，痰质黏稠，胸脘满闷，纳呆呕恶，头晕目眩，或神昏癫狂，喉中痰鸣，或肢体麻木，舌苔白腻，脉滑等。

Clinical manifestations: cough and expectoration, sticky sputum, fullness and oppression in chest and abdomen, anorexia and vomiting, dizziness, faint and epilepsy, wheezing due to retention of phlegm in throat, numbness of limbs, white and greasy tongue coating, slippery pulse, etc.

（三）饮证
3.3 Fluid retention syndrome

饮证是指饮邪停聚于腔隙或胃肠，以胸闷脘痞、呕吐清水、咳吐痰涎清稀、肋间饱满等为主要表现的证候。

Fluid retention syndrome refers to the syndrome of pathogenic fluid gathers in lacuna or gastrointestinal tract, and its main manifestations are fullness and oppression in chest and abdomen, vomiting clear water, coughing of phlegm, thin saliva and water, and fullness in intercostal space.

临床表现：咳嗽气喘，痰多而稀，胸闷心悸，甚则倚息不能平卧，或脘腹痞满，水声辘辘，泛吐清水，或头晕目眩，小便不利，肢体浮肿，沉重酸困，苔白滑，脉弦等。

Clinical manifestations: cough, asthma, excessive and thin phlegm, chest distress, palpitation, and even leaning to rest due to inability to lie on the back, or fullness of abdomen, vomiting of clear water, dizziness, dysuria, edema of limbs, heaviness and soreness, white and slippery coating, stringy pulse, etc.

（四）水停证
3.4 Water retention syndrome

水停证又称水肿，是指体内水液停聚，泛滥肌肤所引起的以面目、四肢、胸腹甚至全身浮肿，小便不利，或腹大胀满，舌质淡胖等为主要临床表现的证候。临床上有阳水、阴水之分。水肿性质属实者，称为阳水；水肿性质属虚者，称为阴水。阳水多发病急，来势猛，眼睑、头面先肿，上半身肿甚；阴水多发病缓，来势徐，水肿先起于足部，腰以下肿为甚。

Water retention syndrome, also known as edema, refers to the syndrome of water retention in the body overflowing to the surface of the body, and the main clinical manifestations include edema of face, limbs, chest and abdomen, and even the entire body, dysuria, fullness of abdomen, pale and bulgy tongue, etc. Clinically, there are yang edema and yin edema. If the nature of edema is excess, it belongs to yang edema; If the nature of edema belongs to deficiency, it is yin edema. Yang edema is characterized by an acute onset of swelling of the face and eyelid, and the upper body is the most swollen part; Yin edema is characterized by a gradual onset of swelling feet or leg swelling, and the part below the waist is the most swollen.

第三节　脏腑辨证

Section 3　Syndrome Differentiation of Zang-Fu Viscera

脏腑辨证是根据脏腑的生理功能和病理变化，对四诊收集的临床资料进行综合分析，以判断疾病的病因病机、确定证候类型的一种辨证方法。

Syndrome differentiation of zang-fu viscera is a syndrome differentiation method which comprehensively analyzes the clinical data collected from the four diagnostic methods, so as to judge the etiology and pathogenesis of diseases and determine the types of syndromes in accordance with the physiological functions and pathological changes of zang-fu viscera.

一、心与小肠病辨证

1 Syndrome differentiation of the heart and small intestine disease

心病常见症状有心悸、心痛、怔忡、失眠、健忘、神志异常、舌疮、脉结或代等。小肠病常见症状有腹胀、腹痛、肠鸣、腹泻、尿赤涩灼痛、尿血等。

Common symptoms of heart disease include palpitation, heart pain, severe palpitation, insomnia, amnesia, abnormal consciousness, tongue sore, regularly or irregularly intermittent pulse, etc. Common symptoms of small intestine disease include abdominal distension, abdominal pain, borborygmus, diarrhea, red and hesitant urine with burning pain, hematuria and so on.

（一）心病辨证

1.1 Syndrome differentiation of heart disease

1. 心气虚证　是指心气不足，推动无力所致的证候。

Syndrome of deficiency of heart qi　It refers to the syndrome caused by deficient of heart qi failing to help with the heart to pump blood.

临床表现：心悸怔忡，胸闷气短，神疲自汗，活动后诸症加重，面白，舌淡，脉虚细等。

Clinical manifestations: palpitation, chest distress, shortness of breath, exhaustion and spontaneous sweating, aggravation of these symptoms after activities, pale complexion, pale tongue, feeble or thready pulse, etc.

2. 心阳虚证 是指心阳虚衰，温运失司，虚寒内生所致的证候。

Syndrome of deficiency of heart yang It refers to the syndrome caused by deficient heart yang failing to warm the body and causing endogenous deficiency-cold.

临床表现：心悸怔忡，胸痛憋闷，畏寒肢冷，神疲乏力，气短自汗，面色㿠白（或青紫），舌淡胖或紫暗，苔白滑，脉细微或结代等。

Clinical manifestations: palpitation, chest pain, oppression, fear of cold and cold limbs, fatigue, shortness of breath, spontaneous sweating, pallid (or blue-purple) complexion, pale and bulgy or dark and bulgy tongue, white and slippery coating, thready and faint or regularly or irregularly intermittent pulse, etc.

3. 心阳暴脱证 是指心阳衰极，阳气暴脱所表现的一种亡阳证。

Syndrome of sudden collapse of heart yang It refers to a kind of yang depletion syndrome characterized by extreme decline of heart yang and sudden collapse of yang qi.

临床表现：素有心阳虚证，突发冷汗淋漓，四肢厥冷，面色苍白，呼吸微弱，心痛剧烈，口唇青紫，神志模糊或昏迷，唇舌紫暗，脉微欲绝等。

Clinical manifestations: syndrome of deficiency of heart yang for a long time, sudden onset of cold sweat, deadly cold limbs, pale complexion, weak breathing, severe heart pain, blue-purple lips, blurred consciousness or coma, dark lips and tongue, faint pulse, etc.

4. 心血虚证 是指心血不足，心失濡养所致的证候。

Syndrome of deficiency of heart blood It refers to the syndrome caused by deficient heart blood failing to nourish the heart.

临床表现：心悸，失眠，多梦，健忘，头晕眼花，面色苍白或萎黄，唇舌色淡，脉细无力等。

Clinical manifestations: palpitation, insomnia, dreaminess, amnesia, dizziness, pale or sallow complexion, pale lips and tongue, thready and weak pulse, etc.

5. 心阴虚证 是指心阴亏虚，心神失养，虚热内扰所致的证候。

Syndrome of deficiency of heart yin It refers to the syndrome caused by deficient heart yin failing to nourish heart spirit and causing internal disturbance of deficiency heat.

临床表现：心悸，心烦，失眠多梦，口干咽燥，形体消瘦，或见五心烦热，潮热盗汗，舌红苔少，脉细数等。

Clinical manifestations: palpitation, disquieted heart spirit, insomnia and dreaminess, dry mouth and throat, emaciation, or dysphoria with feverish sensation in chest, palms and soles, tidal fever and night sweating, red tongue with little coating and thready and rapid pulse.

6. 心火亢盛证 是指火热内炽，扰乱神明，迫血妄行所致的证候。

Syndrome of exuberance of heart fire It refers to the syndrome caused by internal fire–heat disturbing spirit and forcing blood to move out of the vessels.

临床表现：身热面赤，心烦不寐，口渴喜饮，便秘溲黄，舌红苔黄，脉数有力。或口舌生疮，溃烂疼痛；或为小便短赤，灼热涩痛；或见吐血、衄血；或见神志不清、谵语狂躁等。

Clinical manifestations: hot body and red face, insomnia due to disquieted heart spirit, thirst with desire to drink, constipation and yellow urine, red tongue with yellow coating, rapid and strong pulse, or oral ulcers and pain; or deep–colored urine in small amounts, with burning and astringent pain; or hematemesis and epistaxis; or unconsciousness, delirium, mania, etc.

7. 心脉痹阻证 是指瘀血、痰浊、寒邪、气滞等因素痹阻心脉所致的证候。

Syndrome of blockade of heart vessel It refers to the syndrome caused by blood stasis, phlegm turbidity, cold pathogen, qi stagnation and other factors blocking the heart vessels.

临床表现：心悸怔忡，心胸憋闷疼痛，痛引肩背内臂，时发时止。血瘀心脉者，则心痛如刺，舌紫暗（或舌见瘀斑瘀点），脉细涩或结代；痰阻心脉者，则心胸闷痛，身重困倦，体胖痰多，舌苔白腻，脉沉滑；寒凝心脉者，则突发胸部剧痛，遇寒加重，得温则减，形寒肢冷，舌淡苔白，脉沉迟或沉紧；气滞心脉者，则心胸胀痛，善太息，脉弦等。

Clinical manifestations: palpitation, oppression and pain of heart and chest,and intermittent pain perceived by shoulder, back and inner arm. Patients with blood stasis blocking blood vessels may have symptoms of heart pain as if pricked by a needle, purple and dark tongue (or ecchymosis and petechia on the tongue), and thready and hesitant or regularly or irregularly intermittent pulse; Patients with phlegm blocking blood vessels have symptoms of stuffy and painful heart and chest, heavy and sleepy body, fat body with profuse phlegm, white and greasy coating, and deep and slippery pulse; Patients with cold congealing blood vessels have symptoms of severe and sudden chest pain, which will worsen when encountering cold and alleviate with warmth, cold body and limbs, pale tongue and white coating, and deep and slow or deep and tight pulse; Patients with qi stagnating blood vessels have symptoms of distending pain in heart and chest, tendency to sigh, stringy pulse and so on.

8. 痰迷心窍证 是指痰浊蒙蔽心包，以神志昏蒙为主要表现的证候。

Syndrome of phlegm misting the heart spirit It refers to the syndrome of phlegm turbidity misting pericardium and it is mainly manifested by clouding of consciousness.

临床表现：意识模糊，甚则昏不知人；或为精神抑郁，神志痴呆，表情淡漠，喃喃自语，举止失常；或突然昏仆，不省人事，喉中痰鸣，口吐涎沫，手足抽搐，并见胸闷呕恶，苔白腻，脉滑等。

Clinical manifestations: confusion of consciousness, even faint; or depression, dementia, indifferent expression, muttering and abnormal behavior; or sudden faint, unconsciousness, wheezing due to retention of phlegm in throat, spitting of saliva, tetany, chest distress, vomiting, white and greasy coating, slippery pulse, etc.

9. 痰火扰心证 是指痰火扰乱心神，神志异常所致的证候。

Syndrome of phlegm fire disturbing heart It refers to the syndrome of phlegm fire disturbing mind and causing abnormal consciousness.

临床表现：身热气粗，面红目赤，喉间痰鸣，咳痰黄稠，神昏谵狂，舌红，苔黄腻，脉滑数。或见心烦失眠，头晕目眩，胸闷痰多；或见神志不清，言语错乱，哭笑无常，狂言怒骂，打人毁物，属狂证等。

Clinical manifestations: hot body, thick breath, red face and eyes, wheezing due to retention of phlegm in throat, yellow and thick expectoration, faint, delirium, mania, red tongue, yellow and greasy coating and slippery and rapid pulse. Or disquieted heart spirit, insomnia, dizziness, chest distress and profuse phlegm; Or unconsciousness, paraphasia, impermanence in crying and laughing, raving, beating people and destroying things, and so on.

（二）小肠病辨证

1.2 Syndrome differentiation of small intestine disease

小肠实热证是指心火移热小肠，小肠邪热炽盛，泌别清浊失职所致的证候。

Syndrome of excessive heat of small intestine refers to the syndrome caused by heart fire moving heat to the small intestine, which leads to excessive etiological heat of small intestine, and dysfunction of separating the clear from the turbid.

临床表现：心烦口渴，口舌生疮，小便短赤、涩痛，或尿血，舌红苔黄，脉数有力等。

Clinical manifestations: disquieted heart spirit, thirst, sores in mouth and tongue, deep-colored urine in small amounts, with burning and astringent pain, or hematuria, red tongue with yellow coating, rapid and strong pulse, etc.

二、肺与大肠病辨证

2 Syndrome differentiation of lung and large intestine disease

肺病常见症状有咳嗽、气喘、咳痰、胸痛、鼻塞流涕、水肿等。大肠病常见症状有便秘、泄泻、腹胀、腹痛、肠鸣矢气、里急后重、泻下脓血等。

Common symptoms of lung disease include cough, asthma, expectoration, chest pain, nasal obstruction, runny nose, edema and so on. Common symptoms of large intestine disease include constipation, diarrhea, abdominal distension, abdominal pain, borborygmus, flatus, tenesmus, stool with pus and blood and so on.

（一）肺病辨证

2.1 Syndrome differentiation of lung disease

1. 肺气虚证 是指肺气不足，卫外不固，宣降无力所致的证候。

Syndrome of deficiency of lung qi It refers to the syndrome of deficient lung qi failing to secure the body and govern upward and outward diffusion as well as descent and purification.

临床表现：咳喘无力声低，咳痰清稀，少气懒言，动则尤甚，伴面色淡白、神疲乏力、自汗、恶风，易于感冒，舌淡苔白，脉细弱等。

Clinical manifestations: cough and gasping with low voice, spitting of clear and thin phlegm, panting and no desire to speak, aggravation during activities, accompanied by pale complexion, fatigue, spontaneous sweating, aversion to wind, easy to catch a cold, pale tongue with white coating, thready and weak pulse, etc.

2. 肺阴虚证 是指肺阴亏虚，虚火内生所致的证候。

Syndrome of deficiency of lung yin It refers to the syndrome caused by lung yin deficiency and endogenous deficiency fire.

临床表现：干咳无痰，或痰少而黏、不易咳出，甚或痰中带血，声音嘶哑，伴五心烦热、潮热盗汗、形体消瘦、颧红、口燥咽干，舌红少苔，脉细数等。

Clinical manifestations: dry cough without phlegm, or with less and sticky phlegm which is not easy to cough up, or even bloody phlegm, hoarseness, accompanied by dysphoria with feverish sensation in chest, palms and soles, tidal fever and night sweating, emaciation, hectic cheek, dry mouth and throat, red tongue with little coating, and thready and rapid pulse.

3. 风寒束肺证 是指风寒侵袭，肺卫失宣所致的证候。

Syndrome of wind cold attacking lungs It refers to the syndrome caused by wind cold invasion and impairment of diffusion function.

临床表现：咳喘、痰白清稀，恶寒重，发热轻，鼻塞，流清涕，头身痛，无汗，脉浮紧等。

Clinical manifestations: cough and gasping, white and thin phlegm, severe aversion to cold, mild fever, stuffy nose, clear nasal discharge, head and body pain, no sweat, floating and tight pulse, etc.

4. 风热犯肺证 是指风热侵犯，肺卫失宣所致的证候。

Syndrome of wind-heat invading lung It refers to the syndrome caused by wind heat invasion and impairment of diffusion function.

临床表现：咳嗽、咳痰黄稠，发热微恶寒，口微渴，咽喉肿痛，流黄浊涕，舌边尖红，苔黄，脉浮数等。

Clinical manifestations: cough, spitting of yellow and thick phlegm, fever, slight aversion to cold, slight thirst, sore and swollen throat, yellow and turbid nasal discharge, red tongue tip and edges, yellow coating, floating and rapid pulse, etc.

5. 燥邪犯肺证 是指燥邪犯肺，肺卫失宣，肺失清润所致的证候。

Syndrome of dryness invading lung It refers to the syndrome caused by dryness pathogen invading lungs, and impairment of diffusion and clearing function of lungs.

临床表现：干咳无痰，或痰少而黏且不易咳出，轻微恶寒发热，口鼻干燥，或见鼻衄，无汗，苔薄干燥，脉浮紧或浮数等。

Clinical manifestations: dry cough without phlegm, or with little and sticky phlegm which is difficult to cough up, slight aversion to cold with fever, dry nose and mouth, or epistaxis, no sweat, thin and dry coating, floating and tight or floating and rapid pulse, etc.

6. 痰热壅肺证 是指痰热交结，壅滞于肺，肺失宣肃所致的证候。

Syndrome of phlegm–heat obstructing lung It refers to the syndrome caused by phlegm heat intersecting and stagnating in lungs and lungs failing to govern upward and outward diffusion as well as descent and purification.

临床表现：咳喘，呼吸气粗，甚则鼻翼扇动，痰黄稠而量多或为脓血腥臭痰，胸痛，壮热，口渴，尿黄赤，便秘，舌红，苔黄腻，脉滑数等。

Clinical manifestations: cough and gasping, thick breath, even alaenasi flaring, yellow and thick phlegm or purulent and bloody foul phlegm, chest pain, high fever, thirst, yellow and red urine, constipation, red tongue, yellow and greasy coating, slippery and rapid pulse, etc.

7. 寒饮阻肺证 是指素有伏饮，复感寒邪，水饮上逆，肺失宣肃所致的证候。

Syndrome of cold fluid blocking lung It refers to the syndrome caused by fluid retention attacked by cold pathogen and reversing upward, and thus lungs failing to govern upward and outward diffusion as well as descent and purification.

临床表现：咳嗽，痰液清稀量多，背寒肢冷，咳喘倚息不得平卧，舌淡苔白滑或白腻，脉弦紧等。

Clinical manifestations: cough, clear and thin phlegm in large amounts, cold back and limbs, cough and asthma, inability to lie on the back, pale tongue with white and slippery or white and greasy coating, stringy and tight pulse, etc.

8. 肺热炽盛证 是指热邪壅盛于肺，肺失宣肃所致的证候。

Syndrome of excessive lung heat It refers to the syndrome caused by heat pathogen accumulating in the lungs and lungs failing to govern upward and outward diffusion as well as descent and purification.

临床表现：壮热，口渴喜饮，呼吸气粗，咳嗽，痰黄稠，鼻翼扇动，衄血，咳血，便结，尿短赤，舌红苔黄，脉洪数等。

Clinical manifestations: high fever, thirst with desire to drink, coarse breathing sound, cough, yellow and thick phlegm, alaenasi flaring, epistaxis, hemoptysis, dry stool, deep–colored urine in small amounts, red tongue with yellow coating, and surging and rapid pulse.

（二）大肠病辨证

2.2 Syndrome differentiation large intestine disease

1. 大肠湿热证 是指湿热壅阻肠道气机，大肠传导失职所致的证候。

Syndrome of dampness–heat in large intestine It refers to the syndrome caused by dampness–heat blocking intestinal qi movement and impairment of conducting and discharging function.

临床表现：腹痛腹胀，下痢脓血，里急后重，或暴泻黄浊臭水，肛门灼热，尿短赤，舌红，苔黄腻，脉滑数等。

Clinical manifestations: abdominal pain, abdominal distension, diarrhea with pus and blood, tenesmus, or sudden diarrhea with yellow, turbid and smelly water, anus with burning pain, deep–colored urine in small amounts, red tongue, yellow and greasy coating, slippery and rapid pulse, etc.

2. 肠热腑实证 是指热邪与糟粕互结大肠所致的里实热证。

Syndrome of intestine heat and fu–viscera excess It refers to the syndrome of excess heat in the interior caused by the interaction of heat pathogen and faeces in the large intestine.

临床表现：壮热或日晡潮热，口渴，腹满胀痛拒按，大便秘结，或热结旁流，尿短赤，舌红苔黄而焦燥，脉沉实有力等。

Clinical manifestations: high fever or afternoon tidal fever, thirst, abdominal fullness,distending pain which will be amplified when being pressed, constipation, or heat fecaloma with watery discharge, deep–colored urine in small amounts, red tongue with yellow and scorched coating, and deep and excess pulse.

3. 肠燥津亏证 是指大肠津液亏损，肠失濡润，传导失司所致的证候。

Syndrome of intestinal dryness and fluid deficiency It refers to the syndrome caused by deficiency of fluid in large intestine, and impairment of moistening, conducting and discharging functions.

临床表现：大便秘结干燥，难以排出，常数日一行，口干咽燥，或伴口臭、腹胀，舌红少津，脉细涩等。

Clinical manifestations: constipation and dry stool with a frequency of one time in several days, dry mouth and throat, or accompanied by halitosis, abdominal distension, red tongue with little fluid, thready and hesitant pulse, etc.

三、脾与胃病辨证

3 Syndrome differentiation of spleen and stomach disease

脾病常见症状有食欲不振、腹满、便溏、内脏下垂、出血、水肿等。胃病常见症状有胃脘胀痛、恶心、呕吐、嗳气、呃逆等。

Common symptoms of spleen disease include poor appetite, abdominal fullness, loose stool, visceroptosis, bleeding, edema and so on. Common symptoms of stomach disease include epigastric pain, nausea, vomiting, belching, hiccup and so on.

（一）脾病辨证

3.1 Syndrome differentiation of spleen disease

1. 脾气虚证 是指脾气不足，运化失司所致的证候。

Syndrome of deficiency of spleen qi It refers to the syndrome caused by deficiency of spleen qi and impairment of the function of transportation and transformation.

临床表现：腹胀纳呆，食后胀甚，大便溏薄，面色苍白或萎黄，少气懒言，肢体倦怠，或浮肿或消瘦，舌淡苔白，脉缓弱等。

Clinical manifestations: abdominal distension which will aggravate after eating, loose stool, pale or sallow complexion, panting and no desire to speak, flabby muscle, edema or emaciation, pale tongue with white coating, moderate and weak pulse, etc.

2. 脾阳虚证 是指脾阳虚衰，失于温运，阴寒内生所致的证候。

Syndrome of deficiency of spleen yang It refers to the syndrome caused by deficient spleen yang failing to warm and transport food and causing endogenous yin cold.

临床表现：腹胀纳呆，大便稀溏或完谷不化，脘腹冷痛绵绵，喜温喜按，形寒肢冷，神倦气短，小便清长，或尿少浮肿，或妇人带下清稀量多色白，舌淡胖、边有齿痕，苔白滑，脉沉迟无力等。

Clinical manifestations: abdominal distension and anorexia, loose stool or diarrhea with undigested food, cold and dull pain which can be relieved when encountering warmth or being pressed, cold body and limbs, tiredness and shortness of breath, clear urine in large amounts, or little urine with swollen bladder, or clear and thin leucorrhea with a white colour and large amount,, pale and bulgy tongue with teeth compression on the edge of the tongue body, white and slippery coating, deep, slow and weak pulse, etc.

3. 中气下陷证 是指脾气虚弱，升举无力，清阳下陷所致的证候。

Syndrome of sinking of qi due to spleen deficiency It refers to the syndrome caused by deficient spleen qi failing to ascend and clear yang qi sinking.

临床表现：脘腹坠胀，头晕耳鸣，久泻久痢，便意频作，食后尤甚，肛门坠胀，或内脏、子宫下垂，脱肛，伴气短懒言、神疲乏力、面白无华，舌淡苔白，脉缓弱等。

Clinical manifestations: bearing–down sensation in the abdomen, dizziness and tinnitus, chronic diarrhea and dysentery, frequent defecation which will aggravate after eating, bearing–down sensation in the anus, or prolapse of viscera and uterus, anal prolapse, accompanied by shortness of breath and no desire to speak, fatigue, pale complexion without lustre, pale tongue with white coating, moderate and weak pulse, etc.

4. 脾不统血证 是指脾气亏虚不能统摄血液所致的证候，又称气不摄血证。

Syndrome of spleen failing to manage blood It refers to the syndrome caused by deficient spleen qi failing to control blood, which is also called syndrome of qi failing to control blood.

临床表现：鼻衄，齿衄，肌衄，吐血，尿血，便血，或妇女月经过多、崩漏，伴食少便溏、神疲乏力、面色无华、少气懒言，舌淡苔白，脉细弱等。

Clinical manifestations: epistaxis, gum bleeding, sweat pore bleeding, hematemesis, hematuria, hematochezia, or profuse menstruation, metrorrhagia, loose stool with poor appetite, fatigue, pale complexion without lustre, panting and no desire to speak, pale tongue with white coating, thready and weak pulse, etc.

5. 寒湿困脾证 是指寒湿内盛，脾阳受困所致的证候。

Syndrome of cold–dampness disturbing spleen It refers to the syndrome caused by excessive cold–dampness disturbing spleen yang.

临床表现：脘腹痞闷，食欲不振，泛恶欲吐，便溏，头身困重，或身目发黄、色暗如烟熏，或浮肿尿少，或妇人带下色白量多，舌淡胖，苔白腻，脉濡缓或沉细等。

Clinical manifestations: abdominal fullness, loss of appetite, vomiting, loose stool, heavy head and body, yellow body and eyes with the color as dark as smoke, edema and little urine, leucorrhea with a white colour and large amount, pale and bulgy tongue with white and greasy coating, soft and moderate or deep and thready pulse, etc.

6. 湿热蕴脾证 是指湿热中阻，脾失健运所致的证候。

Syndrome of dampness–heat stagnating in spleen It refers to the syndrome caused by dampness–heat stagnation and dysfunction of spleen in transportation.

临床表现：脘痞腹胀，纳呆厌食，口中黏腻，渴不多饮，身重肢倦，大便溏泄不爽，或皮肤瘙痒，或身热不扬，尿短黄，舌红，苔黄腻，脉濡数等。

Clinical manifestations: epigastric fullness, abdominal distension, anorexia, sticky mouth, thirst but lack of drinking, heavy and fatigue body and limbs, loose stool with a sensation of incomplete defecation, itchy skin, hiding fever, yellow urine in small amounts, red tongue with yellow and greasy coating, and soft and rapid pulse, etc.

（二）胃病辨证

3.2 Syndrome differentiation of stomach disease

1. 胃阴虚证 是指胃之津液受损，胃失濡润、和降所表现的证候。

Syndrome of deficiency of stomach yin It refers to the syndrome of deficient fluid failing to nourish the stomach and affecting the descending of stomach qi.

临床表现：胃脘隐隐灼痛，饥不欲食，胃脘嘈杂，干呕呃逆，口燥咽干，便干，尿短少，舌红苔少，脉细数等。

Clinical manifestations: dull burning pain in the epigastric region, hunger but with no desire to eat, noisy sound in epigastric region, retching and hiccup, dry mouth and throat, dry stool, scanty urine, red tongue and little coating, and thready and rapid pulse.

2. 寒滞胃脘证 是指寒邪犯胃，胃气郁滞，胃失和降所致的证候。

Syndrome of retention of cold in stomach It refers to the syndrome caused by cold pathogen invading stomach, stagnation of stomach qi and failure of stomach qi to descend.

临床表现：胃脘冷痛，得温则减，遇寒痛甚，恶心呕吐，或口泛清水，形寒肢冷，舌淡苔白滑，脉沉紧等。

Clinical manifestations: cold pain which will worsen when encountering cold and alleviate with warmth, nausea and vomiting, or clear water flowing out of the mouth, cold body and limbs, pale tongue with white and slippery coating, deep and tight pulse, etc.

3. 胃热炽盛证 是指火热内蕴于胃腑，胃失和降所致的证候。

Syndrome of exuberance heat in stomach It refers to the syndrome caused by accumulated fire heat in the stomach affecting the descending of stomach qi.

临床表现：胃脘灼痛，吞酸嘈杂，渴喜冷饮，口臭，牙龈肿痛溃烂，齿衄，或消谷善饥，便秘，尿短赤，舌红苔黄，脉数有力等。

Clinical manifestations: burning pain in the stomach, acid regurgitation, a noisy sound in epigastric region, thirst with a liking for cold drinks, halitosis, swelling, pain and ulceration of gums, gum bleeding, or rapid digestion of food and polyorexia, constipation, red urine in small amounts, red tongue with yellow coating, strong and rapid pulse, etc.

4. 食滞胃脘证 是指饮食不化，停滞于胃脘，胃气失和所致的证候。

Syndrome of retention of food in stomach It refers to the syndrome caused by stagnation of food in the stomach affecting the descending of stomach qi.

临床表现：胃脘胀满、疼痛拒按，厌食，嗳腐吞酸，呕吐酸腐馊食，便泻不爽，泻下酸腐臭秽，舌苔厚腻，脉弦滑等。

Clinical manifestations: fullness of stomach, pain which will be amplified when being pressed, anorexia, belching and acid regurgitation, vomiting of sour and rotten food, diarrhea of sour, rancid and filthy residues with a sensation of incomplete defecation, thick and greasy tongue coating, stringy and slippery pulse, etc.

四、肝与胆病辨证

4 Syndrome differentiation of liver and gallbladder disease

肝病常见症状有精神抑郁或急躁易怒，头晕目眩，胸胁、少腹胀痛，肢体震颤，四肢抽搐，视物不清，月经不调等。胆病常见症状有口苦，呕胆汁，面目身黄，胆怯等。

Common symptoms of liver disease include depression or irritability, dizziness, hypochondriac and abdominal distending pain, limb tremor, limb convulsion, cloudy vision, menstrual disorders and so on. Common symptoms of gallbladder diseases include bitter taste, vomiting of bile, yellow face, eyeballs and skin, timidity and so on.

（一）肝病辨证

4.1 Syndrome differentiation of liver disease

1. 肝气郁结证 是指肝失疏泄，气机郁滞所表现的证候。

Syndrome of stagnation of liver qi It refers to the syndrome of liver failing to maintain the free flow of qi.

临床表现：情志抑郁易怒，胸胁、少腹胀闷窜痛，喜太息，或咽部有异物感，或见颈部瘿瘤、瘰疬，或胁下肿块，或妇人经前期乳房胀痛、痛经，脉弦等。

Clinical manifestations: emotional depression, irritability, distention and migratory pain of chest, hypochondrium and abdomen, sighing, foreign body sensation in pharynx, goiter, scrofula, or hypochondrium lump, or distending pain of breasts during the early period of menstruation, dysmenorrhea, stringy pulse, etc.

2. 肝火上炎证 是指肝火炽盛，气火上逆所致的证候。

Syndrome of liver fire flaring up It refers to the syndrome caused by exuberance liver fire flowing upward.

临床表现：头晕胀痛，面红目赤，口干口苦，急躁易怒，失眠或噩梦纷纭，耳鸣，或胁肋灼痛，或吐血衄血，便结尿黄，脉弦数等。

Clinical manifestations: dizziness and distending pain, red face and eyes, dry mouth and bitter taste, irritability, insomnia or nightmares, tinnitus, burning pain in hypochondriac ribs, hematemesis, bleeding from five aperture or subcutaneous tissue, yellow urine, dry stool, and stringy and rapid pulse.

3. 肝血虚证 是指肝血亏虚，机体失去濡养所致的证候。

Syndrome of deficiency of liver blood It refers to the syndrome caused by deficient liver blood failing to nourish the body.

临床表现：头晕目眩，视力减退或夜盲，面色无华，夜寐多梦；四肢麻木，关节拘挛，手足震颤，肌肉瞤动，爪甲不荣，或妇人月经量少、色淡，甚则闭经，舌淡苔白，脉细等。

Clinical manifestations: dizziness, visual deterioration or nyctalopia, pale complexion without lustre, dreaminess; limb numbness, joint contraction. hand and foot tremor, muscle tremor, undignified nail, or a woman with small menstrual volume, pale color, even amenorrhea, pale tongue, white fur, thin pulse, etc.

4. 肝阴虚证 是指肝阴亏虚，阴不制阳，虚火内生所致的证候。

Syndrome of deficiency of liver yin It refers to the syndrome caused by liver yin deficiency, yin failure to control yang, and endogenous deficiency fire.

临床表现：头晕眼花，两目干涩，视物不清，面部烘热，或颧红，五心烦热，潮热盗汗，或胁肋灼痛，或手足蠕动，口燥咽干，舌红少苔，脉弦细数等。

Clinical manifestations: dizziness, dry eyes, blurred vision, hot face, or hectic cheek, dysphoria with feverish sensation in chest, palms and soles, hot flashes and night sweating, or burning pain in hypochondrium, or wriggling of limbs, dry mouth and throat, red tongue with little coating, string and thin pulse, etc.

5. 肝阳上亢证 是指肝肾之阴不足，阴不制阳，肝阳亢盛所致的证候。

Syndrome of upper hyperactivity of liver yang It refers to the syndrome caused by insufficient yin in the liver and kidney, inability of yin to control yang, and hyperactivity of liver yang.

临床表现：头目胀痛，眩晕耳鸣，面红目赤，耳鸣耳聋，急躁易怒，腰膝酸软，头重脚轻，舌红少津，脉弦或弦细数等。

Clinical manifestations: head pain, dizziness and tinnitus, red face and red eyes, tinnitus and deafness, irritability, soreness and weakness of waist and knees, top–heavy feet, red tongue with little fluid, stringy or thin pulse, etc.

6. 肝风内动证 是指具有眩晕欲仆、抽搐、震颤等“动摇”特征的一类证候。临床常见肝阳化风、热极生风、阴虚动风、血虚生风等证。

Syndrome of liver wind stirring up internally It refers to a type of syndrome with “shaking” characteristics such as dizziness, convulsions, and tremors. Clinical syndromes such as hyperactive liver yang causing wind, extreme heat generating wind, stirring wind due to yin deficiency, and blood deficiency generating wind are common.

（1）肝阳化风证 是指肝阳上亢无制而引动肝风所致的证候。

The syndrome of hyperactive liver yang causing wind It refers to the syndrome caused by hyperactivity of liver yang and uncontrolled liver wind.

临床表现：头胀头痛，眩晕欲仆，步履不稳，项强肢颤，语言謇涩，手足麻木，或突然昏倒，不省人事，口眼㖞斜，半身不遂，舌强不语，喉中痰鸣，舌红苔白或腻，脉弦滑等。

Clinical manifestations: distention in the head and headache, dizziness, unsteady walking, stiff neck and trembling limbs, dysphasia, numbness of hands and feet, or sudden fainting, unconsciousness, facial paralysis, hemiplegia, strong tongue and silent speech, wheezing due to retention of phlegm in throat, red tongue with white or greasy coating, stringy pulse, etc.

（2）热极生风证 是指热邪亢盛，筋脉失养，引动肝风所致的证候。

The syndrome of extreme heat generating wind It refers to the syndrome caused by excessive heat pathogen, malnutrition of tendons and veins, and stimulation of liver wind.

临床表现：高热口渴，神昏谵妄，颈项强直，四肢抽搐，甚或角弓反张，舌红苔黄燥，脉弦数有力等。

Clinical manifestations: high fever and thirst, unconsciousness and delirium, stiff neck, limb twitching, or even angular arch reflexion, red tongue with yellow dry coating, strong pulse, etc.

（3）阴虚生风证 是指肝肾阴亏，筋脉失养，虚风内动所致的证候。

The syndrome of stirring wind due to yin deficiency　It refers to the syndrome caused by deficiency of liver and kidney yin, malnutrition of tendons and veins, and internal movement of deficiency wind.

临床表现：手足蠕动甚则瘛疭，眩晕耳鸣，两目干涩，视物模糊，五心烦热，潮热盗汗，颧红咽干，形体消瘦，舌红少津，脉弦细数等。

Clinical manifestations: wriggling of limbs, dizziness and tinnitus, dry eyes, blurred vision, dysphoria with feverish sensation in chest, palms and soles, tidal fever and night sweating, hectic cheek and dry throat, body weight loss, red tongue and less fluid, stringy and thin pulse, etc.

（4）血虚生风证　是指肝血亏虚，筋脉失养，虚风内动所致的证候。

The syndrome of blood deficiency generating wind　It refers to the syndrome caused by liver blood deficiency, malnutrition of tendons and veins, and internal movement of deficiency wind.

临床表现：头晕眼花，失眠多梦，肢体震颤，四肢麻木，肌肉瞤动，关节拘急不利，面色无华，爪甲不荣，舌淡苔白，脉细弱等。

Clinical manifestations: dizziness, insomnia and dreaminess, tremor of limbs, numbness of limbs, muscle stoppage, unfavorable joint tightness, dull complexion, disgraceful claws and nails, pale tongue with white coating, thin and weak pulse, etc.

7. 寒凝肝脉证　是指寒邪凝滞肝脉所致的证候。

Syndrome of cold coagulated in liver channel　It refers to the syndrome caused by cold pathogen stagnation of liver pulse.

临床表现：少腹牵引睾丸坠胀冷痛，或阴囊收缩引痛，或颠顶冷痛，形寒肢冷，得温则减，舌淡苔白滑，脉沉紧或弦紧等。

Clinical manifestations: abdominal traction, testicular swelling and cold pain, or scrotal contraction caused pain, or cold pain on top of the head, cold shape and cold limbs, decrease when warm, pale tongue with white and slippery coating, heavy or stringy pulse, etc.

（二）胆病辨证

4.2 Syndrome differentiation of gallbladder disease

胆郁痰扰证　是指胆失疏泄，痰热内扰所致的证候。

The syndrome of stagnated gallbladder qi with disturbing phlegm　It refers to the syndrome caused by the loss of gallbladder drainage and internal disturbance of phlegm and heat.

临床表现：胆怯易惊，惊悸失眠，烦躁不宁，眩晕耳鸣，胸胁胀闷，口苦欲呕，舌红，苔黄腻，脉弦数等。

Clinical manifestations: timidity and fright, palpitations and insomnia, irritability and restlessness, dizziness and tinnitus, distension and tightness of chest and hypochondrium, bitter taste in mouth and vomiting, red tongue, yellow and greasy coating, stringy pulse, etc.

五、肾与膀胱病辨证

5 Syndrome differentiation of kidney and bladder diseases

肾病常见症状有腰膝酸软或疼痛、耳鸣耳聋、齿动发脱、男子阳痿遗精或精少不育、女子经少闭经不孕、水肿、虚喘、二便排泄异常等。膀胱病常见症状有尿频、尿急、尿痛、尿闭、遗尿、小便失禁等。

Common symptoms of kidney disease include soreness or pain in the waist and knees, tinnitus and deafness, tooth movement and loss, male impotence, spermatorrhea or oligospermia infertility, female oligomenorrhea and amenorrhea infertility, edema, deficiency asthma, abnormal stool excretion, etc. Common symptoms of bladder disease include frequent urination, urgency, painful urination, urinary occlusion, enuresis, urinary incontinence, etc.

（一）肾病辨证

5.1 Syndrome differentiation of kidney disease

1. 肾阳虚证　是指肾阳不足，失于温煦，虚寒内生所致的证候。

Syndrome of deficiency of kidney yang　It refers to the syndrome caused by insufficient kidney yang, loss of warmth, and endogenous deficiency and cold.

临床表现：腰膝酸软而冷痛，形寒肢冷，下肢尤甚，神疲乏力，面色㿠白或黧黑，男子阳痿、早泄，女子宫寒不孕，白带清稀量多，五更泄泻，夜尿频多，舌淡胖，苔白滑，脉沉迟无力等。

Clinical manifestations: soreness and cold pain in waist and knees, cold shape and cold limbs, especially lower limbs, fatigue, white or dark complexion, impotence and premature ejaculation in men, infertility with uterine cold in women, clear and thin leucorrhea, diarrhea at five nights, frequent nocturia, pale and fat tongue, white and slippery coating, deep and weak pulse, etc.

2. 肾阴虚证　是指肾阴不足，失于濡养，虚火内扰所致的证候。

Syndrome of deficiency of kidney yin　It refers to the syndrome caused by insufficient kidney yin, loss of nourishment, and internal disturbance of deficiency fire.

临床表现：腰膝酸软而痛，眩晕耳鸣，失眠多梦，男子阳强易举，女子经少或经闭，伴咽干口燥，形体消瘦，五心烦热，潮热盗汗，颧红，舌红少苔，脉细数等。

Clinical manifestations: soreness and pain in waist and knees, dizziness and tinnitus, insomnia and dreaminess, persistent erection of penis in men, oligomenorrhea or amenorrhea in women, accompanied by dry throat and dry mouth, body weight loss, dysphoria with feverish sensation in chest, palms and soles, tidal fever and night sweating, hectic cheek, red tongue with little coating, thin pulse, etc.

3. 肾精不足证　是指肾精亏损，脑与骨、髓失充所致的证候。

The syndrome of insufficiency of kidney qi It refers to the syndrome caused by the loss of kidney essence and the failure of brain, bone and marrow.

临床表现：小儿发育迟缓，囟门迟闭，身材矮小，智力低下，骨骼痿软；成人早衰，发脱齿摇，耳鸣耳聋，腰膝酸软，足痿无力，健忘恍惚，神情呆钝，动作迟钝，男子精少不育，女子经闭不孕，舌淡，脉细弱等。

Clinical manifestations: children's developmental delay, delayed closure of fontanelle, short stature, mental retardation, and weak bones; Premature aging in adults, tooth loss, tinnitus and deafness, soreness and weakness of waist and knees, weakness of feet, forgetfulness and trance, dull expression, dull movements, infertility in men, amenorrhea and infertility in women, pale tongue, thin and weak pulse, etc.

4. 肾气不固证 是指肾气不足，下元失固所致的证候。

The syndrome of non-consolidation of kidney qi It refers to the syndrome caused by insufficient kidney qi and insufficient lower yuan.

临床表现：腰膝酸软，神疲乏力，耳鸣耳聋，小便频数清长，夜尿增多，或尿后余沥不尽，小便失禁，遗尿，男子滑精早泄，女子胎动易滑，舌淡苔白，脉沉细弱等。

Clinical manifestations: soreness and weakness of waist and knees, fatigue, tinnitus and deafness, frequent and clear urination, increased nocturia, or endless leaching after urination, urinary incontinence, enuresis, night emission and premature ejaculation in men, slippery fetal movement in women, pale tongue with white coating, heavy and thin pulse, etc.

5. 肾不纳气证 是指肾气虚衰，气不归元所致的证候。

Deficiency of kidney failing to control respiring qi It refers to the syndrome caused by deficiency of kidney qi and failure of qi to return to its origin.

临床表现：久病咳喘，呼多吸少，气不接续，动则喘甚，腰膝酸软，舌淡苔白，脉沉弱等。

Clinical manifestations: chronic illness, cough and asthma, exhale more and inhale less, breath is not continuous, severe asthma when moving, soreness and weakness of waist and knees, pale tongue with white coating, deep and weak pulse, etc.

（二）膀胱病辨证

5.2 Syndrome differentiation of bladder disease

膀胱湿热证 是指湿热蕴结膀胱，膀胱气化失司所致的证候。

Syndrome of dampness-heat of bladder It refers to the syndrome caused by the accumulation of damp-heat in the bladder and the loss of bladder qi.

临床表现：尿频尿急，尿道灼痛，色黄短少，或尿有砂石，或尿血，小腹胀痛，或腰、腹掣痛，舌红，苔黄腻，脉滑数等。

Clinical manifestations: frequent and urgent urination, burning pain in the urethra, short yellow color, or gravel in the urine, or blood in the urine, lower abdominal distension and pain, or waist and abdominal dragging pain, red tongue, yellow and greasy coating, slippery pulse, etc.

六、脏腑兼病辨证

6 Syndrome differentiation of concurrent Zang-Fu disease

凡同时见到两个或两个以上脏腑的病证，即为脏腑兼病。

Where two or more viscera are seen at the same time, it is concurrent Zang–Fu disease.

（一）心肾不交证

6.1 Syndrome of disharmony between heart and kidney

心肾不交证是指心肾阴虚火旺，水火既济失调所致的证候。

Syndrome of disharmony between heart and kidney refers to the syndrome caused by deficiency of heart–kidney yin and excessive fire, and ataxia of water and fire.

临床表现：心烦不寐，多梦，心悸健忘，头晕耳鸣，腰膝酸软，时有梦遗，潮热盗汗，五心烦热，咽干口燥，舌红苔少，脉细数等。

Clinical manifestations: upset sleeplessness, dreaminess, palpitations and forgetfulness, dizziness and tinnitus, soreness and weakness of waist and knees, sometimes wet dreams, tidal fever and night sweating, dysphoria with feverish sensation in chest, palms and soles, dry throat and dry mouth, red tongue with little coating, thin pulse, etc.

（二）心脾两虚证

6.2 Syndrome of deficiency of both heart and spleen

心脾两虚证是指脾气虚弱与心血不足所致的证候。

Syndrome of deficiency of both heart and spleen refers to the syndrome caused by weakness of spleen and insufficiency of heart and blood.

临床表现：心悸怔忡，失眠多梦，眩晕健忘，食欲不振，腹胀便溏，面色苍白或萎黄，神疲乏力，或见皮下紫斑，或妇人月经量少、色淡、淋漓不尽，舌质淡嫩，脉细弱等。

Clinical manifestations: severe palpitation, insomnia and dreaminess, dizziness and forgetfulness, loss of appetite, abdominal distension and loose stools, pale or sallow complexion, fatigue, or subcutaneous purple spots, or the woman's menstrual flow is low, pale color, inexhaustive drenching, and the tongue is light and tender, and the pulse is thin and weak, etc.

（三）脾肾阳虚证

6.3 Syndrome of yang deficiency of spleen and kidney

脾肾阳虚证是指脾肾两脏阳气虚弱，虚寒内生所致的证候。

Syndrome of yang deficiency of spleen and kidney refers to the syndrome caused by weakness of yang qi in the spleen and kidney and endogenous deficiency and cold.

临床表现：形寒肢冷，面色㿠白，腰膝脘腹冷痛，久泻久痢，或完谷不化，五更泄泻，便质清稀，或面浮肢肿，小便不利，或见腹胀满，舌质淡胖、边有齿痕，苔白滑，脉弱或沉迟无力等。

Clinical manifestations: cold shape and cold limbs, pale complexion, cold pain in the waist, knees, epigastric abdomen, chronic diarrhea and chronic dysentery, or diarrhea with undigested food, morning rush syndrome, clear and thin stool, or swollen limbs on the face, difficult urination, or abdominal distension, pale and fat tongue, tooth marks on the edges, white and slippery coating, weak or deep and weak pulse, etc.

（四）肝肾阴虚证

6.4 Syndrome of yin deficiency of liver and kidney

肝肾阴虚证是指肝肾两脏阴虚，虚火内扰所致的证候。

Syndrome of yin deficiency of liver and kidney refers to the syndrome caused by yin deficiency of both organs of the liver and kidney and internal disturbance of deficiency fire.

临床表现：头晕目眩，耳鸣，健忘，失眠多梦，腰膝酸软，胁肋灼痛，咽干口燥，五心烦热，颧红盗汗，男子遗精，女子经少，舌红少苔，脉细数等。

Clinical manifestations: dizziness, tinnitus, forgetfulness, insomnia and dreaminess, soreness and weakness of waist and knees, burning pain in hypochondrium, dry throat and dry mouth, dysphoria with feverish sensation in chest, palms and soles, hectic cheek and night sweats, nocturnal emission, oligomenorrhea in women, red tongue with little coating, and thin pulse.

（五）肝脾不调证

6.5 Syndrome of disharmony between liver and spleen

肝脾不调证是指肝失疏泄，脾失健运所致的证候，又称肝郁脾虚证。

Syndrome of disharmony between liver and spleen refers to the syndrome caused by liver loss of drainage and dysfunction of spleen in transportation, also known as liver stagnation and spleen deficiency syndrome.

临床表现：胸胁胀满窜痛，喜太息，情志抑郁或急躁易怒，腹痛欲泻，泻后痛减，纳呆腹胀，大便溏而不爽，肠鸣矢气，舌苔白或腻，脉弦等。

Clinical manifestations: fullness and pain in the chest and hypochondrium, excessive joy and breath, emotional depression or irritability, abdominal pain and diarrhea, reduced pain after diarrhea, anorexia and abdominal distension, loose and unpleasant stools, borborygmus and flatus, white or greasy tongue coating, stringy pulse, etc.

（六）肝胃不和证

6.6 Liver and stomach disharmony syndrome

肝胃不和证是指肝失疏泄，横逆犯胃，胃失和降所致的证候。

Liver–stomach disharmony syndrome refers to the syndrome caused by liver loss of drainage, transverse invasion of the stomach, and stomach loss of harmony.

临床表现：胁肋、胃脘胀满窜痛，呃逆嗳气，恶心呕吐，嘈杂吞酸，饮食减少，烦躁易怒，或喜太息，纳呆食少，舌淡红，苔薄黄，脉弦等。

Clinical manifestations: fullness and pain in hypochondrium and epigastric area, hiccups and belching, nausea and vomiting, sour regurgitation, reduced diet, irritability, or excessive breath, poor appetite and indigestion, pale red tongue, thin yellow coating, stringy pulse, etc.

（七）肝火犯肺证

6.7 Syndrome of liver fire invading lung

肝火犯肺证是指肝郁化火，上逆灼肺，肺失肃降所致的证候。

Syndrome of liver fire invading lung refers to the syndrome caused by liver stagnation and turning into fire, upward reverse burning of the lungs, and lung loss and descent.

临床表现：面红目赤，头胀头晕，急躁易怒，胸胁灼痛，口苦而干，咳嗽阵作，痰黄而黏，甚则咯血，舌红苔黄，脉弦数等。

Clinical manifestations: red face and red eyes, distention in the head and dizziness, irritability, burning pain in the chest and hypochondrium, bitter and dry mouth, cough, yellow and sticky phlegm, even hemoptysis, red tongue with yellow coating, stringy pulse, etc.

（八）肝胆湿热证

6.8 Syndrome of dampness-heat of liver and gallbladder

肝胆湿热证是指湿热之邪蕴结肝胆，疏泄失职所致的证候。

Syndrome of dampness–heat of liver and gallbladder refers to the syndrome caused by the accumulation of damp–heat evil in the liver and gallbladder and dereliction of duty.

临床表现：胁肋胀痛，腹胀口苦，厌食油腻，大便不调，小便短赤，或寒热往来，或胁下有痞块，或身目发黄，或阴囊湿疹，或外阴瘙痒难忍，或睾丸灼痛肿胀，或妇人带下黄臭，舌红，苔黄腻，脉弦数等。

Clinical manifestations: hypochondrium distension and pain, abdominal distension and bitter mouth, anorexia and greasy, irregular stool, short and red urine, or cold and heat flow, or ruffians under the hypochondrium, or yellowing eyes, or scrotal eczema, or unbearable vulva itching, or burning pain and swelling of testicles, or the woman's yellow odor, red tongue, yellow greasy coating, stringy pulse, etc.

第四节 外感病辨证
Section 4 Exogenous Diseases Syndrome Differentiation

中医学辨证方法有很多种，除前几节讲述的辨证方法之外，还包括六经辨证、卫气营血辨证、三焦辨证等。

There are many kinds of syndrome differentiation methods in traditional Chinese medicine. In addition to the syndrome differentiation methods described in the previous sections, they also include syndrome differentiation of six meridians, syndrome differentiation of wei qi and blood, syndrome differentiation of sanjiao, etc.

一、六经辨证
1 Six meridians syndrome differentiation

六经辨证是张仲景在《素问·热论》六经分证的基础上，根据外感病的证候特点及传变规律而总结出来的一种外感病的辨证方法。

The syndrome differentiation of the six meridians is a syndrome differentiation method of exogenous diseases summarized by Zhang Zhongjing on the basis of the syndrome differentiation of the six meridians in Su Wen Re Lun, according to the syndrome characteristics and transmission rules of exogenous diseases.

六经即太阳、阳明、少阳、太阴、厥阴、少阴，代表外感病六类证候的名称，故常称“六经病证”。凡病位偏表在腑、正气旺盛、病势亢奋者，为三阳病证；病位偏里在脏、正气不足、病势减退者，为三阴病证。

The six meridians, namely Taiyang, Yangming, Shaoyang, Taiyin, Jueyin and Shaoyin, represent the names of six types of syndromes of exogenous diseases, so they are often called “six meridians syndromes”. If the disease position is partial to the internal organs, the righteousness is vigorous, and the disease is excited, it is the syndrome of three yang diseases; If the disease location is partial to the internal organs, the righteousness is insufficient, and the disease condition is decreased, it is the syndrome of three yin diseases.

六经辨证将外感病的各种证候以阴阳为纲加以概括，作为论治的依据。其三阳病证以六腑及阳经病变为主，三阴病证以五脏阴经病变为主。可见，六经病证实质上是对十二经脉、五脏六腑病理变化的归纳，且贯穿了八纲辨证的内容。因此，六经辨证不仅可作为外感病的辨证纲领，而且可指导内伤杂病的辨证。

The syndrome differentiation of the six meridians summarizes the various syndromes of exogenous diseases with yin and yang as the key link, which is the basis for treatment. The three–yang disease syndrome is mainly characterized by the lesions of the six internal organs and the yang meridian, and the three–yin disease syndrome is mainly characterized by the lesions of the five internal organs and the yin meridian. It can be seen that the confirmation of the six meridians disease is a qualitative summary of the pathological changes of the twelve meridians and internal organs, and runs through the content of syndrome differentiation of the eight principles. Therefore, the syndrome differentiation of the six meridians can not only be used as the syndrome differentiation program of exogenous diseases, but also guide the syndrome differentiation of internal injuries and miscellaneous diseases.

二、卫气营血辨证

2 Wei Qi Ying Blood Syndrome Differentiation

卫气营血辨证是清代叶天士在《温热论》中阐述的一种诊治外感温热病的辨证方法，是将外感温热病发展过程中不同病理阶段所反映的证候分为卫分证、气分证、营分证、血分证四类，用以说明病位的深浅、病情的轻重和传变规律，并指导临床治疗。具体而言，卫分主表，病位在肺及体表，病情轻浅；气分主里，病位在肺、胸膈、胆、三焦、胃、肠，病情较重；营分为热邪进入心营，病位在心与心包络，病情深重；血分为热邪深入心、肝、肾，已经动血耗血，病情危极。

The syndrome differentiation of Wei Qi and Ying Xue is a syndrome differentiation method for the diagnosis and treatment of exogenous warm–heat diseases described by Ye Tianshi in “On Warm–heat” in Qing Dynasty. It divides the syndromes reflected in different pathological stages in the development of exogenous warm–heat diseases into four categories: Wei Fen Syndrome, Qi Fen Syndrome, Ying Fen Syndrome and Blood Fen Syndrome, which is used to explain the depth of the disease location, the severity of the disease and the transmission law, and to guide clinical treatment. Specifically, Wei is divided into the main surface, the disease is located in the lungs and body surface, and the disease is mild and shallow; Qi is divided into the main body, and the disease is located in the lungs, chest and diaphragm, gallbladder, triple burner, stomach and intestines, and the disease is serious; The camp is divided into heat pathogen entering the heart camp, and the disease is located in the heart and pericardium, and the condition is deep; Blood is divided into heat pathogens that penetrate deeply into the heart, liver and kidney. Blood has been moved and consumed, and the condition is extremely critical.

三、三焦辨证

3 Sanjiao syndrome differentiation

三焦辨证是将外感温热病的证候归纳为上焦病证、中焦病证、下焦病证，用以阐明三焦所属脏腑在外感温热病中各个不同阶段的病理变化、临床表现及其传变规律。上焦病证包括手太阴肺经和手厥阴心包经的病变，中焦病证包括手阳明大肠经、足阳明胃经和足太阴脾经的病变，下焦病证包括足少阴肾经和足厥阴肝经的病变。

Sanjiao syndrome differentiation is to summarize the syndromes of exogenous warmth and heat into upper jiao syndrome, middle jiao syndrome and lower jiao syndrome, so as to clarify the pathological changes, clinical manifestations and transmission rules of the viscera belonging to the sanjiao in different stages of exogenous warmth and heat. The upper Jiao disease syndrome includes the lesions of the lung meridian of the hand Taiyin and the pericardial meridian of the hand Jueyin, the middle Jiao disease syndrome includes the lesions of the large intestine meridian of the hand Yangming, the stomach meridian of the foot Yangming and the spleen meridian of the foot Taiyin, and the lower Jiao disease syndrome includes the lesions of the kidney meridian of the foot Shaoyin and the liver meridian of the foot Jueyin.

第十章　中药基本知识
Chapter 10　Basic Knowledge of Chinese Medicine

中药是指在中医中药理论指导下，用以防病、治病的一部分天然药（植物药、矿物药、动物药）及其加工品，以及部分化学、生物制品类药物。中药学是专门研究中药基本理论和中药来源、产地、采集、炮制、性能、功效及临床应用规律等知识的一门学科。

Traditional Chinese medicine refers to some natural medicines (botanical medicines, mineral medicines, animal medicines) and their processed products, as well as some chemical and biological products, which are used to prevent and treat diseases under the guidance of traditional Chinese medicine theory. Chinese material medica refers to a discipline that specializes in the basic theory of traditional Chinese medicine and the knowledge of the source, origin, collection, processing, performance, efficacy and clinical application rules of traditional Chinese medicine.

所谓道地药材，又称地道药材，是指历史悠久、产地适宜、品种优良、产量宏丰、炮制考究、疗效突出、带有地域特点的药材。

The so-called genuine medicinal materials, also known as authentic medicinal herbs, refer to medicinal materials with a long history, suitable origin, excellent varieties, great yield, exquisite processing, outstanding curative effect and regional characteristics.

炮制，古时又称“炮炙”“修事”“修治”，指药物在应用或制各种剂型前，根据医疗、调制、制剂的需要而进行必要的加工处理的过程。炮制方法是历代逐步发展和充实起来的，一般来讲，可以分为以下 5 类。①修治：包括纯净、粉碎、切制药材三道工序，为进一步的加工贮存、调剂、制剂和临床用药做好准备。②水制：用水或其他辅料处理药材的方法称为水制法。其目的主要是清洁药物、除去杂质、软化药物、便于切制、降低毒性及调整药性等。常见的方法有漂洗、焖、润、浸泡、喷洒、水飞等。③火制：将药物经火加热处理的方法称为火制法。根据加热的温度、时间和方法的不同，分为炒、炙、烫、煅、煨、炮、燎、烘等。④水火共制：既要用水又要用火，有些药物还必须加入其他辅料进行炮制，包括蒸、煮、炖、潬、淬等方法。⑤其他制法：不包括在以上 4 种之内的炮制法，常见的有制霜、发芽、发酵、精制、药拌等方法。

Processing, also known as "cannon–roasting", "processing" and "repairing" in ancient times, refers to the process of necessary processing according to the needs of medical treatment, preparation and preparation before medicine is applied or prepared in various dosage forms. Processing methods have been gradually developed and enriched in the past dynasties. Generally speaking, they can be divided into the following five categories. ① Treatment: including three processes of purification, crushing, and cutting pharmaceutical materials, so as to prepare for further processing, storage, dispensing, preparation and clinical medication. ② Water preparation: The method of treating medicinal materials with water or other auxiliary materials is called water preparation method. Its main purpose is to clean drugs, remove impurities, soften drugs, facilitate cutting, reduce toxicity and adjust medicinal properties. Common methods include rinsing, simmering, moistening, soaking, spraying, water flying, etc. ③ Fire preparation: The method of heating drugs by fire is called fire preparation method. According to the different heating temperature, time and method, it is divided into stir–frying, roasting, scalding, calcining, simmering, cannon, burning, baking, etc. ④ Co–production of water and fire: both water and fire are required, and some drugs must be processed by adding other auxiliary materials, including steaming, boiling, stewing, quenching and other methods. ⑤ Other preparation methods: the processing methods not included in the above four methods, the common ones include frosting, germination, fermentation, refining, medicine mixing and other methods.

第一节 中药的性能、配伍及用量用法

Section 1 Performance, Compatibility, Dosage and Usage of Traditional Chinese Medicine

一、中药的性能

1 Performance of traditional Chinese medicine

（一）四气

1.1 Four nature of drugs

四气是指寒、热、温、凉四种不同的药性，又称四性。它反映了药物对人体阴阳盛衰、寒热变化的作用倾向。

Four nature of drugs refers to the four different medicinal properties of cold, heat, warm and cool, also known as the four properties. It reflects the effect tendency of drugs on the ups and downs of yin and yang and the changes of cold and heat in human body.

药性的寒、热、温、凉是由药物作用于人体所产生的不同反应和所获得的不同疗效而总结出来的，它与所治疗疾病的性质是相对而言的。

The medicinal properties of cold, heat, warm and cold are summarized by the different reactions and different curative effects of drugs acting on the human body, and they are relative to the nature of the diseases being treated.

一般而言，寒凉药分别具有清热泻火、凉血解毒、滋阴除蒸、泄热通便、清热利尿、清化热痰、清心开窍、凉肝息风等作用，而温热药则分别具有温里散寒、暖肝散结、补火助阳、温阳利水、温经通络、引火归原、回阳救逆等作用。

Generally speaking, cold and cooling medicines have the functions of clearing away heat and purging fire, cooling blood and detoxifying, nourishing yin and removing steam, releasing heat and laxative, clearing away heat and diuresis, clearing away heat and phlegm, clearing the heart and opening orifices, cooling the liver and restlessing wind, while warming medicines have the functions of warming the inside and dispelling cold, warming the liver and dispelling stagnation, tonifying fire and helping yang, warming meridians and dredging collaterals, returning fire to the original, returning yang and rescuing adverse effects.

（二）五味

1.2 Five flavors

五味是指药物有辛、甘、酸、苦、咸五种不同的味道，因而具有不同的治疗作用。有些药物还具有淡味或涩味，因而实际上不止五种。但五味是最基本的五种滋味，所以仍称为五味。五味所代表药物的作用及主治病证分述如下。

The five flavors mean that the medicine has five different tastes: pungent, sweet, sour, bitter and salty, so it has different therapeutic effects. Some medicines also have a light or astringent taste, so there are actually more than five kinds. But the five flavors are the most basic five flavors, so they are still called the five flavors. The effects of the medicines represented by the five flavors and the main diseases and syndromes are described as follows.

1. 辛 辛味药有发散、行气、行血等作用。多用于表证及气血阻滞之证。

Pungent Pungent medicines has the functions of diverging, promoting qi, and promoting blood. It is mostly used for exterior syndrome and syndrome of qi and blood blockade.

2. 甘 甘味药有补益、和中、调和药性和缓急止痛的作用。多用于正气虚弱、身体诸痛及调和药性、中毒解救等方面。

Sweet Sweet medicines have the effects of tonifying, harmonizing, harmonizing medicinal properties and relieving pain. It is mostly used for weakness of righteousness, physical pains, reconciliation of medicinal properties, poisoning rescue, etc.

3. 酸 酸味药有收敛、固涩的作用。多用于体虚多汗、肺虚久咳、久泻肠滑、遗精滑精、遗尿尿频、崩漏不止等。

Sour Sour medicines have astringent and astringent effects. It is mostly used for physical weakness and hyperhidrosis, chronic cough due to lung deficiency, chronic diarrhea and slippery intestine, nocturnal emission and slippery spermatorrhea, frequent enuresis, metrorrhagia, etc.

4. 苦 苦味药有清泄、通泄、降泄、燥湿、坚阴、坚厚肠胃的作用。多用于热证、火证、喘证、呕恶、便秘、湿证、阴虚火旺等。

Bitter Bitter medicines has the functions of clearing discharge, dredging discharge, lowering discharge, drying dampness, strengthening yin, and thickening the intestines and stomach. It is mostly used for heat syndrome, fire syndrome, asthma syndrome, vomiting, constipation, dampness syndrome, yin deficiency and excessive fire, etc.

5. 咸 咸味药有软坚散结、泻下通便的作用。多用于大便燥结、痰核、瘰疬、瘿瘤、癥瘕痞块等。

Salty Salty medicines has the effects of softening hard and dispersing stagnation, purging and laxative. It is mostly used for dry stool, sputum nucleus, scrofula, gall tumor, symptomatic mass, etc.

6. 淡 淡味药有渗湿、利小便的作用。多用于水肿、脚气、小便不利之证。

Tasteless Tasteless medicines has the effects of soaking dampness and promoting urination. It is mostly used for edema, athlete's foot, and unfavorable urination.

7. 涩 涩味药与酸味药的作用相似，有收敛固涩的作用。多用于虚汗、泄泻、尿频、遗精、滑精、出血等。

Astringent Astringent and astringent medicines have similar effects to sour drugs, and have astringent and astringent effects. It is mostly used for deficiency sweating, diarrhea, frequent urination, nocturnal emission, spermatorrhea, bleeding, etc.

（三）归经

1.3 Channel tropism

归经，是指药物对于机体某部分的选择性作用，即某药对某些脏腑经络有特殊的亲和作用，因而对这些部位的病变起着主要或特殊的治疗作用。

Channel tropism refers to the selective effect of drugs on certain parts of the body, that is, a certain drug has a special affinity for certain viscera and meridians, so it plays a main or special therapeutic effect on the lesions of these parts.

中药归经理论的形成是在中医基本理论指导下，以脏腑经络学说为基础，以药物所治疗的具体病证为依据，经过长期临床实践总结出来的用药理论。

The formation of the theory of channel tropism of traditional Chinese medicine is a medication theory summarized through long-term clinical practice under the guidance of the basic theory of traditional Chinese medicine, based on the theory of zang-fu organs and meridians, and based on the specific diseases and syndromes treated by drugs.

运用归经理论指导临床用药，还要依据脏腑经络相关学说，注意脏腑病变的相互影响，恰当选择用药。

To use the theory of channel tropism to guide clinical medication, we should also pay attention to the mutual influence of viscera lesions and choose medication appropriately according to the relevant theories of viscera and meridians.

（四）毒性

1.4 Toxicity

1. 广义毒性的概念 古代常把毒药看作一切药物的总称，毒性就是药物的偏性；古代还把毒性看作药物毒副作用大小的标志。因此，古代药物毒性的含义较广。

The concept of toxicity in a broad sense In ancient times, poison was often regarded as the general term for all drugs, and toxicity was the bias of drugs; In ancient times, toxicity was also regarded as a sign of the toxic side effects of drugs. Therefore, the toxicity of ancient drugs has a broad meaning.

2. 狭义毒性的概念 指药物对机体所产生的不良影响及损害性。“物之害人即为毒。”毒性反应与副作用不同，它对人体的危害性较大，甚至可危及生命。

The concept of toxicity in a narrow sense It refers to the adverse effects and damage caused by drugs on the body. Toxic reaction is different from side effects, it is more harmful to human body, even life-threatening. “Things that harm others are poisonous.” Toxic reaction is different from side effects. It is more harmful to human body and even life-threatening.

二、中药的配伍

2 Compatibility of traditional Chinese medicine

药物单独或配合应用主要有单行、相须、相使、相畏、相杀、相恶、相反七种情况，称为中药的“七情”配伍。

The application of drugs alone or in combination mainly includes seven situations: single line, mutual whisker, mutual envoy, mutual fear, mutual killing, mutual evil, and opposite, which is called the “seven emotions” compatibility of traditional Chinese medicine.

1. 单行 指单用一味药物治疗某种病情单一的疾病。对病情比较单纯的病证，往往选择一种针对性强的药物即可达到治疗目的，如独参汤。

Drug used singly It refers to the treatment of a single disease with a single drug alone. For relatively simple disease syndromes, a highly targeted drug can often be selected to achieve the purpose of treatment, such as Dushen Decoction.

2. 相须 指两种功效相似的药物配合应用，可以增强原有药物的疗效。

Mutual promotion It refers to the combined application of two drugs with similar efficacy, which can enhance the efficacy of the original drug.

3. 相使 指以一种药物为主，另一种药物为辅，两种药物合用，辅药可以提高主药的功效。

Mutual enhancement It refers to one drug as the main drug and the other as the supplement. The two drugs are used together, and the auxiliary drugs can improve the efficacy of the main drug.

4. 相畏　指一种药物的毒副作用能被另一种药物所抑制。

Incompatibility It means that the toxic and side effects of one drug can be inhibited by another drug.

5. 相杀　指一种药物能够减轻或消除另一种药物的毒副作用。

Counteract toxicity of another drug It means that one drug can reduce or eliminate the toxic and side effects of another drug.

6. 相恶　指两药合用，一种药物能破坏另一种药物的功效。

Mutual inhibition It refers to the combination of two drugs, one drug can destroy the efficacy of the other drug.

7. 相反　指两种药物同用能产生或增强毒性或副作用。如甘草反甘遂、贝母反乌头等，详见用药禁忌“十八反”“十九畏”。“十八反”的内容：甘草反甘遂、大戟、海藻、芫花；乌头反贝母、瓜蒌、半夏、白蔹、白及；藜芦反人参、沙参、丹参、玄参、细辛、芍药。“十九畏”的内容：硫黄畏朴硝，水银畏砒霜，狼毒畏密陀僧，巴豆畏牵牛，丁香畏郁金，川乌、草乌畏犀角，牙硝畏三棱，官桂畏赤石脂，人参畏五灵脂。

Clashing It means that means that the combined use of two drugs can produce or enhance toxicity or side effects. For example, licorice is anti-kansui, Fritillaria is anti-aconitum, etc. For details, please refer to the medication contraindications “Eighteen anti-fears” and “Nineteen fears”. Contents of “Eighteen Anti-Glycyrrhiza uralensis”: Glycyrrhiza uralensis, Euphorbia euphorbia, seaweed and coriander flower; Fritillaria aconitum, Trichosanthes kirilowii, Pinellia ternata, Ampelopsis ampelopsis, Baiji; Veratrum antiginseng, adenophora, salvia miltiorrhiza, scrophulariaceae, asarum and peony lactiflora. The contents of “Nineteen Fears”: sulfur is afraid of plain nitrate, mercury is afraid of arsenic, wolfsbane is afraid of lithargite, croton is afraid of morning glory, clove is afraid of turmeric, Chuan Wutou (Aconite) is afraid of Rhinoceros Horn. Cao Wutou (Aconite) is afraid of Rhinoceros Horn. Tooth Nitre (Nitrate) is afraid of Sanling (Curcuma zedoaria). Cassia Bark (Cinnamomum) is afraid of Red Stone Grease (Haematite). Ginseng is afraid of Wulingzhi (Salvia miltiorrhiza).

三、中药的用量及用法

3 Dosage and usage of traditional Chinese medicine

（一）中药剂量

3.1 Dosage of traditional Chinese medicine

中药剂量是指中药临床应用时的分量。它主要指明了每味药的成人一日量（按：本书每味药物标明的用量，除特别注明以外，都是指干燥后的生药在汤剂中成人一日内用量），其次指方剂中每味药之间的比较分量，即相对剂量。

The dosage of traditional Chinese medicine refers to the weight of traditional Chinese medicine in clinical application. It mainly indicates the daily dosage of each medicine for adults (note: the dosage indicated for each medicine in this book, unless otherwise specified, refers to the daily dosage of the dried crude medicine in the decoction for adults), and secondly refers to the comparative weight between each medicine in the prescription, that is, the relative dose.

（二）中药的用法

3.2 Usage of traditional Chinese medicine

1. 煎煮方法 先将药材浸泡 30 ～ 60 分钟，用水量以高出药面为度。一般中药煎煮两次，第二煎加水量为第一煎的 1/3 ～ 1/2。两次煎液去渣滤净，混合后分 2 次服用。煎煮的火候和时间要根据药物性能而定。一般来讲，解表药、清热药宜武火煎煮，时间宜短，煮沸后煎 3 ～ 5 分钟即可；补养药需用文火慢煎，时间宜长，煮沸后再续煎 30 ～ 60 分钟。某些药物因其质地不同，煎法比较特殊，处方上需加以注明，归纳起来包括先煎、后下、包煎、另煎、溶化、泡服、冲服、煎汤代水等不同煎煮法。

Decoction method First soak the medicinal materials for 30 to 60 minutes, and the water consumption should be higher than the medicinal surface. Generally, traditional Chinese medicine is decocted twice, and the amount of water added to the second decoction is 1/3–1/2 of the first decoction. Remove the residue and filter the decoction twice, mix and take it twice. The temperature and time of decoction depend on the performance of the drug. Generally speaking, exterior–relieving drugs and heat–clearing drugs should be decocted with strong fire, and the time should be short. After boiling, they can be decocted for 3–5 minutes; The tonic medicine should be decocted slowly with slow fire, and the time should be long. After boiling, it should be decocted for 30–60 minutes. Because of their different textures, some drugs have special decoction methods, which need to be indicated on the prescription. To sum up, they include different decoction methods such as first decoction, then decoction, wrapping decoction, separate decoction, melting, soaking, washing, decoction instead of water, etc.

2. 服药时间 汤剂一般每日 1 剂，煎 2 次分服，两次间隔时间为 4 ～ 6 小时。临床用药时可根据病情增减，如急性病、热性病可 1 日 2 剂。至于饭前还是饭后服，则主要取决于病变部位和性质。一般来讲，病在胸膈以上者，如眩晕、头痛、目疾、咽痛等宜饭后服；如病在胸膈以下，如胃、肝、肾等疾患，则宜饭前服。某些对胃肠有刺激性的药物宜饭后服；补益药多滋腻碍胃，宜空腹服；驱虫药、泻下药也宜空腹服；治疟药宜在疟疾发作前的两小时服用；安神药宜睡前服；慢性病要定时服；急性病、呕吐、惊厥及石淋、咽喉病须煎汤代茶饮者，均可不定时服。

Taking time The decoction is generally taken once a day, decocted twice and taken separately, with an interval of 4 to 6 hours. Clinical medication can be increased or decreased according to the condition, such as acute disease and febrile disease can be used 2 doses a day. As for whether to take it before or after meals, it mainly depends on the location and nature of the lesion. Generally speaking, those with diseases above the chest and diaphragm, such as dizziness, headache, eye disease, sore throat, etc., should be taken after meals; If the disease is below the chest and diaphragm, such as stomach, liver, kidney and other diseases, it should be taken before meals. Some drugs that are irritating to the gastrointestinal tract should be taken after meals; Tonic drugs are too nourishing and greasy to hinder the stomach, so they should be taken on an empty stomach; Anthelmintics and laxative drugs should also be taken on an empty stomach; Malaria drugs should be taken two hours before the onset of malaria; Tranquilizing medicine should be taken before going to bed; Chronic diseases should be taken regularly; Those with acute illness, vomiting, convulsions, stone stranguria, and throat disease who need to decoct instead of tea can take it from time to time.

第二节　常用中药
Section 2　Commonly used Chinese medicines

一、解表药
1 Superficies relieving drugs

凡以发散表邪，解除表证为主要功效，主要用于外感表证的药物，称为解表药。

Drugs that are mainly used for exogenous exterior syndromes with the main effect of diverging exterior pathogens and relieving exterior syndromes are called exterior-relieving drugs.

解表药多味辛质轻，性分温、凉，大多归肺、膀胱经。功能发散解表。主要用于外感表证，症见恶寒、发热、头痛、身痛、无汗或有汗。

Exterior-relieving drugs are multi-taste, pungent and light, warm and cool in nature, and most of them belong to the lung and bladder meridians. It can diverge and relieve the surface. It is mainly used for exogenous symptoms, such as aversion to cold, fever, headache, body pain, anhidrosis or sweating.

发汗力较强的药物，使用时用量不宜过大，以免发汗太过，耗伤阳气，损及津液。表虚自汗、阴虚盗汗，以及疮疡日久、淋证、失血患者，虽有表证，也应慎用。解表药多属辛散轻扬之品，入汤剂不宜久煎。

Drugs with strong sweating power should not be used in too large dosage, so as to avoid excessive sweating, consuming yang qi and damaging body fluids. Patients with spontaneous sweating due to superficial deficiency, night sweats due to yin deficiency, and chronic sores, stranguria, and blood loss should be used with caution although they have superficial syndromes. Exterior-relieving drugs are mostly pungent and light medicinals, and they should not be decocted for a long time in decoction.

（一）发散风寒药

1.1 Dispersing wind-cold medicine

本类药物味多辛，性多温燥，主归肺、膀胱经，具有发散风寒邪气之功。主治风寒表证，症见恶寒发热、鼻塞流涕、舌苔薄白、脉浮紧。常见药物包括麻黄、桂枝、荆芥、防风、白芷等（表 10–1）。

This kind of medicine is pungent in taste, warm and dry in nature, mainly belongs to the lung and bladder meridians, and has the function of dispersing wind–cold evil qi. Indications of wind–cold symptoms, including aversion to cold and fever, nasal congestion and runny nose, thin and white tongue coating, and tight pulse. Common drugs include ephedra, cinnamon twig, schizonepeta, parsnip, angelica dahurica, etc. (Table 10–1).

表 10–1　常见发散风寒药

Table 10–1　Common divergent wind–cold drugs

药名 Drug name	药性 Medicinal properties	功效 Efficacy	主治 Indications	用法用量 Usage and Dosage
麻黄 ephedra	辛、微苦，温。归肺、膀胱经 Pungent, slightly bitter, warm. Return to lung and bladder meridian	发汗散寒，宣肺平喘，利水消肿 Sweating and dispelling cold, ventilating lung qi and relieving asthma, diuresis and reducing swelling	风寒感冒；胸闷喘咳；风水浮肿；风寒痹证，阴疽，痰核 Wind-cold cold; Chest tightness, wheezing and cough; Feng Shui Puffy; Wind-cold arthralgia syndrome, yin gangrene, phlegm nucleus	煎服，2～10g Decoction, 2-10g
桂枝 cinnamon twig	辛、甘，温。归心、肺、膀胱经 Pungent, sweet, warm. Return to the heart, lung and bladder meridian	发汗解肌，温通经脉，助阳化气，平冲降气 Sweating and relieving muscles, warming and dredging meridians, helping yang to transform qi, leveling and lowering qi	风寒表证；脘腹冷痛、血寒经闭，关节痹痛；痰饮、水肿；心悸、奔豚 Wind-cold exterior syndrome; Cold abdominal pain, blood cold amenorrhea, joint arthralgia; Phlegm drinking, edema; Heart palpitations, renal mass disease	煎服，3～10g Decoction, 3-10g
荆芥 Schizonepeta	辛，微温。归肺、肝经 Pungent, lukewarm. Return to lung and liver meridians	解表散风，透疹消疮，止血 Relieve exterior and disperse wind, penetrate rash and eliminate sores, and stop bleeding	外感表证；风疹瘙痒，麻疹不透；疮疡初起兼有表证；吐衄下血，炒炭止血 Exogenous exterior syndrome; Rubella itchy, measles impenetrable; The initial onset of sores and ulcers has both superficial syndromes; Vomiting epistaxis and bleeding, stir-fry charcoal to stop bleeding	煎服，5～10g，不宜久煎 Decoction, 5-10g, not suitable for long-term decoction

续表

药名 Drug name	药性 Medicinal properties	功效 Efficacy	主治 Indications	用法用量 Usage and Dosage
防风 windproof	辛、甘，微温。归膀胱、肝、脾经 Pungent, sweet, slightly warm. Return to bladder, liver and spleen meridians	祛风解表，胜湿止痛，止痉 Dispelling wind and relieving exterior symptoms, overcoming dampness and relieving pain, relieving spasm	感冒头痛；风湿痹痛；风疹瘙痒；破伤风证 Cold headaches; rheumatic arthralgia; Rubella pruritus; Tetanus syndrome	煎服，5～10g Decoction, 5-10g
白芷 Angelica dahurica	辛，温。归胃、大肠、肺经 Pungent, Wen. Return to stomach, large intestine and lung meridians	解表散寒，祛风止痛，宣通鼻窍，燥湿止带，消肿排脓 Relieve exterior and dispel cold, dispel wind and relieve pain, dispel nasal orifices, dry dampness and stop belt, reduce swelling and discharge pus	感冒头痛，眉棱骨痛；鼻塞流涕，鼻鼽，鼻渊，牙痛；带下；疮痈肿痛 Cold headache, brow bone pain; Nasal congestion and runny nose, allergic nose, nasal abyss, toothache; Tape Under; Sore, carbuncle, swelling and pain	煎服，3～10g Decoction, 3-10g

（二）发散风热药

1.2 Divergent wind-heat medicine

本类药物性味多辛凉，有发散风热之功。主治风热感冒及温病初起邪在卫分，症见发热、微恶风寒、咽干口渴、头痛目赤、舌边尖红、苔薄黄、脉浮数。常见药物包括薄荷、牛蒡子、菊花、柴胡、葛根等（表 10–2）。

This class of drugs is pungent and cool in nature and taste, and has the function of dispersing wind and heat. Indications of wind-heat cold and febrile disease at the beginning of pathogenic disease in Weifen, with symptoms such as fever, slight aversion to wind-cold, dry throat and thirst, headache, red eyes, sharp red tongue, thin yellow coating, and floating pulse. Common drugs include peppermint, burdock seed, chrysanthemum, bupleurum, kudzu root, etc. (Table 10–2).

表 10–2　常见发散风热药

Table 10–2　Common divergent wind–heat drugs

药名 Drug name	药性 Medicinal properties	功效 Efficacy	主治 Indications	用法用量 Usage and Dosage
薄荷 Peppermint	辛，凉。归肺、肝经 Pungent, cool. Return to lung and liver meridians	疏散风热，清利头目，利咽透疹，疏肝行气 Evacuate wind-heat, clear and benefit leaders, relieve throat and rash, soothe liver and promote qi	风热感冒，风温初起；头痛目赤，喉痹口疮；麻疹不透，风疹瘙痒；肝气郁滞，胸胁胀闷 Wind-heat cold, wind-temperature initial onset; Headache, red eyes, throat paralysis and aphtha; Measles is impenetrable, rubella itchy; Stagnation of liver qi, distension and tightness of chest and hypochondrium	煎服，3～6g，宜后下 Decoction, 3-6g, preferably later
牛蒡子 Burdock seed	辛、苦，寒。归肺、胃经 Pungent, bitter, cold. Return to lung and stomach meridians	疏散风热，宣肺透疹，解毒利咽 Evacuate wind-heat, ventilating lung qi, detoxify and soothe throat	风热感冒，温病初起，咳嗽痰多；麻疹不透，风疹瘙痒；咽喉肿痛，痄腮丹毒，痈肿疮毒 Wind-heat cold, febrile disease at the beginning, cough with excessive phlegm; Measles is impenetrable, rubella itchy; Sore throat, mumps and erysipelas, carbuncle and sore	煎服，6～12g Decoction, 6-12g
菊花 Chrysanthemum	甘、苦，微寒。归肺、肝经 Sweet, bitter, slightly cold. Return to lung and liver meridians	散风清热，平肝明目，清热解毒 Dispersing wind and clearing away heat, calming liver and improving eyesight, clearing away heat and detoxifying	风热感冒；肝阳上亢，头痛眩晕；目赤肿痛，眼目昏花；疮痈肿毒 Wind-heat cold; Hyperactivity of liver yang, headache and dizziness; Red, swollen and painful eyes, dizzy eyes; Sore carbuncle swelling poison	煎服，5～10g Decoction, 5-10g
柴胡 Bupleurum	辛、苦，微寒。归肝、胆、肺经 Pungent, bitter, slightly cold. Return to liver, gallbladder and lung meridians	疏散退热，疏肝解郁，升举阳气 Evacuate and reduce fever, soothe liver and relieve depression, and raise yang qi	感冒发热，寒热往来，少阳证；肝郁气滞，胸胁胀痛，月经不调；子宫脱垂，脱肛，疟疾寒热 Cold and fever, cold and heat exchanges, Shaoyang syndrome; Liver stagnation and qi stagnation, chest and hypochondrium distension and pain, irregular menstruation; Uterine prolapse, anal prolapse, malaria cold and heat	煎服，3～10g Decoction, 3-10g

续表

药名 Drug name	药性 Medicinal properties	功效 Efficacy	主治 Indications	用法用量 Usage and Dosage
葛根 Pueraria lobata	甘、辛，凉。归脾、胃、肺经 Sweet, pungent and cool. Return to spleen, stomach and lung meridians	解肌退热，生津止渴，透疹，升阳止泻，通经活络，解酒毒 Relieve muscles and reduce fever, produce body fluid and quench thirst, penetrate rash, ascend yang and stop diarrhea, dredge meridians and activate collaterals, relive alcohol and toxicity	外感发热头痛，项背强痛；口渴，消渴；麻疹不透；热痢，泄泻；眩晕头痛，中风偏瘫，胸痹心痛；酒毒伤中 Exogenous fever, headache, strong pain in the neck and back; Thirst, quenching; Measles is impenetrable; Fever dysentery, diarrhea; Dizziness and headache, stroke and hemiplegia, chest impediment and heartache; Injured by alcohol poisoning	煎服，10～15g Decoction, 10-15g

二、清热药

2 Heat-clearing medicine

凡以清泄里热为主要功效，主要用于里热证的药物，称为清热药。

All drugs that have the main effect of clearing away internal heat and are mainly used for internal heat syndrome are called heat–clearing drugs.

本类药物多属寒凉，功效是清热泻火、解毒、凉血、清虚热等。

Most of these drugs are cold and cool, and the effects are to clear away heat and purge fire, detoxify, cool blood, clear away deficiency and heat, etc.

清热药主要用于里热证，症见热病高热、热痢、痈肿疮毒及阴虚内热等所致各种里热证候。

Heat–clearing medicine is mainly used for internal heat syndrome, and the symptoms include various internal heat syndromes caused by fever, high fever, heat dysentery, carbuncle and sore toxin, and internal heat caused by yin deficiency.

本类药物性多寒凉，易伤脾胃，故脾胃气虚，食少便溏者慎用；苦寒药物易化燥伤阴，热证伤阴或阴虚患者慎用；清热药禁用于阴盛格阳或真寒假热之证。

This kind of drug is often cold and easily damages the spleen and stomach, so it should be used with caution in patients with deficiency of spleen and stomach qi, who eat less and with loose stools; Bitter cold drugs are easy to change dryness and damage yin, and patients with heat syndrome damage yin or yin deficiency should be used with caution; Heat–clearing medicine is forbidden for the syndrome of yin excessive geyang or true winter holiday heat.

（一）清热泻火药

2.1 Heat-clearing and purgative gunpowder

本类药物多属苦寒或甘寒，具有清热泻火之功。主治急性热病，症见高热、汗出、烦渴、谵语、发狂、小便短赤、舌苔黄燥、脉洪实。常见清热泻火药包括石膏、知母、栀子等（表 10–3）。

Most of these drugs belong to bitter cold or sweet cold, and have the function of clearing away heat and purging fire. Indications of acute fever, with symptoms such as high fever, sweating, polydipsia, delirium, madness, short and red urine, yellow and dry tongue coating, and flood and solid pulse. Common heat–clearing and purgative powders include gypsum, anemarrhena, gardenia jasminoides, etc. (Table 10–3).

表 10–3 常见清热泻火药

Table 10–3 Common heat–clearing and purgative gunpowder

药名 Drug name	药性 Medicinal properties	功效 Efficacy	主治 Indications	用法用量 Usage and Dosage
石膏 gypsum	甘、辛，大寒。归肺、胃经 Sweet, pungent, great cold. Return to lung and stomach meridians	清热泻火，除烦止渴 Clear away heat and purge fire, eliminate vexation and quench thirst	外感热病，高热烦渴；肺热喘咳；胃火亢盛，头痛，牙痛 Exogenous fever, high fever and polydipsia; lung heat asthma cough; Hyperactivity of stomach fire, headache, toothache	煎服，15～60g，先煎 Decoction, 15-60g, decoct first
知母 Anemarrhena	苦、甘，寒。归肺、胃、肾经。 Bitter, sweet, cold. Returns to the lung, stomach and kidney meridians.	清热泻火，滋阴润燥 Clearing away heat and purging fire, nourishing yin and moistening dryness	外感热病，高热烦渴；肺热燥咳；骨蒸潮热；内热消渴；肠燥便秘 Exogenous fever, high fever and polydipsia; Dry cough due to lung heat; Bone steaming and tidal fever; Internal heat quenches thirst; Intestinal dryness and constipation	煎服，6～12g Decoction, 6-12g
栀子 Gardenia jasminoides	苦，寒。归心、肺、三焦经 Bitter, cold. Return to heart, lung and sanjiao meridians	泻火除烦，清热利湿，凉血解毒；外用消肿止痛 Purge fire and eliminate annoyance, clear away heat and dampness, cool blood and detoxify; External use to reduce swelling and relieve pain	热病心烦；湿热黄疸；淋证涩痛；血热吐衄；目赤肿痛；扭挫伤痛 Fever upset; damp-heat jaundice; Stranguria syndrome astringent pain; Blood heat vomiting epistaxis; Red, swollen and painful eyes; Pain from sprain and contusion	煎服，6～10g；外用生品适量 Decoction, 6-10g; Appropriate amount of raw products for topical use

（二）清热燥湿药

2.2 Heat-clearing and dampness-drying medicine

本类药物多苦寒，苦能燥湿，寒能清热，具有清热燥湿之功，主治湿热证。常见清热燥湿药包括黄芩、黄连、黄柏等（表 10–4）。

This class of drugs is mostly bitter and cold, bitter can dry dampness, cold can clear away heat, has the function of clearing away heat and drying dampness, and is mainly used to treat damp–heat syndrome. Common heat–clearing and dampness–drying drugs include Scutellaria baicalensis, Coptis chinensis, Phellodendron cork, etc. (Table 10–4).

表 10–4　常见清热燥湿药

Table 10–4　Common heat–clearing and dampness–drying drugs

药名 Drug name	药性 Medicinal properties	功效 Efficacy	主治 Indications	用法用量 Usage and Dosage
黄芩 Scutellaria baicalensis	苦，寒。归肺、胆、脾、大肠、小肠经 Bitter, cold. Returns to lung, gallbladder, spleen, large intestine and small intestine meridians	清热燥湿，泻火解毒，止血安胎 Clearing away heat and drying dampness, purging fire and detoxifying, stopping bleeding and preventing fetus	湿温、暑湿，胸闷呕恶，湿热痞满，泻痢，黄疸；肺热咳嗽，高热烦渴；血热吐衄，痈肿疮毒；胎动不安 Damp-temperature, summer dampness, chest tightness, vomiting, damp-heat fullness, diarrhea, jaundice; Lung heat cough, high fever and polydipsia; Blood heat vomiting epistaxis, carbuncle swelling and sore poison; Fetal restlessness	煎服，3 ～ 10g Decoction, 3-10g
黄连 Coptis chinensis	苦，寒。归心、脾、胃、肝、胆、大肠经 Bitter, cold. Return to the heart, spleen, stomach, liver, gallbladder and large intestine meridians	清热燥湿，泻火解毒 Clear away heat and dry dampness, purge fire and detoxify	湿热痞满，呕吐吞酸，泻痢，黄疸；高热神昏，心火亢盛，心烦不寐，心悸不宁，血热吐衄；痈肿疮毒，湿疹湿疮，耳道流脓；胃火炽盛，烦渴消渴 Damp-heat fullness, vomiting and swallowing acid, diarrhea, jaundice; High fever, unconsciousness, excessive heart fire, upset and insomnia, palpitations and restless heart, blood heat and vomiting; Carbuncle swelling sore poison, eczema wet sore, ear canal pus discharge; Flaming stomach fire, polydipsia and thirst	煎服，2 ～ 5g Decoction, 2-5g

续表

药名 Drug name	药性 Medicinal properties	功效 Efficacy	主治 Indications	用法用量 Usage and Dosage
黄柏 Phellodendron cork	苦，寒。归肾、膀胱经 Bitter, cold. Return to kidney and bladder meridian	清热燥湿，泻火除蒸，解毒疗疮 Clearing away heat and drying dampness, purging fire and removing steam, detoxifying and treating sores	湿热泻痢，黄疸尿赤，带下阴痒，热淋涩痛；疮疡肿毒，湿疹瘙痒，脚气脚痿；阴虚火旺，盗汗骨蒸，遗精滑精 Damp-heat diarrhea, jaundice, red urine, yin itching, heat stranguria astringent pain; Sores, swelling and toxicity, eczema and itching, Beriberi, foot flaccidity; Yin deficiency and excessive fire, night sweats and bone steaming, nocturnal emission and spermatorrhea	煎服，3～12g Decoction, 3-12g

（三）清热解毒药

2.3 Heat-clearing and detoxification drugs

本类药物多属寒凉，清热之中更长于解毒，具有清解火热毒邪功效。主治痈肿疮毒、丹毒、温毒发斑、痄腮、咽喉肿痛、热毒下痢、虫蛇咬伤、癌肿、水火烫伤及其他急性热病。常见清热解毒药包括金银花、连翘、板蓝根、蒲公英、鱼腥草、白头翁等（表 10–5）。

Most of these drugs are cold and cold, and they are longer in clearing away heat than detoxifying, and have the effect of clearing away fire and toxic pathogens. It is mainly used to treat carbuncle and sore poison, erysipelas, warm poison spots, mumps, sore throat, diarrhea due to heat poison, insect and snake bites, cancer, water and fire burns and other acute febrile diseases. Common heat–clearing and detoxifying drugs include honeysuckle, forsythia suspensa, Radix isatidis, dandelion, houttuynia, pulsatilla, etc. (Table 10–5).

表 10–5 常见清热解毒药

Table 10–5 Common heat–clearing and detoxification drugs

药名 Drug name	药性 Medicinal properties	功效 Efficacy	主治 Indications	用法用量 Usage and Dosage
金银花 honeysuckle	甘，寒。归肺、心、胃经 Sweet, cold. Return to lung, heart and stomach meridians	清热解毒，疏散风热 Clear away heat and detoxify, evacuate wind and heat	痈肿疔疮，喉痹，丹毒；风热感冒，温病发热；热毒血痢 Carbuncle and furuncle, throat paralysis, erysipelas; Wind-heat cold, febrile disease and fever; Heat toxic blood dysentery	煎服，6～15g；炒炭宜用于热毒血痢 Decoction, 6-15g; Fried charcoal is suitable for heat-poisoned blood dysentery

续表

药名 Drug name	药性 Medicinal properties	功效 Efficacy	主治 Indications	用法用量 Usage and Dosage
连翘 Forsythia suspensa	苦，微寒。归肺、心、小肠经 Bitter, slightly cold. Return to lung, heart and small intestine meridians	清热解毒，消肿散结，疏散风热 Clear away heat and toxic materials, reduce swelling and dissipate stagnation, and evacuate wind-heat	痈疽，瘰疬，乳痈，丹毒；风热感冒，温病初起，温热入营，高热烦渴，神昏发斑；热淋涩痛 Carbuncle, scrofula, breast carbuncle, erysipelas; Wind-heat cold, febrile disease at the beginning, warm heat entering the camp, high fever and polydipsia, unconsciousness and spots; Heat stranguria astringent pain	煎服，6～15g Decoction, 6-15g
板蓝根 Radix isatidis	苦，寒。归心、胃经 Bitter, cold. Return to heart and stomach meridian	清热解毒，凉血利咽 Clearing away heat and toxic materials, cooling blood and relieving throat	温疫时毒，发热咽痛；温毒发斑，丹毒痄腮，烂喉丹痧，大头瘟疫，痈肿疮毒 Poison during febrile epidemic, fever and sore throat; Warm poison spots, erysipelas mumps, rotten throat Dan sha, big head plague, carbuncle swelling and sore poison	煎服，9～15g Decoction, 9-15g
蒲公英 Dandelion	苦、甘，寒。归肝、胃经 Bitter, sweet, cold. Return to liver and stomach meridians	清热解毒，消肿散结，利湿通淋 Clear away heat and toxic materials, reduce swelling and dissipate stagnation, relieve dampness and dredge stranguria	疔疮肿毒，乳痈瘰疬，目赤咽痛，肺痈肠痈；湿热黄疸，热淋涩痛 Furuncle swelling and poison, breast carbuncle scrofula, red eyes and sore throat, lung carbuncle and intestinal carbuncle; Damp-heat jaundice, heat stranguria astringent pain	煎服，10～15g Decoction, 10-15g
鱼腥草 Houttuynia cordata	辛，微寒。归肺经 Pungent, slightly cold. Return to lung meridian	清热解毒，消痈排脓，利尿通淋 Clearing heat and detoxification, eliminating carbuncle and discharging pus, diuretic and Tonglin	肺痈吐脓，痰热喘咳；痈肿疮毒；热淋，热痢 Pulmonary carbuncle vomiting pus, phlegm-heat asthma and cough; Carbuncle swelling sore poison; Hot stranguria, heat dysentery	煎服，15～25g Decoction, 15-25g
白头翁 Pulsatilla	苦，寒。归胃、大肠经 Bitter, cold. Return to stomach and large intestine meridian	清热解毒，凉血止痢 Clearing away heat and toxic materials, cooling blood and stopping dysentery	热毒血痢；痈肿疮毒，阴痒带下 Heat toxic blood dysentery; Carbuncle, swelling, sore, vaginal itching	煎服，9～15g Decoction, 9-15g

（四）清热凉血药

2.4 Heat-clearing and blood-cooling medicine

本类药物多属苦甘咸寒，入血分，具有清解营分、血分热邪的功效。主治血分实热证，温热病热入营血，血热妄行，症见斑疹和各种出血（如鼻衄、牙龈出血、吐血、便血等）及舌绛、烦躁，甚至神昏谵语等。常见清热凉血药包括生地黄、玄参、牡丹皮、赤芍等（表 10–6）。

Most of these drugs are bitter, sweet, salty and cold, enter the blood component, and have the effects of clearing the camp component and blood component heat pathogen. Indications of blood division and excess heat syndrome, warm fever disease with heat entering the ying blood, blood heat moving wildly, symptoms such as macular rash and various bleeding (such as epistaxis, gum bleeding, vomiting blood, hematochezia, etc.), crimson tongue, irritability, and even unconsciousness and delirium, etc. Common medicines for clearing away heat and cooling blood include Rehmannia glutinosa, Scrophulariae, Peony Bark, Red Paeony Root, (Table 10–6).

表 10–6 常见清热凉血药

Table 10–6 Common heat–clearing and blood–cooling drugs

药名 Drug name	药性 Medicinal properties	功效 Efficacy	主治 Indications	用法用量 Usage and Dosage
生地黄 Rehmannia glutinosa	甘、苦，寒。归心、肝、肾经 Sweet, bitter, cold. Return to the heart, liver and kidney meridians	清热凉血，养阴生津 Clearing away heat and cooling blood, nourishing yin and promoting fluid production	热入营血，温毒发斑，吐血衄血；阴虚内热，骨蒸潮热；热病伤阴，舌绛烦渴，津伤口渴，内热消渴，津伤便秘 Heat enters the ying blood, warm poison spots, vomiting blood and epistaxis; Yin deficiency internal heat, bone steaming and tidal fever; Fever injury yin, tongue crimson polydipsia, thirst due to fluid injury, internal heat quenching thirst, fluid injury constipation	煎服，10 ～ 15g Decoction, 10-15g
玄参 Scrophulariae	甘、苦、咸，微寒。归肺、胃、肾经 Sweet, bitter, salty, slightly cold. Return to lung, stomach and kidney meridians	清热凉血，滋阴降火，解毒散结 Clearing away heat and cooling blood, nourishing yin and lowering fire, detoxifying and dispersing stagnation	热入营血，温毒发斑；热病伤阴，舌绛烦渴，津伤便秘，骨蒸劳嗽；目赤咽痛，白喉瘰疬，痈肿疮毒 Heat enters the ying blood, and warm poison causes spots; Fever injuries yin, tongue crimson and polydipsia, body fluid injury constipation, bone steaming and cough; Red eyes and sore throat, diphtheria scrofula, carbuncle swelling and sore poison	煎服，9 ～ 15g Decoction, 9-15g

续表

药名 Drug name	药性 Medicinal properties	功效 Efficacy	主治 Indications	用法用量 Usage and Dosage
牡丹皮 Peony bark	苦、辛，微寒。归心、肝、肾经 Bitter, pungent, slightly cold. Return to the heart, liver and kidney meridians	清热凉血，活血化瘀 Clearing away heat and cooling blood, promoting blood circulation and removing blood stasis	热入营血，温毒发斑，吐血衄血；夜热早凉，无汗骨蒸；血滞经闭，痛经癥瘕；痈肿疮毒，肠痈初起 Heat enters the ying blood, warm poison spots, vomiting blood and epistaxis; Hot at night and cool in the morning, no sweat and bone steaming; Blood stagnation, amenorrhea, dysmenorrhea; Carbuncle swelling and sore toxin, initial onset of intestinal carbuncle	煎服，6～12g Decoction, 6-12g
赤芍 Red peony	苦、微寒。归肝经 Bitter and slightly cold. Return to liver meridian	清热凉血，散瘀止痛 Clearing away heat and cooling blood, dispersing blood stasis and relieving pain	热入营血，温毒发斑，吐血衄血；肝郁胁痛，经闭痛经，癥瘕腹痛，跌仆损伤；痈肿疮疡，目赤肿痛 Heat enters the ying blood, warm poison spots, vomiting blood and epistaxis; Liver stagnation and hypochondriac pain, amenorrhea and dysmenorrhea, abdominal pain, fall and servant injury; Carbuncle, swelling and sore, red eyes, swelling and pain	煎服，6～12g Decoction, 6-12g

（五）清虚热药

2.5 Medicine for clearing deficiency and heat

本类药物多属寒凉，主入阴分，具有清虚热、退骨蒸功效。主治肝肾阴虚，虚火内扰所致的骨蒸潮热、午后发热及温热病后期，邪热未尽，伤阴劫液，而致夜热早凉等虚热证。常见清虚热药包括青蒿、地骨皮等（表 10–7）。

Most of these drugs are cold and cool, mainly enter yin, and have the effects of clearing deficiency and heat and reducing bone steaming. It is mainly used to treat deficiency–heat syndromes such as bone steaming and tidal fever, afternoon fever and late stage of warm–heat disease caused by liver and kidney yin deficiency, internal disturbance of deficiency–fire, unexhausted evil heat, damaging yin and robbing liquid, resulting in night heat and early cooling. Common drugs for clearing deficiency and heat include Artemisia annua, Cortex lycii radicis, etc. (Table 10–7).

表 10–7　常见清虚热药

Table 10–7　Common drugs for clearing deficiency and heat

药名 Drug name	药性 Medicinal properties	功效 Efficacy	主治 Indications	用法用量 Usage and Dosage
青蒿 Artemisia annua	苦、辛，寒。归肝、胆经 Bitter, pungent, cold. Return to the liver and gallbladder meridians.	清虚热，除骨蒸，解暑热，截疟，退黄 Clearing deficiency heat, removing bone steaming, relieving summer heat, intercepting malaria, and reducing yellowness	疟疾；温邪伤阴，夜热早凉；阴虚发热，劳热骨蒸；暑邪发热 Malaria; Warm evil hurts yin, night hot and early cold; Yin deficiency fever, fatigue heat bone steaming; Summer pathogen fever	煎服，6～12g Decoction, 6-12g
地骨皮 Cortex lycii radicis	甘，寒。归肺、肝、肾经 Gan, Han. Return to lung, liver and kidney meridians	凉血除蒸，清肺降火 Cooling blood, removing steam, clearing lung and reducing fire	阴虚潮热，骨蒸盗汗；肺热咳嗽；吐血衄血；内热消渴 Yin deficiency tidal fever, bone steaming night sweats; Cough due to lung heat; Hematemesis and epistaxis; Internal heat quenching thirst	煎服，9～15g Decoction, 9-15g

三、泻下药

3 Purgative drugs

凡能引起腹泻，或润滑大肠，促进排便，主要用于大便不通的药物，称为泻下药。

Any drugs that can cause diarrhea, or lubricate the large intestine and promote bowel movement are mainly used for bowel blockage, which are called laxative drugs.

本类药物为沉降之品，主归大肠经。主要功效：①泻下通便，以排除胃肠积滞和燥屎等。②清热泻火，使实热壅滞之邪通过泻下而清解，起到“上病治下”“釜底抽薪”的作用。③逐水退肿，使水湿停饮随大小便排除，达到祛除停饮、消退水肿的目的。

This class of drugs are sedimentation medicinals, which mainly belongs to the large intestine meridian. Main effects: ① Diarrhea and laxative to eliminate gastrointestinal stagnation and dry feces. ② Clear away heat and purge fire, so that the evil of excess heat stagnation can be cleared through purging, and it plays the role of “treating the disease from the upper side” and “drawing the salary from the bottom of the pot”. ③ Remove water to reduce swelling, so that water dampness can be eliminated with urination and defecation, so as to achieve the purpose of eliminating stopping drinking and subsiding edema.

泻下药主要适用于大便秘结、胃肠积滞、实热内结及水肿停饮等里实证，部分药物还可用于疮痈肿毒及瘀血证。常见泻下药包括大黄、芒硝、番泻叶、火麻仁、甘遂等（表 10–8）。

Purgative drugs are mainly suitable for internal cases such as constipation, gastrointestinal stagnation, excess heat internal knot and edema stopping drinking. Some drugs can also be used for sore, carbuncle, swelling and blood stasis syndrome. Common purgatire medicines includes rhubarb, Glauber's salt, etc. (Table 10–8).).

表 10–8 常见泻下药

Table 10–8 Common purgatire drugs

药名 Drug name	药性 Medicinal properties	功效 Efficacy	主治 Indications	用法用量 Usage and Dosage
大黄 Rhubarb	苦，寒。归脾、胃、大肠、肝、心包经 Bitter, cold. Returns to the spleen, stomach, large intestine, liver and pericardium meridians	泻下攻积，清热泻火，凉血解毒，逐瘀通经，利湿退黄 Purging and attacking accumulation, clearing away heat and purging fire, cooling blood and detoxifying, removing blood stasis and dredging menstruation, promoting dampness and reducing yellowness	积滞便秘；血热吐衄，目赤咽肿；热毒疮疡，烧烫伤；瘀血诸证；湿热痢疾，黄疸，淋证 Stagnation constipation; Blood heat vomiting epistaxis, red eyes and swollen throat; Heat sores, burns and scalds; Syndromes of blood stasis; Damp-heat dysentery, jaundice, stranguria syndrome	煎服，5～15g Decoction, 5-15g
芒硝 Glauber's salt	咸、苦，寒。归胃、大肠经 Salty, bitter, cold. Return to stomach and large intestine meridian	泻下攻积，润燥软坚，清火消肿 Purge and attack accumulation, moisten dryness and soften firmness, clear fire and reduce swelling	积滞便秘；咽痛，口疮，目赤，痈疮肿痛 Stagnation constipation; Sore throat, aphtha, red eyes, swelling and pain of carbuncle	6～12g，冲入药汁内或开水溶化后服 6-12g, flush into medicinal juice or dissolve in boiling water before taking

四、祛风湿药

4 Rheumatism removal medicine

凡以祛除风寒湿邪为主要功效，主要用于风湿痹证的药物，称为祛风湿药。

All drugs that have the main effect of eliminating wind–cold–dampness pathogens and are mainly used for rheumatism syndrome are called rheumatism–eliminating drugs.

本类药物味多辛苦，性或温或凉，能祛除留着于肌肉、经络、筋骨的风湿之邪，有的还兼有散寒、舒筋、通络、止痛、活血或补肝肾、强筋骨等作用。

This kind of medicine is hard in taste, warm or cool in nature, and can remove rheumatism pathogens that remain in muscles, meridians, muscles and bones. Some of them also have the functions of dispelling cold, relaxing tendons, dredging collaterals, relieving pain, promoting blood circulation or tonifying liver and kidney, and strengthening muscles and bones.

祛风湿药主要用于风湿痹证之肢体疼痛，关节不利、肿大，筋脉拘挛等症。部分药物还适用于腰膝酸软、下肢痿弱等。

Rheumatism-dispelling drugs are mainly used for limb pain, joint disadvantages, swelling, tendons and veins constriction and other symptoms of rheumatism and arthralgia syndrome. Some drugs are also suitable for soreness and weakness of waist and knees, weakness of lower limbs, etc.

祛风湿药易伤阴耗血，阴血亏虚者应慎用。痹证多属慢性疾病，为服用方便，可制成酒或丸散剂。常见祛风湿药包括独活、木瓜、秦艽、防己、桑寄生、五加皮等（表10–9）。

Dispelling rheumatism drugs are easy to damage yin and consume blood, and those with yin and blood deficiency should use them with caution. Bi syndrome is mostly a chronic disease, which can be made into wine or pills for convenience. Common rheumatism-eliminating drugs include Duhuo, Papaya, Gentiana macrophylla, Fangji, Mulberry parasitism, etc. (Table 10–9).

表 10–9 常见祛风湿药

Table 10–9 Common rheumatism–eliminating drugs

药名 Drug name	药性 Medicinal properties	功效 Efficacy	主治 Indications	用法用量 Usage and Dosage
独活 Live alone	辛、苦，微温。归肾、膀胱经 Pungent, bitter, slightly warm. Return to kidney and bladder meridian	祛风湿，通痹止痛 Dispel rheumatism, relieve arthralgia and relieve pain	风寒湿痹；风寒夹湿表证；少阴头痛，皮肤湿痒 Wind-cold-dampness arthralgia; Exterior syndrome of wind-cold mixed with dampness; Shaoyin headache, wet and itchy skin	煎服，3～10g Decoction, 3-10g
木瓜 Papaya	酸，温。归肝、脾经 Sour, warm. Return to liver and spleen meridians	舒筋活络，和胃化湿 Relax tendons and activate collaterals, harmonize the stomach and resolve dampness	风湿痹证；脚气水肿；吐泻转筋 Rheumatism arthralgia syndrome; Athlete's foot edema; Vomiting and diarrhea	煎服，6～9g Decoction, 6-9g
秦艽 Gentiana macrophylla	辛、苦，平。归胃、肝、胆经 Pungent, bitter, flat. Return to stomach, liver and gallbladder meridians	祛风湿，清湿热，止痹痛，退虚热 Dispelling rheumatism, clearing dampness and heat, relieving arthralgia and pain, and reducing deficiency and heat	风湿痹证；中风不遂；骨蒸潮热，疳积发热；湿热黄疸 Rheumatism arthralgia syndrome; Failure of stroke; Bone steaming and tidal fever, malnutrition and fever; Damp-heat jaundice	煎服，3～10g Decoction, 3-10g
防己 Fangji	苦、辛，寒。归膀胱、肺经 Bitter, pungent, cold. Return to bladder and lung meridians	祛风湿，止痛，利水消肿 Dispel rheumatism, relieve pain, promote diuresis and reduce swelling	风湿痹证；水肿脚气，小便不利，湿疹疮毒 Rheumatism arthralgia syndrome; Edema, athlete's foot, difficulty urinating, eczema and sores	煎服，5～10g Decoction, 5-10g

续表

药名 Drug name	药性 Medicinal properties	功效 Efficacy	主治 Indications	用法用量 Usage and Dosage
桑寄生 Mulberry parasitism	苦、甘，平。归肝、肾经 Bitter, sweet, flat. Return to liver and kidney meridians	祛风湿，补肝肾，强筋骨，安胎 Dispelling rheumatism, tonifying liver and kidney, strengthening muscles and bones, and preventing fetus	风湿痹证；崩漏经多，妊娠漏血，胎动不安 Rheumatism arthralgia syndrome; Metrorrhagia, blood leakage during pregnancy, uneasy fetal movement	煎服，9～15g Decoction, 9-15g

五、化湿药
5 Dampness-removing medicine

凡气味芳香，性偏温燥，以化湿运脾为主要功效，主要用于中焦湿阻证的药物，称为化湿药。

All drugs with fragrant smell, warm and dry nature, with the main effect of removing dampness and transporting the spleen, are mainly used for the syndrome of dampness obstruction in middle jiao, and are called dampness-removing drugs.

本类药物辛香温燥，主归脾、胃经。主要用于湿浊内阻，脾为湿困，运化失常所致的脘腹痞满、呕吐泛酸、大便溏薄、食少体倦、口甘多涎、舌苔白腻等。此外，化湿药还有芳香解暑之功，湿温、暑湿等证亦可选用。

This kind of medicine is spicy, warm and dry, and mainly belongs to the spleen and stomach meridians. It is mainly used for internal resistance of dampness and turbidity, dampness of the spleen, abdominal fullness, vomiting pantothenic acid, loose stools, poor appetite and body tiredness, sweet mouth and excessive salivation, white and greasy tongue coating, etc. caused by abnormal transportation and transformation. In addition, dampness-removing medicine has the function of aromatic and summer-relieving, and it can also be used for syndromes such as dampness-temperature and summer-dampness.

本类药物气味芳香，多含挥发油，入汤剂宜后下，且不宜久煎，以免其挥发性有效成分逸失而降低疗效。常见的化湿药包括广藿香、苍术、厚朴等（表 10-10）。

This kind of medicine has a fragrant smell and contains volatile oil. It should be put into the decoction later, and it should not be decocted for a long time, so as to avoid the loss of its volatile active ingredients and reduce the curative effect. Common dampness-removing drugs include patchouli, atractylodes, magnolia officinalis, etc. (Table 10-10).

表 10–10 常见化湿药

Table 10–10 Common humidification drugs

药名 Drug name	药性 Medicinal properties	功效 Efficacy	主治 Indications	用法用量 Usage and Dosage
广藿香 Patchouli	辛，微温。归脾、胃、肺经 Pungent, lukewarm. Return to spleen, stomach and lung meridians	化湿，止呕，解暑 Remove dampness, stop vomiting, relieve summer heat	湿阻中焦；呕吐；暑湿或湿温初起 Wet resistance medium coke; Vomiting; Summer dampness or humidity at the beginning of humidity temperature	煎服，5～10g Decoction, 5-10g
苍术 Atractylodes	辛，苦，温。归脾、胃、肝经 Pungent, bitter, warm. Return to spleen, stomach and liver meridians	燥湿健脾，祛风散寒，明目 Dry dampness and strengthen spleen, dispel wind and cold, improve eyesight	湿阻中焦证；风湿痹证，风寒夹湿表证；夜盲症及眼目昏涩 Dampness resistance middle jiao syndrome; Rheumatism arthralgia syndrome arthralgia syndrome, wind-cold mixed with dampness exterior syndrome; Night blindness and dizzy eyes	煎服，3～9g Decoction, 3-9g
厚朴 Magnolia officinalis	苦、辛，温。归脾、胃、肺、大肠经 Bitter, pungent, warm. Returns to the spleen, stomach, lung and large intestine meridians	燥湿消痰，下气除满 Dry dampness and eliminate phlegm, lower qi and remove fullness	湿阻中焦，脘腹胀满；食积气滞，腹胀便秘；痰饮喘咳；痰气互阻之梅核气 Dampness blocks the middle burner, and the abdominal distension is full; Food accumulation and qi stagnation, abdominal distension and constipation; Phlegm drinking, asthma and cough; Globus hysteriocus caused by mutual obstruction of phlegm and qi	煎服,3～10g，或入丸散 Decoction, 3-10g, or into pill powder

六、利水渗湿药

6 Diuretic and dampness-infiltrating drugs

凡能通利水道、渗泄水湿，主要用于水湿内停病证的药物，称为利水渗湿药。

Any drugs that can clean the waterway and discharge water and dampness, and are mainly used for the syndrome of internal arrest of water and dampness, are called diuretic and dampness-infiltrating drugs.

本类药物味多甘淡，主归膀胱、小肠经，具有利水消肿、利尿通淋、利湿退黄等功效，主要用于小便不利、水肿、泄泻、痰饮、淋证、黄疸、湿疮、带下、湿温等水湿所致的各种病证。

This kind of medicine is sweet and light in taste, mainly belongs to the bladder and small intestine meridians, and has the effects of diuresis and swelling, diuresis and stranguria, diuresis and yellowing, etc. It is mainly used for various diseases caused by water and dampness such as dysuria, edema, diarrhea, phlegm drinking, stranguria, jaundice, damp sore, stranguria, and dampness temperature.

利水渗湿药易耗伤津液，对阴亏津少、肾虚遗精遗尿者，宜慎用或忌用。有些药物有较强的通利作用，孕妇应慎用。常见利水渗湿药包括茯苓、薏苡仁、泽泻、车前子、茵陈、金钱草等（表 10–11）。

Diuretic and dampness–infiltrating drugs are easy to consume body fluids, and should be used with caution or avoidance for those with yin deficiency and fluid deficiency, kidney deficiency, nocturnal emission and enuresis. Some drugs have strong beneficial effects, so pregnant women should use them with caution. Common diuretic and dampness–infiltrating drugs include Poria cocos, Coix seed, Alisma orientalis, Plantago seed, Artemisia chinensis, Lysimachia, etc. (Table 10–11).

表 10–11　常见利水渗湿药

Table 10–11　Common diuretic and dampness–infiltrating drugs

药名 Drug name	药性 Medicinal properties	功效 Efficacy	主治 Indications	用法用量 Usage and Dosage
茯苓 Poria cocos	甘、淡，平。归心、肺、脾、肾经 Sweet, light, flat. Return to the heart, lung, spleen and kidney meridians	利水，渗湿，健脾，宁心 Diuresis, soaking dampness, invigorating spleen, calming heart	水肿；痰饮；脾虚泄泻；心悸，失眠 Edema; Phlegm drink; Diarrhea due to spleen deficiency; Palpitations, insomnia	煎服，10 ～ 15g Decoction, 10-15g
薏苡仁 Coix seed	甘、淡，凉。归脾、胃、肺经 Sweet, light and cool. Return to spleen, stomach and lung meridians	利水消肿，健脾止泻，除痹，排脓，解毒散结 Diuresis and swelling, invigorating spleen and stopping diarrhea, removing paralysis, draining pus, detoxifying and dispersing stagnation	水肿，小便不利，脚气；脾虚泄泻；湿痹拘挛；肺痈，肠痈；赘疣，癌肿 Edema, poor urination, athlete's foot; Diarrhea due to spleen deficiency; Dampness arthralgia convulsion; Pulmonary carbuncle, intestinal carbuncle; Verruca, cancer	煎服，9 ～ 30g Decoction, 9-30g
泽泻 Alisma orientalis	甘，淡，寒。归肾、膀胱经 Sweet, light, cold. Return to kidney and bladder meridian	利水渗湿，泄热，化浊降脂 Diuresis, discharge dampness, release heat, dissolve turbidity and reduce lipid	水肿，小便不利，泄泻；淋证，遗精；高脂血症 Edema, poor urination, diarrhea; Stranguria syndrome, nocturnal emission; hyperlipidemia	煎服，5 ～ 10g Decoction, 5-10g

续表

药名 Drug name	药性 Medicinal properties	功效 Efficacy	主治 Indications	用法用量 Usage and Dosage
车前子 Plantago seed	甘，微寒。归肝、肾、肺、小肠经 Sweet, slightly cold. Returns to liver, kidney, lung and small intestine meridians	清热利尿通淋，渗湿止泻，明目，祛痰 Clearing away heat, diuresis, dredging stranguria, seeping dampness, stopping diarrhea, improving eyesight, expectorant	淋证，水肿；泄泻；目赤肿痛，目暗昏花，翳障；痰热咳嗽 Stranguria syndrome, edema; diarrhea; Red, swollen and painful eyes, dark and dim eyes, and blurred eyes; phlegm-heat cough	煎服，9～15g包煎 Decoction, 9-15g package decoction
茵陈 Artemisia chinensis	苦、辛，微寒。归脾、胃、肝、胆经 Bitter, pungent, slightly cold. Return to the spleen, stomach, liver and gallbladder meridians	清利湿热，利胆退黄 Clearing dampness and heat, promoting gallbladder and reducing yellowness	黄疸；湿疮瘙痒 jaundice; Pruritus wet sores	煎服，6～15g；外用适量 Decoction, 6-15g; Appropriate amount for external use
金钱草 Lysimachia	甘、咸，微寒。归肝、胆、肾、膀胱经 Sweet, salty, slightly cold. Returns to liver, gallbladder, kidney and bladder meridians	利湿退黄，利尿通淋，解毒消肿 Diuresis and yellowness, diuresis and stranguria, detoxification and swelling	湿热黄疸；石淋，热淋；痈肿疔疮，毒蛇咬伤 damp-heat jaundice; Stone drenching, hot drenching; Carbuncle and furuncle, snake bite	煎服，9～15g Decoction, 9-15g

七、温里药

7 Warming medicine

凡以温里祛寒为主要功效，主要用于里寒证的药物，称为温里药。

Any medicine whose main effect is to warm the interior and dispel cold, and is mainly used for internal cold syndrome, is called warming medicine.

本类药物均味辛而性温热，辛能散、行，温能通，善走脏腑而能温里祛寒、温经止痛，故可用于里寒证，尤以里寒实证为主。个别药物尚能助阳、回阳，用以治疗虚寒证、亡阳证。

These drugs are pungent in taste but warm in nature. The pungent can disperse and move, and the warm can circulate. They are good at moving the internal organs and can warm the internal organs to dispel cold, warm the menstruation and relieve pain. Therefore, they can be used for internal cold syndrome, especially for internal cold syndrome. Individual drugs can still help and restore yang, and are used to treat deficiency–cold syndrome and death–yang syndrome.

温里药因其主要归经的不同而有多种效用。主归脾、胃经者，能温中散寒止痛，可用于外寒入侵，直中脾胃或脾胃虚寒证，症见脘腹冷痛、呕吐泄泻、舌淡苔白等。主归肺经者，能温肺化饮，用于肺寒痰饮证，症见痰鸣咳喘、痰白清稀、舌淡苔白滑等。主归肝经者，能暖肝散寒止痛，用于寒侵肝经的少腹痛、寒疝腹痛或厥阴头痛等。主归肾经者，能温肾助阳，用于肾阳不足证，症见阳痿宫冷、腰膝冷痛、夜尿频多、滑精遗尿等。主归心、肾两经者，能温阳通脉，用于心肾阳虚证，症见心悸怔忡、畏寒肢冷、小便不利、肢体浮肿等；或回阳救逆，用于亡阳厥逆证，症见畏寒蜷卧、汗出神疲、四肢厥逆、脉微欲绝等。

Warming medicine has many effects because of its different channel tropism. It mainly belongs to the spleen and stomach meridians. It can warm the middle, dispel cold and relieve pain. It can be used for external cold invasion, straight to the spleen and stomach or spleen and stomach deficiency and cold syndrome. The symptoms include cold pain in the epigastric abdomen, vomiting and diarrhea, pale tongue and white coating, etc. Those who mainly return to the lung meridian can warm the lungs and dissolve drinks. It is used for lung cold phlegm drinking syndrome. The symptoms include phlegm cough and asthma, white and thin phlegm, pale tongue and white and slippery coating, etc. Mainly belonging to the liver meridian, it can warm the liver, dispel cold and relieve pain. It is used for less abdominal pain, cold hernia abdominal pain or Jueyin headache caused by cold invasion of the liver meridian. Mainly belonging to the kidney meridian, it can warm the kidney and help yang, and is used for the syndrome of kidney yang deficiency. The symptoms include impotence, uterine cold, cold pain in the waist and knees, frequent nocturia, spermatozoa and enuresis, etc. Those who mainly return to the heart and kidney meridians can warm yang and dredge the meridians. It is used for the syndrome of heart and kidney yang deficiency. The symptoms include palpitations, cold limbs, difficult urination, edema of limbs, etc.; Or return to yang to save rebellion, it is used for the syndrome of dead yang jue rebellion. The symptoms include chills and lying curled up, sweating and fatigue, limbs jue rebellion, slight pulse, etc.

本类药物多辛热燥烈，易耗阴动火，故天气炎热时或素体火旺者当减少用量；真热假寒证禁用；凡实热证、阴虚火旺、津血亏虚者忌用；孕妇慎用。常见温里药包括附子、干姜、肉桂、吴茱萸等（表 10–12）。

This kind of medicine is pungent, hot, dry and strong, and it is easy to consume yin and stir fire. Therefore, when the weather is hot or if the body fire is excessive, the dosage should be reduced; True heat and false cold syndrome is forbidden; Those with excessive heat syndrome, yin deficiency and excessive fire, and fluid and blood deficiency should be avoided; Use with caution in pregnant women. Common warming medicines include aconite, dried ginger, cinnamon, Evodia rutaecarpa, etc. (Table 10–12).

表 10–12 常见温里药

Table 10–12 Common warming drugs

药名 Drug name	药性 Medicinal properties	功效 Efficacy	主治 Indications	用法用量 Usage and Dosage
附子 Aconite	辛、甘，大热；有毒。归心、肾、脾经 Pungent, sweet, big heat; Toxic. Return to the heart, kidney and spleen meridians	回阳救逆，补火助阳，散寒止痛 Return Yang to relieve rebellion, replenish fire and aid yang, dispel cold and relieve pain	亡阳证；阳虚证；寒痹疼痛 Dead Yang syndrome; Yang deficiency syndrome; Cold paralysis pain	煎服，3 ～ 15g Decoction, 3–15g
干姜 Dried ginger	辛，热。归脾、胃、肾、心、肺经 Pungent, Hot. Returns to the spleen, stomach, kidney, heart and lung meridians	温中散寒，回阳通脉，温肺化饮 Warming the middle and dispelling cold, returning yang and dredging pulse, warming lung and transforming drink	脘腹冷痛，呕吐泄泻；亡阳证；寒饮喘咳 Cold abdominal pain, vomiting and diarrhea; Dead Yang syndrome; Cold drink, asthma and cough	煎服，3 ～ 10g Decoction, 3-10g
肉桂 cinnamon	辛、甘，大热。归肾、脾、心、肝经 Pungent, sweet, major hot. Returns to kidney, spleen, heart and liver meridians	补火助阳，引火归原，散寒止痛，温通经脉 Tonifying fire and helping yang, causing fire to return to its original origin, dispelling cold and relieving pain, warming and dredging meridians	阳痿宫冷；寒凝诸痛证；寒滞血脉诸证；虚阳上浮；久病体虚，气血不足者 Impotence uterine cold; Cold coagulation of various pain syndromes; Syndromes of cold stagnation of blood vessels; Virtual Yang rises; Patients with long-term illness and physical weakness, deficiency of qi and blood	煎服，1 ～ 5g，宜后下或焗服；研末冲服，每次 1 ～ 2g Decoction, 1-5g, should be taken later or baked; Grind the powder and take it, 1-2g each time
吴茱萸 Evodia rutaecarpa	辛、苦，热；有小毒。归肝、脾、胃、肾经 Pungent, bitter, hot; Small poison. Returns to liver, spleen, stomach and kidney meridians	散寒止痛，降逆止呕，助阳止泻 Dispels cold and relieves pain, reduces adverse regression and relieves vomiting, helps yang and relieves diarrhea	寒凝疼痛；胃寒呕吐；虚寒泄泻 Cold coagulation pain; stomach cold and vomiting; Diarrhea due to deficiency and cold	煎服，2 ～ 5g；外用适量 Decoction, 2-5g; Appropriate amount for external use

八、理气药

8 Qi-regulating medicine

凡以疏理气机为主要功效，主要用于气滞或气逆证的药物，称为理气药。

Any medicine with the main effect of dispelling qi and regulating qi machine and mainly used for qi stagnation or qi adverse syndrome is called qi regulating medicine.

本类药物味多辛苦温而芳香。其味辛能行，味苦能泄，芳香能走窜，性温能通行，主归脾、胃、肝、肺经。以其性能不同，而分别具有理气健脾、疏肝解郁、理气宽胸、行气止痛、破气散结等功效。

This kind of medicine has a lot of hard taste, warm and fragrant taste. Its pungent taste can be moved, its bitter taste can be released, its aromatic smell can travel, and its warm nature can pass through. It mainly belongs to the spleen, stomach, liver and lung meridians. Because of their different properties, they have the effects of regulating qi and strengthening the spleen, soothing the liver and relieving depression, regulating qi and widening the chest, promoting qi and relieving pain, breaking qi and dispersing stagnation, etc.

理气药主要用于脾胃气滞所致脘腹胀痛、恶心呕吐、腹泻或便秘等；肝气郁滞所致胁肋胀痛、抑郁不乐、疝气疼痛、乳房胀痛、月经不调等；肺气壅滞所致胸闷胸痛、咳嗽气喘等。

Qi–regulating medicines are mainly used for abdominal distension and pain, nausea and vomiting, diarrhea or constipation caused by spleen and stomach qi stagnation; Hypochondrium distension and pain, depression and unhappiness, hernia pain, breast distension and pain, irregular menstruation, etc. caused by liver qi stagnation; Chest tightness, chest pain, cough and asthma caused by lung qi stagnation.

本类药物性多辛温香燥，易耗气伤阴，故气阴不足者慎用。常见理气药包括陈皮、枳实、木香、香附等（表 10–13）。

This kind of drug is pungent, warm, fragrant and dry, and it is easy to consume qi and damage yin, so it should be used with caution for those with insufficient qi and yin. Common qi–regulating drugs include dried tangerine peel, Fructus aurantii, wood incense, Cyperi Rhizoma, etc. (Table 10–13).

表 10–13 常见理气药

Table 10–13 Common qi–regulating drugs

药名 Drug name	药性 Medicinal properties	功效 Efficacy	主治 Indications	用法用量 Usage and Dosage
陈皮 Tangerine peel	辛、苦，温。归脾、肺经 Pungent, bitter, warm. Return to spleen and lung meridians	理气健脾，燥湿化痰 Regulating qi and strengthening spleen, drying dampness and resolving phlegm	脾胃气滞证；湿痰、寒痰咳嗽 Spleen and stomach qi stagnation syndrome; Damp phlegm, cold phlegm cough	煎服，3 ～ 10g Decoction, 3-10g

续表

药名 Drug name	药性 Medicinal properties	功效 Efficacy	主治 Indications	用法用量 Usage and Dosage
枳实 Fructus aurantii	苦、辛、酸，温。归脾、胃、大肠经 Bitter, pungent, sour, warm. Return to spleen, stomach and large intestine meridians	破气除痞，化痰消积 Break qi and eliminate ruffian, resolve phlegm and eliminate accumulation	胃肠积滞，湿热泻痢；胸痹，结胸；气滞胸胁疼痛；胃扩张、胃下垂、子宫脱垂、脱肛等脏器下垂病证 Gastrointestinal stagnation, damp-heat diarrhea; Chest paralysis, chest knot; Qi stagnation chest and hypochondriac pain; Gastric dilatation, gastroptosis, uterine prolapse, anal prolapse and other organ ptosis syndromes	煎服，3～10g，大量可用至30g Decoction, 3-10g, a large amount can be used to 30g
木香 Woody incense	辛、苦，温。归脾、胃、大肠、三焦、胆经 Pungent, bitter, warm. Returns to the spleen, stomach, large intestine, triple burner and gallbladder meridians	行气止痛，健脾消食 Promoting qi and relieving pain, invigorating spleen and digesting food	脾胃气滞证；泻痢里急后重；腹痛胁痛，黄疸，疝气疼痛；胸痹；减轻补益药的碍胃和滞气之弊，有助于消化吸收 Spleen and stomach qi stagnation syndrome; Diarrhea and dysentery tenesmus; Abdominal pain hypochondriac pain, jaundice, hernia pain; Chest paralysis; Reduce the disadvantages of tonic drugs that hinder the stomach and stagnate qi, and help digestion and absorption	煎服，3～6g Decoction, 3-6g
香附 Cyperi Rhizoma	辛，微苦，微甘，平。归肝、脾、三焦经 Pungent, slightly bitter, slightly sweet, flat. Return to liver, spleen and sanjiao meridians	疏肝解郁，理气宽中，调经止痛 Soothe liver and relieve depression, regulate qi and broaden the middle, regulate menstruation and relieve pain	肝郁气滞胁痛、腹痛；月经不调，痛经，乳房胀痛；气滞腹痛 Hypochondriac pain and abdominal pain due to liver stagnation and qi stagnation; Irregular menstruation, dysmenorrhea, breast distension and pain; qi stagnation abdominal pain	煎服，6～10g Decoction, 6-10g

九、消食药

9 Digestive medicine

凡以消化食积为主要功效，主要用于食积证的药物，称为消食药。

All drugs that have the main effect of digesting food accumulation and are mainly used for food accumulation syndrome are called digestive medicines.

消食药多味甘、性平，主归脾、胃二经。功能消食化积，部分消食药又兼有行气、祛痰、活血等功效。

Digestive medicine is sweet in taste and flat in nature, and mainly belongs to the spleen and stomach meridians. Some digestive drugs have the effects of promoting qi, eliminating phlegm, promoting blood circulation, etc., and some digestive drugs have the effects of promoting qi, eliminating phlegm and promoting blood circulation.

本类药物主要用于食积停滞证，症见脘腹胀满、嗳气吞酸、恶心呕吐、不思饮食、大便失常等，以及脾胃虚弱、消化不良者。

This class of drugs is mainly used for the syndrome of food stagnation, such as epigastric abdominal distension, belching and swallowing acid, nausea and vomiting, lack of thinking about eating, stool abnormalities, etc., as well as spleen and stomach weakness and indigestion.

消食药虽多数效缓，但仍不乏耗气之弊，故气虚而无积滞者慎用。常见消食药包括山楂、神曲、麦芽等（表 10–14）。

Although most digestive medicines have slow effects, they still have the disadvantages of consuming qi, so those with qi deficiency and no stagnation should use them with caution. Common digestive drugs include hawthorn, divine comedy, malt, etc. (Table 10–14).

表 10–14 常见消食药

Table 10–14 Common digestive drugs

药名 Drug name	药性 Medicinal properties	功效 Efficacy	主治 Indications	用法用量 Usage and Dosage
山楂 Hawthorn	酸、甘，微温。归脾、胃、肝经 Sour, sweet, slightly warm. Return to spleen, stomach and liver meridians	消食健胃，行气散瘀，化浊降脂 Digesting food and invigorating stomach, promoting qi and dispersing blood stasis, resolving turbidity and lowering lipid	饮食积滞证；泻痢腹痛，疝气疼痛；瘀血证；高脂血症 Diet stagnation syndrome; Diarrhea, abdominal pain, hernia pain; Blood stasis syndrome; hyperlipidemia	煎服，9～12g Decoction, 9-12g
神曲 Divine Comedy	甘、辛，温。归脾、胃经 Sweet, pungent, warm. Return to spleen and stomach meridians	消食化积，健脾和胃 Digest food and resolve accumulation, strengthen spleen and stomach	饮食积滞证；食积兼外感发热 Diet stagnation syndrome; Food accumulation and exogenous fever	煎服，6～15g Decoction, 6-15g
麦芽 malt	甘，平。归脾、胃经 Gan, Ping. Return to spleen and stomach meridians	行气消食，健脾开胃，回乳消积 Promoting qi and digesting food, strengthening spleen and appetizing, returning milk and eliminating accumulation	饮食积滞证，脾虚食滞证；断乳，乳房胀痛；肝郁胁痛，肝胃气痛 Food stagnation syndrome, spleen deficiency and food stagnation syndrome; Weaning, breast distension and pain; Liver stagnation and hypochondriac pain, liver and stomach qi pain	煎服，10～15g；回乳炒用 60g Decoction, 10-15g; 60g for returning milk and frying

十、驱虫药
10 Anthelmintics

凡以驱除或杀灭人体内肠道寄生虫为主要功效，主要用于虫证的药物，称为驱虫药。

Any drug whose main function is to repel or kill intestinal parasites in human body and is mainly used for insect syndrome is called anthelmintics.

驱虫药大多归大肠、脾、胃经，部分药物具有一定的毒性。功能驱虫或杀虫，特别是对肠道内寄生虫的杀灭、麻痹作用尤为明显；部分药物兼能行气、消积、润肠、疗癣等。

Anthelmintics mostly belong to the large intestine, spleen and stomach meridians, and some drugs have certain toxicity. Functional anthelmintic or insecticidal, especially for killing and paralyzing parasites in the intestinal tract; Some drugs can also promote qi, eliminate accumulation, moisten intestines, treat ringworm, etc.

本类药物主要用于肠道内寄生虫，包括蛔虫、绦虫、蛲虫、钩虫等，症见绕脐腹痛且时发时止，不思饮食或多食善饥，嗜食异物，肛门、耳、鼻瘙痒，迁延日久则面色萎黄，形体消瘦，腹大且青筋暴露，毛发枯槁，浮肿等。部分药物兼治食积气滞、小儿疳积、便秘、疥癣瘙痒等。

This class of drugs is mainly used for intestinal parasites, including roundworms, tapeworms, pinworms, hookworms, etc. The symptoms include abdominal pain around the umbilical cord that occurs and stops from time to time, not thinking about eating or eating more and making hunger, eating foreign bodies, itching of anus, ears, and nose, which leads to yellow complexion, emaciation of body, large abdomen and exposed veins, withered hair, edema, etc. Some drugs can also treat food accumulation and qi stagnation, malnutrition in children, constipation, mange itching, etc.

驱虫药需控制剂量，防止用量过大中毒或损伤正气；对素体虚弱、年老体衰及孕妇，更当慎用。驱虫药一般应在空腹时服用，以保疗效。对发热或腹痛剧烈者，不宜急于驱虫，待症状缓解后，再施用驱虫药物。常见驱虫药包括槟榔、使君子、苦楝皮等（表 10–15）。

The dosage of anthelmintics should be controlled to prevent excessive dosage from poisoning or damaging righteousness; It should be used with caution for weak, elderly and pregnant women. Anthelmintics should generally be taken on an empty stomach to ensure curative effect. For those with fever or severe abdominal pain, it is not advisable to rush to deworming, and then apply deworming drugs after the symptoms are relieved. Common anthelmintics include Areca nut, Quisqualis indica, neem bark, etc. (Table 10–15).

表 10–15 常见驱虫药

Table 10–15 Common anthelmintics

药名 Drug name	药性 Medicinal properties	功效 Efficacy	主治 Indications	用法用量 Usage and Dosage
槟榔 Areca nut	苦、辛，温。归胃、大肠经 Bitter, pungent, warm. Return to stomach and large intestine meridian	杀虫，消积，行气，利水，截疟 Killing insects, eliminating accumulation, promoting qi, diuresis, intercepting malaria	多种肠道寄生虫病；食积气滞，泻痢后重；水肿，脚气肿痛；疟疾 Multiple intestinal parasitic diseases; Food accumulation and qi stagnation, severe diarrhea and dysentery; Edema, swelling and pain of athlete's foot; malaria	煎服，3～10g。驱绦虫、姜片虫 30～60g Decoction, 3-10g. Repellent tapeworm and ginger worm 30-60g
使君子 Quisqualis indica	甘，温。归脾、胃经 Sweet, warm. Return to spleen and stomach meridians	治蛔虫病、蛲虫病、小儿疳积 Treat ascariasis, enterobiasis, malnutrition in children	蛔虫病，蛲虫病；小儿疳积 Ascariasis, Enterobiasis; malnutrition in children	煎服，9～12g，捣碎；使君子仁，6～9g，小儿每岁 1～1.5 粒，取仁炒香嚼服，一日总量不超过 20 粒。空腹服用，每日 1 次，连用 3 日 Decoction, 9-12g, mashed; Semen quisqualis, 6-9g, 1-1.5 capsules per year for children, stir-fry the kernels and chew them, and the total daily amount should not exceed 20 capsules. Take on an empty stomach, once a day for 3 consecutive days
苦楝皮 Neem bark	苦，寒；有毒。归肝、脾、胃经 Bitter, cold; Toxic. Return to liver, spleen and stomach meridians	杀虫，疗癣 Killing insects, treating ringworm	蛔虫病，蛲虫病，虫积腹痛；疥癣瘙痒 Ascariasis, enterobiasis, worm accumulation abdominal pain; mange pruritus	煎服，3～6g；鲜品 15～30g，外用适量 Decoction, 3-6g; Fresh product 15-30g, appropriate amount for external use

十一、止血药

11 Hemostatic drugs

凡以制止体内外出血为主要功效，主要用于各种出血病证的药物，称为止血药。

Drugs whose main function is to stop internal and external bleeding and are mainly used for various hemorrhagic diseases are called hemostatic drugs.

凉血止血药性多苦寒，化瘀止血药、温经止血药性多辛温，收敛止血药多为平性。

止血药大多归心、肝经。功能止血，因其兼有作用不同，而分别具有收敛止血、凉血止血、化瘀止血、温经止血等作用。

Blood-cooling hemostatic drugs are mostly bitter and cold, blood stasis-removing hemostatic drugs and meridian-warming hemostatic drugs are mostly pungent and warm, and astringent hemostatic drugs are mostly flat. Most hemostatic drugs return to the heart and liver meridians. Functional hemostasis, because of its different functions, has the functions of astringent hemostasis, cooling blood and hemostasis, removing blood stasis and hemostasis, warming meridian and hemostasis, etc.

止血药主要用于咯血、咳血、衄血、吐血、便血、尿血、崩漏及外伤出血等体内外各种出血病证。常见止血药包括白及、地榆、三七、茜草、艾叶等（表 10-16）。

Hemostatic drugs are mainly used for various hemorrhagic diseases in and out of vivo such as hemoptysis, hemoptysis, epistaxis, vomiting blood, hematochezia, hemuria, metrorrhagia and traumatic bleeding. Common hemostatic drugs include Baiji, Sanguisorba, Panax notoginseng, Rubia, Mugwort leaves, etc. (Table 10-16).

表 10-16　常见止血药

Table 10-16　Common hemostatic drugs

药名 Drug name	药性 Medicinal properties	功效 Efficacy	主治 Indications	用法用量 Usage and Dosage
白及 Baiji	苦、甘、涩，微寒。归肺、肝、胃经 Bitter, sweet, astringent, slightly cold. Return to lung, liver and stomach meridians	收敛止血，消肿生肌 Astringing to stop bleeding, reduction of swelling and muscle growth	出血证；疮疡肿毒，皮肤皲裂，水火烫伤疮疡者 Bleeding syndrome; Sores, swollen and poisonous, chapped skin, scalded sores by water and fire	煎服，6～15g；大剂量可用至 30g；研末吞服，每次 3～6g，外用适量 Decoction, 6-15g; Large doses can be up to 30g; Grind the powder and swallow, 3-6g each time, appropriate amount for external use
地榆 Sanguisorba	苦、酸、涩，微寒。归肝、大肠经 Bitter, sour, astringent, slightly cold. Return to liver and large intestine meridian	凉血止血，解毒敛疮 Cool blood to stop bleeding, detoxify and restrain sores	血热出血证；水火烫伤，痈疮肿毒 Blood heat hemorrhage syndrome; Water and fire burns, carbuncle, swelling and poison	煎服，9～15g；或入丸、散，外用适量。止血多炒炭用，解毒敛疮多生用 Decoction, 9-15g; Or into pills or powders, appropriate amount for external use. Stir-fried charcoal for hemostasis, detoxification and sores for raw life

续表

药名 Drug name	药性 Medicinal properties	功效 Efficacy	主治 Indications	用法用量 Usage and Dosage
三七 Panax notoginseng	甘、微苦，温。归肝、胃经 Sweet, slightly bitter, warm. Return to liver and stomach meridians	散瘀止血，消肿定痛，补虚强壮 Dispersing blood stasis and stopping bleeding, reducing swelling and relieving pain, tonifying deficiency and strengthening	出血证；瘀血证；虚损劳伤 Bleeding syndrome; Blood stasis syndrome; Virtual strain injury	多研末吞服，1～3g；煎服，3～9g，亦入丸散。外用适量，研末外掺或调敷 Grind more powder and swallow, 1-3g; Decoction, 3-9g, also into pill powder. Appropriate amount for external use, grind into powder and mix externally or adjust application
茜草 Rubia	苦，寒。归肝经 Bitter, cold. Return to liver meridian	凉血，祛瘀，止血，通经 Cooling blood, removing blood stasis, stopping bleeding, dredging menstruation	出血证；瘀阻经闭，跌仆肿痛，关节痹痛 Bleeding syndrome; Blood stasis amenorrhea, swelling and pain, joint arthralgia	煎服，6～10g。亦入丸散 Decoction, 6-10g. Yiru Pill Powder
艾叶 Mugwort leaves	辛、苦，温；有小毒。归肝、脾、肾经 Pungent, bitter, warm; Small poison. Return to liver, spleen and kidney meridians	温经止血，散寒调经；外用祛湿止痒 Warm the menstruation to stop bleeding, dispel cold and regulate menstruation; External use to remove dampness and relieve itching	出血证；月经不调、痛经；胎动不安；湿疹、疥癣。此外，将本品捣绒，制成艾条、艾炷等，用以熏灸体表穴位，能温煦气血、透达经络，为温灸的主要原料 Bleeding syndrome; Irregular menstruation, dysmenorrhea; Fetal restlessness; Eczema, mange. In addition, the product is pounded into velvet and made into moxa sticks, moxa sticks, etc., which are used for fumigating and moxibusting acupoints on the body surface, warming qi and blood, penetrating meridians and collaterals, and are the main raw materials for warm moxibustion	煎服，3～9g；外用适量。温经止血宜炒炭用，余生用 Decoction, 3-9g; Appropriate amount for external use. To warm the menstruation and stop bleeding, it should be fried with charcoal and used for the rest of the life

十二、活血化瘀药

12 Drugs for promoting blood circulation and removing blood stasis

凡以畅通血脉、促进血行、消散瘀血为主要功效，主要用于瘀血病证的药物，称为活血化瘀药，或活血祛瘀药，简称活血药、祛瘀药或化瘀药。其中活血化瘀作用强者，又称为破血药。

All drugs with the main functions of unblocking blood vessels, promoting blood circulation, and dissipating blood stasis, and mainly used for blood stasis diseases and syndromes, are called blood-activating and stasis-removing drugs, or blood-activating and stasis-removing drugs, referred to as blood-activating drugs, stasis-removing drugs or stasis-removing drugs for short. Among them, those with strong effects on promoting blood circulation and removing blood stasis are also called blood-breaking drugs.

活血化瘀药多具辛味，部分动物、昆虫类药物多味咸，药性偏温，部分药性寒凉，多归心、肝两经。通过活血化瘀作用而分别具有止痛、调经、消肿、疗伤、消痈、消癥等功效。其中药力和缓且活血作用较弱者，称为和血、和营；药力峻猛且活血较强者，称为破血、逐瘀。

Drugs for promoting blood circulation and removing blood stasis are mostly pungent, some animal and insect drugs are mostly salty and have warm properties, and some drugs are cold and cold, and mostly return to the heart and liver meridians. By promoting blood circulation and removing blood stasis, it has the effects of relieving pain, regulating menstruation, reducing swelling, healing wounds, eliminating carbuncle and eliminating symptoms. Among them, those with mild medicine power and weak blood circulation activation effect are called Hexue and Heying; If the medicine is strong and strong in promoting blood circulation, it is called breaking blood and removing blood stasis.

本类药物主要用于各种瘀血证，症见患处刺痛、痛处拒按且固定不移、夜间加重，青紫色包块，出血反复不止，血色紫暗或夹血块，面黑唇紫，舌有紫色斑点，脉多细涩或结代等。

This class of drugs is mainly used for various blood stasis syndromes. The symptoms include tingling pain in the affected area, pain refusing to be pressed and fixed, aggravated at night, blue-purple mass, repeated bleeding, dark purple blood or blood clots, black face and purple lips, purple spots on the tongue, fine and astringent pulse or knots, etc.

活血化瘀药行散走窜，活血动血，应注意防其破泄太过，做到化瘀而不伤正，故月经过多、血虚经闭者忌用；破血药孕妇忌用；破血药更易伤人正气，故体虚而兼瘀血者亦应慎用。常见活血化瘀药包括川芎、延胡索、郁金、丹参、牛膝、桃仁、红花、益母草、土鳖虫、莪术等（表 10-17）。

The medicine for promoting blood circulation and removing blood stasis is scattered and running, promoting blood circulation and moving blood, and attention should be paid to prevent it from breaking too much, so as to remove blood stasis without hurting the right body, so it is avoided for patients with menorrhagia and blood deficiency and amenorrhea; Blood-breaking drugs are contraindicated for pregnant women; Blood-breaking drugs are more likely to hurt people's righteousness, so those with physical weakness and blood stasis should also use them with caution. Common drugs for promoting blood circulation and removing blood stasis include Chuanxiong, Corydalis, Curcuma, Salvia miltiorrhiza, Achyranthes bidentata, Peach Kernel, Safflower, Motherwort, Earth beetle, Curcuma zedoary, etc. (Table 10–17).

表 10–17　常见活血化瘀药

Table 10–17　Common drugs for promoting blood circulation and removing blood stasis

药名 Drug name	药性 Medicinal properties	功效 Efficacy	主治 Indications	用法用量 Usage and Dosage
川芎 Chuanxiong	辛，温。归肝、胆、心包经 Pungent, warm. Return to liver, gallbladder and pericardium meridians	活血行气，祛风止痛 Promoting blood circulation and promoting qi, dispelling wind and relieving pain	血瘀气滞痛证；头痛，风湿痹痛 Blood stasis and qi stagnation pain syndrome; Headache, rheumatic arthralgia	煎服，3～10g Decoction, 3-10g
延胡索 Corydalis	辛、苦，温。归肝、脾经 Pungent, bitter, warm. Return to liver and spleen meridians	活血，行气，止痛 Promoting blood circulation, promoting qi, relieving pain	气血瘀滞诸痛 Qi and blood stasis and various pain	煎服，3～10g，研末吞服，每次 1.5～3g Decoction, 3-10g, grind into powder and swallow, 1.5-3g each time
郁金 Curcuma	辛、苦，寒。归肝、胆、心经 Pungent, bitter, cold. Return to liver, gallbladder and heart meridians	活血止痛，行气解郁，清心凉血，利胆退黄 Activating blood to relieve pain, Qi to relieve depression, clear heart to cool blood, gallbladder to withdraw yellow	气滞血瘀，胸胁刺痛、胸痹心痛，月经不调、经闭痛经、乳房胀痛；热病神昏、癫痫、癫狂；血热吐衄、妇女倒经；湿热黄疸，胆道结石 Qi stagnation and blood stasis, tingling pain in the chest and hypochondrium, chest impediment and heartache, irregular menstruation, amenorrhea and dysmenorrhea, breast distension and pain; Fever, unconsciousness, epilepsy, madness; Blood heat vomiting epistaxis, menstruation in women; Damp-heat jaundice, biliary stones	煎服，5～10g，研末服，2～5g Decoction, 5-10g, grind into powder, 2-5g

续表

药名 Drug name	药性 Medicinal properties	功效 Efficacy	主治 Indications	用法用量 Usage and Dosage
丹参 Salvia miltiorrhiza	苦，微寒。归心、肝经 Bitter, slightly cold. Return to heart and liver meridian	活血祛瘀，通经止痛，清心除烦，凉血消痈。 Promoting blood circulation and removing blood stasis, dredging menstruation and relieving pain, clearing the heart and eliminating annoyance, cooling blood and eliminating carbuncle	瘀血阻滞，月经不调，经闭痛经，产后瘀滞腹痛；血瘀胸痹心痛，脘腹胁痛，癥瘕积聚，风湿痹痛；疮痈肿痛；热入营血，烦躁神昏，心悸失眠 Blood stasis blockade, irregular menstruation, amenorrhea and dysmenorrhea, postpartum stasis and abdominal pain; Blood stasis, chest arthralgia, heartache, epigastric and hypochondriac pain, accumulation of symptoms, rheumatic arthralgia; Sores, carbuncles, swelling and pain; Heat into ying blood, irritability, unconsciousness, palpitations and insomnia	煎服，5～15g，活血化瘀宜酒炙用 Decoction, 5-15g, activating blood circulation and removing blood stasis, suitable for wine roasting
牛膝 Achyranthes	苦、甘、酸，平。归肝、肾经 Bitter, sweet, sour, flat. Return to liver and kidney meridians	逐瘀通经，补肝肾，强筋骨，利水通淋，引血下行 Expelling blood stasis and dredging menstruation, tonifying liver and kidney, strengthening muscles and bones, promoting diuresis and dredging stranguria, and drawing blood down	月经不调，痛经，经闭；淋证，水肿，小便不利；头痛，眩晕，吐血，衄血，口舌生疮；腰膝酸痛，筋骨无力 Irregular menstruation, dysmenorrhea, amenorrhea; Stranguria syndrome, edema, difficult urination; Headache, dizziness, vomiting blood, epistaxis, sores in the mouth and tongue; Soreness of waist and knees, weakness of muscles and bones	煎服，6～15g Decoction, 6-15g
桃仁 Peach kernel	苦、甘，平；有小毒。归心、肝、大肠经 Bitter, sweet, flat; Small poison. Return to the heart, liver and large intestine meridian	活血祛瘀，润肠通便，止咳平喘 Promoting blood circulation and removing blood stasis, moistening intestines and relaxing constipation, relieving cough and asthma	瘀血阻滞之经闭、痛经、产后瘀滞腹痛，癥瘕积聚，跌打损伤；肺痈；肠痈，肠燥便秘；咳嗽气喘 Amenorrhea, dysmenorrhea, postpartum stasis, abdominal pain, accumulation of symptoms, bruises and injuries caused by blood stasis; Pulmonary carbuncle; Intestinal carbuncle, intestinal dryness and constipation; Cough and asthma	煎服，5～10g，捣碎；桃仁霜入汤剂宜包煎 Decoction, 5-10g, mashed; Peach kernel cream should be decocted in decoction

续表

药名 Drug name	药性 Medicinal properties	功效 Efficacy	主治 Indications	用法用量 Usage and Dosage
红花 Safflower	辛，温。归心、肝经 Pungent, warm. Guixin and liver meridian	活血通经，祛瘀止痛 Activating blood circulation, dredging menstruation, removing blood stasis and relieving pain	瘀血阻滞之经闭、痛经，产后瘀滞腹痛；瘀阻胸痛、腹痛、胁痛；跌打损伤，瘀滞肿痛；瘀滞斑疹色暗 Amenorrhea and dysmenorrhea caused by blood stasis, postpartum stasis and abdominal pain; Stasis chest pain, abdominal pain, hypochondriac pain; bruises, stagnation, swelling and pain; Stasis macula dark color	煎服，3～10g；外用适量 Decoction, 3-10g; Appropriate amount for external use
益母草 Motherwort	苦、辛，微寒。归肝、心包、膀胱经 Bitter, pungent, slightly cold. Return to liver, pericardium and bladder meridians	活血调经，利尿消肿，清热解毒 Promoting blood circulation and regulating menstruation, diuresis and swelling, clearing away heat and detoxifying	瘀滞之月经不调，经闭、痛经，产后瘀阻腹痛，恶露不尽；水肿尿少；疮痈肿毒 Irregular menstruation due to stasis, amenorrhea, dysmenorrhea, postpartum stasis, abdominal pain, and endless lochia; edema oliguria; Sore carbuncle swelling poison	煎服，10～30g；或熬膏，入丸剂；外用适量捣敷或煎汤外洗 Decoction, 10-30g; Or boil ointment and put it into pills; Appropriate amount for external use: pound and apply or decoct and wash externally
土鳖虫 Earth beetle	咸，寒；有小毒。归肝经 Salty, cold; Small poison. Return to liver meridian	破血逐瘀，续筋接骨 Breaking blood and removing blood stasis, continuing tendons and connecting bones	跌打损伤，筋伤骨折，瘀肿疼痛；血瘀经闭，产后瘀滞腹痛，癥瘕痞块 Bruises, tendon injuries and fractures, bruises and pain; Blood stasis and amenorrhea, postpartum stasis and abdominal pain, symptoms and masses	煎服，3～10g；研末服，1～1.5g，黄酒送服；外用适量 Decoction, 3-10g; Grind the powder and take it, 1-1.5g, and take it with yellow rice wine; Appropriate amount for external use
莪术 Curcuma zedoary	辛、苦，温。归肝、脾经 Pungent, bitter, warm. Return to liver and spleen meridians	行气破血，消积止痛 Promoting qi and breaking blood, eliminates accumulation and relieves pain	气滞血瘀之癥瘕痞块、经闭及胸痹心痛；食积胀痛 Symptoms of qi stagnation and blood stasis: mass, amenorrhea and chest impediment and heartache; Food accumulation distension and pain	煎服，3～15g。醋制后可加强祛瘀止痛作用。外用适量 Decoction, 3-15g. Vinegar can strengthen the effect of removing blood stasis and relieving pain. Appropriate amount for external use

十三、化痰药与止咳平喘药

13 Phlegm-resolving drugs and cough-relieving and antiasthmatic drugs

凡以祛痰或消痰为主要功效，主要用于痰证的药物，称为化痰药；凡以制止或减轻咳嗽和喘息为主要功效，主要用于咳喘证的药物，称为止咳平喘药。因部分化痰药兼止咳、平喘功效；而止咳平喘药也常兼化痰之功，病证上痰、咳、喘三者相互兼杂，故将化痰药与止咳平喘药合并介绍。

Drugs with expectorant or eliminating phlegm as their main effects and mainly used for phlegm syndrome are called phlegm-resolving drugs; Drugs whose main effect is to stop or alleviate cough and wheezing, and are mainly used for cough and asthma syndrome, are called antitussive and antiasthmatic drugs. Because some phlegm-resolving drugs have cough-relieving and asthmatic effects; Cough-relieving and antiasthmatic drugs often have the function of resolving phlegm, and phlegm, cough, and asthma are mixed with each other on the disease syndrome. Therefore, phlegm-relieving drugs and cough-relieving and antiasthmatic drugs are combined and introduced.

化痰药与止咳平喘药味多辛、苦或甘，大多归肺经。功能化痰、止咳、平喘等。部分药物兼能降气、宣肺、润肺、润肠通便、利水消肿、清利湿热等。

Phlegm-resolving drugs and cough-relieving and asthmatic drugs taste pungent, bitter or sweet, and most of them belong to the lung meridian. Function: Resolving phlegm, relieving cough, relieving asthma, etc. Some drugs can also lower qi, ventilate lung qi, moisten lung, moisten intestines, relieve constipation, promote diuresis and reduce swelling, clear dampness and heat, etc.

此两类药物主要用于外感或内伤所致的痰多、咳嗽、气喘，以及因痰所致的眩晕、瘰疬瘿瘤、癫痫惊厥、阴疽流注等。

These two types of drugs are mainly used for excessive phlegm, cough, and asthma caused by exogenous or internal injuries, as well as dizziness, scrofula gall tumor, epileptic convulsions, vaginal gangrene injection, etc. caused by phlegm.

使用化痰与止咳平喘药，应注意温燥性烈的刺激性化痰药，热痰、燥痰及有吐血、咯血倾向者当忌用或慎用；麻疹初起兼表证咳嗽者，不宜单用止咳药，当以疏解清宣透疹为主，以免恋邪而影响麻疹透发，对于收敛及温燥之品，尤为忌用。

When using phlegm-resolving and cough-relieving and antiasthmatic drugs, attention should be paid to irritating phlegm-resolving drugs that are warm and dry. Those with hot phlegm, dry phlegm and tendency to vomit blood and hemoptysis should be avoided or used with caution; Patients with superficial cough at the beginning of measles should not use cough medicine alone. It should be mainly used to relieve clear and clear rash, so as to avoid evil love and affect measles penetration. It is especially contraindicated for astringent and warm dryness medicinals.

（一）化痰药

13.1 Phlegm-resolving medicine

本类药物味多辛、苦，主归肺、脾、肝经，具有化痰之功，因药性不同，又有温化寒痰与清化热痰之别。温化寒痰药性多温燥，具有温肺散寒、燥湿化痰之功，主治寒痰、湿痰证；清化热痰药性寒凉，能清热化痰，主治热痰、燥痰证。部分药物兼治疮痈肿毒、癫痫、中风惊厥、瘰疬瘿瘤等。常见化痰药包括半夏、桔梗、贝母、瓜蒌、竹茹等（表 10–18）。

This kind of medicine has a pungent and bitter taste, mainly belongs to the lung, spleen and liver meridians, and has the function of resolving phlegm. Due to different medicinal properties, it also has the difference between warming and resolving cold phlegm and clearing away hot phlegm. The medicinal properties of warming and resolving cold phlegm are mostly warm and dry, and it has the functions of warming the lungs and dispelling cold, drying dampness and resolving phlegm. It is mainly used to treat cold phlegm and damp phlegm syndrome; The medicinal properties of clearing away heat and phlegm are cold and cool, can clear away heat and resolve phlegm, and mainly treat hot phlegm and dry phlegm syndromes. Some drugs can also treat sore carbuncle swelling poison, epilepsy, stroke convulsion, scrofula gall tumor, etc. Common phlegm–resolving drugs include Pinellia ternata, Platycodon grandiflorum, Fritillaria, Trichosanthes, etc. (Table 10–18).

表 10–18 常见化痰药

Table 10–18 Common phlegm–resolving drugs

药名 Drug name	药性 Medicinal properties	功效 Efficacy	主治 Indications	用法用量 Usage and Dosage
半夏 Pinellia ternata	辛，温；有毒。归脾、胃、肺经 Pungent, warm; Toxic. Return to spleen, stomach and lung meridians	燥湿化痰，降逆止呕，消痞散结 Dry dampness and resolve phlegm, reduce adverse regression and stop vomiting, eliminate ruffians and dissipate stagnation	湿痰、寒痰证；呕吐；胸脘痞闷，梅核气；痈疽肿毒，瘰疬痰核，毒蛇咬伤 Damp phlegm and cold phlegm syndrome; Vomiting; Chest and epigastric stuffiness, Globus hysteriocus; Carbuncle swollen poison, scrofula sputum nucleus, snake bite	煎服，3～10g，一般宜制用 Decoction, 3-10g, generally suitable for preparation
桔梗 Platycodon grandiflorum	苦、辛，平。归肺经 Bitter, pungent, flat. Return to lung meridian	宣肺，祛痰，利咽，排脓 Ventilating lung qi, expectorant, soothing throat, discharge pus	咳嗽痰多，胸闷不畅；咽喉肿痛，失音；肺痈吐脓 Cough with excessive phlegm and chest tightness; Sore throat, aphonia; Pulmonary carbuncle vomiting pus	煎服，3～10g；或入丸、散 Decoction, 3-10g; Or into pills or powders

续表

药名 Drug name	药性 Medicinal properties	功效 Efficacy	主治 Indications	用法用量 Usage and Dosage
川贝母 Fritillaria chuan	苦、甘，微寒。归肺、心经 Bitter, sweet, slightly cold. Return to lung and heart meridian	清热润肺，化痰止咳，散结消痈 Clearing away heat and moistening lung, resolving phlegm and relieving cough, dispersing stagnation and eliminating carbuncle	肺热燥咳，干咳少痰，阴虚劳嗽，痰中带血；瘰疬、乳痈、肺痈 Dry cough due to lung heat, dry cough with less phlegm, cough due to yin deficiency and fatigue, and blood in phlegm; Scrofula, breast carbuncle, lung carbuncle	煎服，3 ～ 10g；研粉冲服，每次1 ～ 2g Decoction, 3-10g; Grind the powder and take it, 1-2g each time
浙贝母 Fritillaria zhejiang	苦，寒。归肺、心经 Bitter, cold. Return to lung and heart meridian	清热化痰止咳，解毒散结消痈 Clearing away heat, resolving phlegm, relieving cough, detoxifying, dispersing stagnation and eliminating carbuncle	风热咳嗽及痰火咳嗽，燥热咳嗽；瘰疬、乳痈、肺痈、痈肿疮毒等 Wind-heat cough, phlegm-fire cough, dry-heat cough; Scrofula, breast carbuncle, lung carbuncle, carbuncle swelling and sore poison, etc.	煎服，5 ～ 10g Decoction, 5-10g
瓜蒌 Trichosanthes	甘，微苦，寒。归肺、胃、大肠经 Sweet, slightly bitter, cold. Return to lung, stomach and large intestine meridians	清热涤痰，宽胸散结，润燥滑肠 Clearing away heat and clearing phlegm, widening chest and dispersing stagnation, moistening dryness and smoothing intestines	肺热咳嗽，痰浊黄稠；胸痹心痛，结胸痞满；肺痈、肠痈、乳痈；大便秘结 Cough due to lung heat, turbid yellow and thick phlegm; Chest paralysis, heartache, chest fullness; Pulmonary carbuncle, intestinal carbuncle, breast carbuncle; Large constipation knot	煎服，全瓜蒌9～15g，瓜蒌皮6～10g，瓜蒌子9～15g，瓜蒌子打碎入煎剂 Decoction, 9-15g of whole Trichosanthes trichosanthes, 6-10g of Trichosanthes trichosanthes peel, 9-15g of Trichosanthes trichosanthes

（二）止咳平喘药

13.2 Antitussive and antiasthmatic drugs

本类药物味多辛苦或甘，主归肺经，具有止咳平喘之功，有的药物偏于止咳，有的偏于平喘，或兼而有之。部分药物兼有润肠通便、利水消肿、清利湿热等作用。主要用于咳喘证。部分药物还可用于肠燥便秘、水肿、胸腹积水、湿热黄疸、癫痫等病证。常见止咳平喘药包括苦杏仁、紫苏子、百部、桑白皮、葶苈子等（表 10–19）。

This kind of drugs taste hard or sweet, mainly belong to the lung meridian, and have the effect of relieving cough and asthma. Some drugs are biased towards relieving cough, some are biased towards relieving asthma, or both. Some drugs have the effects of moistening the intestines and laxative bowels, diuresis and swelling, and clearing away dampness and heat. Mainly used for cough and asthma syndrome. Some drugs can also be used for intestinal dryness, constipation, edema, thoracic and abdominal hydrops, damp–heat jaundice, epilepsy and other diseases. Common antitussive and antiasthmatic drugs include bitter almond, perilla seed, sessile stemona root, mulberry bark, pepperweed seed, etc. (Table 10–19).

表 10–19　常见止咳平喘药

Table 10–19　Common antitussive and antiasthmatic drugs

药名 Drug name	药性 Medicinal properties	功效 Efficacy	主治 Indications	用法用量 Usage and Dosage
苦杏仁 Bitter almond	苦，微温；有小毒。归肺、大肠经 Bitter, slightly warm; Small poison. Return to lung and large intestine meridian	降气止咳平喘，润肠通便 Lowering qi, relieving cough and asthma, moistening intestines and laxative	咳嗽气喘，胸满痰多；肠燥便秘 Cough and asthma, chest full of phlegm; Intestinal dryness and constipation	煎服，5～10g；生品入煎剂宜后下 Decoction, 5-10g; The raw product should be put into the decoction later
紫苏子 Perilla seed	辛，温。归肺经 Pungent, warm. Return to lung meridian	降气化痰，止咳平喘，润肠通便 Lowering qi and resolving phlegm, relieving cough and asthma, moistening intestines and laxative	痰多气逆，咳嗽气喘；肠燥便秘 Excessive phlegm and reverse qi, cough and asthma; Intestinal dryness and constipation	煎服，3～10g；或煮粥食，或入丸、散 Decoction, 3-10g; Or cook porridge, or add pills or powder
百部 Sessile stemona root	甘、苦，微温。归肺经 Sweet, bitter, slightly warm. Return to lung meridian	润肺下气止咳，杀虫灭虱 Moistening lung qi, relieving cough, killing insects and lice	新久咳嗽、百日咳、肺痨咳嗽；蛲虫、头虱、体虱 New cough, whooping cough, tuberculosis cough; Pinworms, head lice, body lice	3～9g；外用适量，水煎或酒浸；久咳虚嗽宜蜜炙用，杀虫灭虱宜生用 3-9g; Appropriate amount for external use, decocted in water or soaked in wine; Chronic cough and deficiency cough should be used with honey, and raw use should be used to kill insects and lice
桑白皮 Mulberry white bark	甘，寒。归肺经 Sweet, cold. Return to lung meridian	泻肺平喘，利水消肿 Purge lung and relieve asthma, diuresis and reduce swelling	肺热喘咳；水肿 Lung heat asthma cough; edema	煎服，6～12g；泻肺利水、清肺火宜生用，肺虚咳喘宜蜜炙用 Decoction, 6-12g; It is suitable for purging lung diuresis and clearing lung fire, and it is suitable for honey burning for cough and asthma due to lung deficiency

续表

药名 Drug name	药性 Medicinal properties	功效 Efficacy	主治 Indications	用法用量 Usage and Dosage
葶苈子 Pepperweed seed	辛、苦，大寒。归肺、膀胱经 Pungent, bitter, cold. Return to lung and bladder meridian	泻肺平喘，行水消肿 Purge lung and relieve asthma, circulate water and reduce swelling	痰涎壅肺，喘咳痰多，胸胁胀满，不得平卧；胸腹水肿，小便不利 Phlegm and saliva obstruct the lungs, wheezing and coughing, excessive phlegm, full chest and hypochondrium, and not lie down; Thoracic and abdominal edema, difficulty urinating	煎服，3～10g，包煎；研末服，3～6g Decoction, 3-10g, wrapped and decocted; Grind into powder and take, 3-6g

十四、安神药
14 Tranquilizing medicine

凡以安定神志为主要功效，主要用于心神不宁病证的药物，称为安神药。

Drugs whose main effect is to calm the mind and are mainly used for restless diseases are called tranquilizing medicines.

本类药物主归心、肝经，多具沉降之性。功能宁心安神。部分药物兼能平肝潜阳、纳气平喘、解毒、活血、敛汗、润肠、祛痰等。

This class of drugs mainly return to the heart and liver meridians, and most of them have sedimentation properties. Function Calms the mind and calms the nerves. Some drugs can calm the liver and suppress yang, absorb qi and relieve asthma, detoxify, activate blood circulation, restrain sweat, moisten intestines, expectorant, etc.

安神药主要用于心神不宁证，症见心悸、怔忡、失眠、多梦、健忘；亦可作为惊风、癫痫、癫狂等病证的辅助药物。部分安神药尚可用于肝阳上亢、肾虚气喘、疮疡肿毒、瘀血、自汗盗汗、肠燥便秘、痰多咳喘等。

Tranquilizing medicines are mainly used for restless syndrome, which includes palpitations, palpitations, insomnia, dreaminess, and forgetfulness; It can also be used as an auxiliary drug for convulsion, epilepsy, madness and other diseases. Some tranquilizing drugs can still be used for hyperactivity of liver yang, kidney deficiency and asthma, sores and swelling, blood stasis, spontaneous sweating and night sweats, intestinal dryness and constipation, cough and asthma with excessive phlegm, etc.

本类药物中有部分需入丸、散剂服用，应适当配伍健运脾胃之品，不宜久服；入煎剂宜打碎久煎。个别药物有毒，当控制用量，以防中毒。安神药多为治标之品，故应配伍消除病因治本之品。常见安神药包括酸枣仁、远志、龙骨等（表 10–20）。

Some of these drugs need to be taken in pills and powders, which should be appropriately compatible with medicinals that strengthen the spleen and stomach, and should not be taken for a long time; The decoction should be broken and decocted for a long time. Individual drugs are toxic, so the dosage should be controlled to prevent poisoning. Tranquilizing drugs are mostly symptomatic medicinals, so they should be combined with medicinals that eliminate the cause and cure the root cause. Common tranquilizing drugs include Ziziphus jujube kernel, Polygala, Keel, etc. (Table 10–20).

表 10–20　常见安神药

Table 10–20　Common tranquilizing drugs

药名 Drug name	药性 Medicinal properties	功效 Efficacy	主治 Indications	用法用量 Usage and Dosage
酸枣仁 Ziziphus jujube kernel	甘、酸，平。归肝、胆、心经 Sweet, sour, flat. Return to liver, gallbladder and heart meridians	养心补肝，宁心安神，敛汗，生津 Nourish the heart and tonify the liver, calm the heart and calm the nerves, restrain sweat, promote fluid production	虚烦不眠，惊悸多梦；体虚多汗；津伤口渴 Annoyance, sleeplessness, palpitations and dreams; Physical weakness and excessive sweating; Fluid injury thirst	煎服，10～15g Decoction, 10-15g
远志 Polygala	苦、辛，温。归心、肾、肺经 Bitter, pungent, warm. Return to the heart, kidney and lung meridians	安神益智，交通心肾，祛痰，消肿 Tranquilize the nerves and improve intelligence, communicate the heart and kidney, expectorant, reduce swelling	失眠，心悸；咳嗽痰多；疮疡肿毒，乳房肿痛 Insomnia, palpitations; Cough with excessive phlegm; Sores, swelling and poison, breast swelling and pain	煎服，3～10g Decoction, 3-10g
龙骨 Keel	甘、涩，平。归心、肝、肾经 Sweet, astringent, flat. Return to the heart, liver and kidney meridians	镇惊安神，平肝潜阳，收敛固涩 Calm the nerves, calm the liver and diminish yang, converge and solidify astringency	心神不安，心悸失眠，惊痫癫狂；肝阳上亢，头晕目眩；滑脱诸证；湿疮湿疹，疮疡溃后不敛 Restlessness, palpitations, insomnia, epilepsy and madness; Hyperactivity of liver yang, dizziness; Slipping away from all kinds of syndromes; Wet sore eczema, the sore does not converge after ulceration	煎服，15～30g，宜先煎；外用适量 Decoction, 15-30g, it is advisable to decoct first; Appropriate amount for external use

十五、平肝息风药

15 Medicine for calming the liver and calming the wind

凡以平肝潜阳、息风止痉为主要功效，主要用于肝阳上亢或肝风内动病证的药物，称为平肝息风药。

All drugs that have the main effects of calming the liver and suppressing yang, calming wind and relieving spasm, and are mainly used for hyperactivity of liver yang or internal movement of liver wind, are called calming liver and calming wind drugs.

本类药物皆归肝经，药性多寒凉，少数药性平或偏温，功效为平肝潜阳（或平抑肝阳）、息风止痉。

These drugs all belong to the liver meridian, and the medicinal properties are mostly cold and cold, while a few are mild or warm. The efficacy is to calm the liver and suppress the yang (or calm the liver yang), calm wind and stop spasm.

平肝息风药主要用于肝阳上亢，头晕目眩，以及肝风内动，痉挛抽搐证。

Pinggan Xifeng medicine is mainly used for hyperactivity of liver yang, dizziness, internal movement of liver wind, spasm and convulsion syndrome.

本类药物有性偏寒凉或性偏温燥之不同，故应区别使用。如脾虚慢惊者，不宜使用寒凉之品；阴虚血亏者，当忌温燥之品；阳气下陷者，亦忌用本类药物。

This class of drugs has different sex cold or sex warm and dry, so they should be used differently. For example, those with spleen deficiency and slow shock should not use cold medicinals; those with yin deficiency and blood deficiency should avoid warm and dry medicinals; those with depression of yang qi should also avoid using this kind of drugs.

（一）平抑肝阳药

15.1 Medicine to calm liver yang

本类药物多为质重之介类或矿石类药物，部分为植物药，具有平肝潜阳或平抑肝阳功效，主治肝阳上亢证，症见头晕、头痛、目胀、舌质红、舌苔黄或少苔、脉弦数。常见平抑肝阳药如石决明、牡蛎、代赭石等（表 10–21）。

Most of these drugs are heavy intermediate or mineral drugs, some of which are botanical drugs, which have the effect of calming the liver and suppressing the liver yang. They are mainly used to treat the syndrome of hyperactivity of liver yang, including dizziness, headache, eye swelling, red tongue, yellow tongue coating or less coating, and stringy pulse. Common drugs to calm liver yang such as concha haliotidis, oyster, ochre, etc. (Table 10–21).

表 10–21　常见平抑肝阳药

Table 10–21　Common drugs for stabilizing liver yang

药名 Drug name	药性 Medicinal properties	功效 Efficacy	主治 Indications	用法用量 Usage and Dosage
石决明 Concha haliotidis	咸，寒。归肝经 Salty, cold. Return to liver meridian	平肝潜阳，清肝明目 Calming the liver and diminishing yang, clearing the liver and improving eyesight	肝阳上亢，头痛眩晕；目赤翳障，视物昏花，青盲雀目 Hyperactivity of liver yang, headache and dizziness; The eyes are red and blind, the vision is dim, and the eyes of the bird are blue and blind	煎服，6～20g Decoction, 6-20g
牡蛎 Oyster	咸、微寒。归肝、胆、肾经 Salty and slightly cold. Return to liver, gallbladder and kidney meridians	潜阳补阴，重镇安神，软坚散结 Hidden yang and tonify yin, calm the nerves, soften hardness and dissipate stagnation	肝阳上亢，头晕目眩；心神不安，惊悸失眠；痰核，瘰疬，瘿瘕积聚；滑脱诸症；胃痛泛酸 Hyperactivity of liver yang, dizziness; Uneasiness, palpitations and insomnia; Phlegm nucleus, scrofula, accumulation of symptoms; Symptoms of spondylolisthesis; Stomach pain Pantothenic acid	煎服，9～30g Decoction, 9-30g
代赭石 Ochre	苦，寒。归肝、心、肺、胃经 Bitter, cold. Return to liver, heart, lung and stomach meridians	平肝潜阳，重镇降逆，凉血止血 Calming the liver and suppressing yang, reducing adverse, cooling blood and stopping bleeding	肝阳上亢，头晕目眩；呕吐，呃逆，噫气；气逆喘息；血热吐衄，崩漏 Hyperactivity of liver yang, dizziness; vomiting, hiccups, breathing; Breathing reverse; Blood heat vomiting epistaxis, metrorrhagia	煎服，9～30g Decoction, 9-30g

（二）息风止痉药

15.2 Wind-relieving and antispasmodic drugs

本类药物主归肝经，多系虫类药，以息肝风、止痉挛抽搐为主要功效。用于温热病热极生风证、肝阳化风证及血虚肝风内动等所致眩晕欲仆、痉挛抽搐、项强肢颤、口眼㖞斜、半身不遂、癫痫、惊风抽搐及破伤风。常见息风止痉药包括羚羊角、牛黄、钩藤、天麻等（表 10–22）。

This kind of drugs mainly belong to the liver meridian, and are mostly worm–like drugs. Its main effects are to relieve liver wind and stop spasms and convulsions. It is used for dizziness, cramps and convulsions, stiff neck and limb tremors, facial paralysis, hemiplegia, epilepsy, convulsions and tetanus caused by warm fever disease, syndrome of extreme heat generating wind, syndrome of hyperactive liver yang causing wind, and internal movement of liver wind due to blood deficiency. Common wind–relieving and antispasmodic drugs include antelope horn, bezoar, uncaria, gastrodia elata, etc. (Table 10–22).

表 10–22 常见息风止痉药

Table 10–22 Common wind-relieving and antispasmodic drugs

药名 Drug name	药性 Medicinal properties	功效 Efficacy	主治 Indications	用法用量 Usage and Dosage
羚羊角 Antelope horn	咸，寒。归肝、心经 Salty, cold. Return to liver and heart meridian	平肝息风，清肝明目，散血解毒 Calming the liver and relieving wind, clearing the liver and improving eyesight, dispersing blood and detoxifying	肝风内动，惊痫抽搐；肝阳上亢，头晕目眩；肝火上炎，目赤头痛，温热病壮热神昏，温毒发斑 Internal movement of liver wind, epilepsy and convulsions; Hyperactivity of liver yang, dizziness; Inflammation of liver fire, red eyes and headache, warm fever disease, strong heat and unconsciousness, warm toxin spots	煎服，1～3g，单煎2小时以上，取汁服；磨汁或研粉服，每次0.3～0.6g Decoction, 1-3g, single decoction for more than 2 hours, take the juice and take it; Grind juice or powder, 0.3-0.6g each time
牛黄 bezoar	甘，凉。归心、肝经 Sweet, cool. Guixin and liver meridian	清心豁痰，开窍凉肝，息风解毒 Clear the heart and eliminate phlegm, open the resuscitation and cool the liver, calm wind and detoxify	壮热神昏、惊厥抽搐；神昏、口噤、痰鸣；咽喉肿痛、溃烂及痈疽疔毒 Strong heat, unconsciousness, convulsions and convulsions; Daze, silence of the mouth, phlegm; Throat swelling, ulceration and carbuncle furunculosis	入丸散，每次0.15～0.35g Pill or powder, 0.15-0.35 g each time
钩藤 Uncaria	甘，凉。归肝、心包经 Sweet, cool. Return to liver and pericardium meridian	息风定惊，清热平肝 Calm wind and calm shock, clear away heat and calm liver	肝风内动，惊痫抽搐；头痛，眩晕；风热表证 Internal movement of liver wind, epilepsy and convulsions; Headache, dizziness; wind-heat exterior syndrome	煎服，3～12g，不宜久煎 Decoction, 3-12g, not suitable for long-term decoction
天麻 Gastrodia elata	甘，平，趋向沉降。归肝经 Sweet, flat, tends to settle. Return to liver meridian	息风止痉，平抑肝阳，祛风通络 Relieving wind and relieving spasm, calming liver yang, dispelling wind and dredging collaterals	肝风内动，惊痫抽搐；眩晕，头痛；中风手足不遂，风湿痹痛 Internal movement of liver wind, epilepsy and convulsions; Vertigo, headache; Stroke hand and foot insufficiency, rheumatic arthralgia	煎服，3～10g Decoction, 3-10g

十六、开窍药

16 Resuscitation drugs

凡具辛香走窜之性，以开窍醒神为主要作用，主要用于闭证神昏的药物，称为开窍药。

All drugs with pungent fragrance and wandering nature, which have the main function of enlightening the resuscitation and refreshing the mind, are mainly used for closed syndrome and unconsciousness, and are called resuscitation drugs.

本类药物气多辛香而善走窜，药性或温或凉，皆归心经，具有开窍醒神的作用。

This kind of medicine is spicy and fragrant, and it is good to walk, and its medicinal properties are either warm or cool, all of which return to the heart meridian, and it has the effect of enlightening the resuscitation and refreshing the mind.

开窍药主要治疗外感六淫之邪陷心包，或痰饮、湿浊、瘀血等蒙蔽心窍所致的神昏病证，症见谵语、惊风、癫痫、中风等猝然昏厥、痉挛抽搐等。

The resuscitation medicine mainly treats the syndrome of unconsciousness caused by exogenous pathogens of six obscenities trapped in the pericardium, or blinding the resuscitation caused by phlegm, dampness, blood stasis, etc. The symptoms include sudden fainting, spasm and convulsion such as delirium, convulsion, epilepsy, and stroke.

本类药物多为救急、治标之品，且能耗气而伤阴，故只宜暂服，不可久用。因本类药物气多辛香，其有效成分易于挥发，内服宜入丸、散剂，不宜入煎剂。常见开窍药包括麝香、石菖蒲等（表 10–23）。

Most of these drugs are emergency and palliative medicinals, and they consume energy and damage yin, so they should only be taken temporarily and not used for a long time. Because this kind of medicine is spicy and fragrant, its active ingredients are easy to volatilize, so it should be taken orally in pills and powders, not in decoction. Common resuscitation drugs include musk, Acorus calamus, etc. (Table 10–23).

表 10–23 常见开窍药

Table 10–23 Common resuscitation drugs

药名 Drug name	药性 Medicinal properties	功效 Efficacy	主治 Indications	用法用量 Usage and Dosage
麝香 Musk	辛，温。归心、脾经 Pungent, warm. Return to heart and spleen meridian	开窍醒神，活血通经，消肿止痛 Opening resuscitation and refreshing mind, promoting blood circulation and dredging menstruation, reducing swelling and relieving pain	闭证神昏；胸痹心痛，癥瘕积聚，血瘀经闭，跌打损伤，风湿痹痛；疮疡肿毒，瘰疬痰核，咽喉肿痛；难产，死胎，胞衣不下 Closed syndrome of unconsciousness; Chest paralysis and heartache, accumulation of symptoms, blood stasis and amenorrhea, bruises and injuries, rheumatic paralysis; Sores, swelling and poison, scrofula, phlegm nucleus, sore throat; Dystocia, stillbirth, placenta retension	入丸散，不宜入煎剂，每次 0.03～0.1g Pill or powder, not decoction, 0.03-0.1g each time

续表

药名 Drug name	药性 Medicinal properties	功效 Efficacy	主治 Indications	用法用量 Usage and Dosage
石菖蒲 Acorus calamus	辛、苦，温。归心、胃经 Pungent, bitter, warm. Return to heart and stomach meridian	开窍豁痰，醒神益智，化湿开胃 Opening the resuscitation and eliminating phlegm, refreshing the mind and improving intelligence, removing dampness and appetizing	痰迷心窍，神昏癫痫；健忘，失眠，心悸，眩晕，嗜睡；耳鸣，耳聋，失音；霍乱，腹痛，痞满，带下，下利 Phlegm obsesses with the heart orifices, unconsciousness and epilepsy; Forgetfulness, insomnia, palpitations, dizziness, lethargy; Tinnitus, deafness, aphonia; Cholera, abdominal pain, fullness, abnormal vaginal discharge, diarrhea	煎服，3 ~ 10g Decoction, 3-10g

十七、补虚药
17 Tonic medicine

凡以补虚扶弱，纠正人体气血阴阳虚衰为主要功效，主要用于虚证的药物，称为补虚药。

Drugs that are mainly used for deficiency syndrome are called tonic drugs with the main effects of tonifying deficiency and strengthening the weak and correcting the deficiency and failure of qi, blood, yin and yang in the human body.

本类药物味多甘，性分温、寒，补气药大多归脾、肺经，补阳药多归肾经，补血药多归心、肝经，补阴药多归肺、胃、肝、肾经。功能补虚扶弱，具体又有补气、补阳、补血、补阴之别。

This class of drugs is sweet in taste, warm and cold in nature. Most of the qi–tonifying drugs belong to the spleen and lung meridians, the yang–tonifying drugs belong to the kidney meridians, the blood–tonifying drugs belong to the heart and liver meridians, and the yin–tonifying drugs belong to the lung, stomach, liver and kidney meridians. The function of tonifying the deficiency and strengthening the weak is specifically divided into tonifying qi, yang, blood and yin.

补虚药主要用于虚证。虚证的临床表现比较复杂，但就其“证型”概括起来，不外气虚、阳虚、血虚、阴虚 4 类。

Tonic drugs are mainly used for deficiency syndrome. The clinical manifestations of deficiency syndrome are complicated, but in terms of its “syndrome types”, there are only four categories: qi deficiency, yang deficiency, blood deficiency and yin deficiency.

本类药物原为虚证而设，凡身体健康，并无虚弱表现者，不宜滥用，以免导致阴阳平衡失调，气血不和，“误补益疾”。实邪方盛，正气未虚者，以祛邪为要，亦不宜用本类药物，以免“闭门留寇”。

This class of drugs was originally designed for deficiency syndrome. Those who are healthy and have no symptoms of weakness should not be abused, so as not to lead to imbalance of yin and yang, disharmony of qi and blood, and "mistakenly tonifying diseases". If the actual evil prescription is abundant and the righteousness is not deficient, it is important to eliminate the evil, and it is not appropriate to use this kind of drugs to avoid "closed doors and keeping bandits".

（一）补气药

17.1 Qi-tonifying medicine

本类药物性味多甘温或平，主归肺、脾经，以补脾气和补肺气为主，部分药物能补心气、补肾气，个别药物能补元气，主要治疗脾气虚证、肺气虚证、心气虚证、肾气虚证等。常见补气药包括人参、党参、黄芪、白术、甘草等（表 10–24）。

These drugs are sweet, warm or flat in nature and taste, mainly belong to the lung and spleen meridians, and mainly replenish spleen qi and lung qi. Some drugs can replenish heart qi and kidney qi, and some drugs can replenish vitality qi. They mainly treat spleen qi deficiency syndrome, lung qi deficiency syndrome, heart qi deficiency syndrome, kidney qi deficiency syndrome, etc. Common qi–invigorating drugs include Panax ginseng, Codonopsis pilosula, Astragalus membranaceus, Atractylodes macrocephala, licorice, etc. (Table 10–24).

表 10–24 常见补气药

Table 10–24 Common qi–tonifying drugs

药名 Drug name	药性 Medicinal properties	功效 Efficacy	主治 Indications	用法用量 Usage and Dosage
人参 Panax ginseng	甘、微苦，微温。归脾、肺、心、肾经 Sweet, slightly bitter, slightly warm. Returns to the spleen, lung, heart and kidney meridians	大补元气，复脉固脱，补脾益肺，生津养血，安神益智 Greatly tonify vitality, restore pulse and solidify detoxification, tonify spleen and lung, promote fluid production and nourish blood, tranquilize nerves and improve intelligence	元气虚极欲脱证；脾肺气虚证；热病气虚津伤口渴及消渴证；心悸，失眠，健忘；阳痿，宫冷 Yuan qi deficiency is extremely desirable to get rid of the syndrome; Spleen and lung qi deficiency syndrome; Fever disease, qi deficiency and fluid injury, thirst and diabetes syndrome; Palpitations, insomnia, forgetfulness; Impotence, uterine cold	另煎兑服，3～9g；也可研粉吞服，1 次 2g，1 日 2 次 Decoction and take separately, 3-9g; It can also be swallowed as powder, 2g once, 2 times a day
党参 codonopsis pilosula	甘，平。归脾、肺经 Sweet, flat. Return to spleen and lung meridians	补脾益肺，养血生津 Tonifying spleen and lung, nourishing blood and promoting fluid production	脾肺气虚证；气津两伤证；气血两虚证 Spleen and lung qi deficiency syndrome; Syndrome of injury of qi and fluid; Syndrome of deficiency of both qi and blood	煎服，9～30g Decoction, 9-30g

续表

药名 Drug name	药性 Medicinal properties	功效 Efficacy	主治 Indications	用法用量 Usage and Dosage
黄芪 Astragalus	甘，微温。归脾、肺经 Sweet, slightly warm. Return to spleen and lung meridians	补气升阳，固表止汗，利水消肿，生津养血，行滞通痹，托毒排脓，敛疮生肌 Invigorate qi and ascend yang, solidify surface and stop perspiration, promote diuresis and reduce swelling, promote fluid production and nourish blood, promote stagnation and dredge arthralgia, support poison and discharge pus, restrain sores and develop muscles	脾胃气虚及中气下陷诸证；肺气虚及表虚自汗；气虚外感诸证，气虚浮肿，小便不利；血虚证，气血两虚证；消渴证；关节痹痛，肢体麻木或半身不遂；痈疽难溃或久溃不敛 Syndromes of spleen and stomach qi deficiency and middle qi depression; Lung qi deficiency and spontaneous sweating due to superficial deficiency; Exogenous syndromes of qi deficiency, qi deficiency and edema, and difficult urination; Blood deficiency syndrome, qi and blood deficiency syndrome; Diabetes syndrome; Joint pain, numbness or hemiplegia of limbs; Carbuncle is difficult to collapse or does not collapse for a long time	煎服，9～30g Decoction, 9-30g
白术 Atractylodes macrocephala	甘，苦，温。归脾、胃经 Sweet, bitter, warm. Return to spleen and stomach meridians	健脾益气，燥湿利水，止汗，安胎 Invigorating spleen and replenishing qi, drying dampness and diuresis, antiperspirant, and preventing fetal fetus	脾气虚证；痰饮水肿；气虚自汗；胎动不安 Syndrome of spleen qi deficiency; Sputum and drinking swelling; Spontaneous sweating due to qi deficiency; Fetal restlessness	煎服，6～12g Decoction, 6-12g
甘草 licorice	甘，平。归心、肺、脾、胃经 Sweet, flat. Return to the heart, lung, spleen and stomach meridians	补脾益气，清热解毒，祛痰止咳，缓急止痛，调和诸药 Tonifying spleen and replenishing qi, clearing away heat and toxic materials, eliminating phlegm and relieving cough, relieving urgency and pain, and reconciling various medicines	心气不足的心动悸，脉结代；脾气虚证；痰多咳嗽；脘腹及四肢挛急作痛；热毒疮疡，咽喉肿痛及药物、食物中毒 Heart palpitations due to insufficient heart qi, pulse knot generation; Syndrome of spleen qi deficiency; Cough with excessive phlegm; Acute cramps and pain in the epigastric abdomen and limbs; Heat toxin sore, sore throat and drug and food poisoning	煎服，2～10g Decoction, 2-10g

（二）补血药

17.2 Blood-tonifying drugs

本类药物性味多甘温质润，主归心、肝经，具有滋补阴血功效，主要用于血虚证，症见面色苍白无华或萎黄，心悸怔忡，失眠，健忘，眩晕，耳鸣，双目干涩，月经愆期、量少色淡，唇甲色淡，舌淡苔白，脉细等。常见补血药包括当归、熟地黄、阿胶、何首乌、白芍等（表 10–25）。

The main body is to be used for the mainstream of the globe of the Common blood–tonic drugs include Angelica sinensis, Rehmannia glutinosa, donkey–hide gelatin, Polygonum multiflorum, Radix paeoniae alba, etc. (Table 10–25).

表 10–25 常见补血药

Table 10–25 Common blood–tonifying drugs

药名 Drug name	药性 Medicinal properties	功效 Efficacy	主治 Indications	用法用量 Usage and Dosage
当归 Angelica sinensis	甘、辛，温。归肝、心、脾经 Sweet, pungent, warm. Return to liver, heart and spleen meridians	补血活血，调经止痛，润肠通便 Enriching blood and promoting blood circulation, regulating menstruation and relieving pain, moistening intestines and relaxing constipation	血虚萎黄，眩晕心悸；月经不调，经闭痛经；虚寒腹痛，风湿痹痛，跌仆损伤，痈疽疮疡；肠燥便秘 Blood deficiency and chlorosis, dizziness and palpitations; Irregular menstruation, amenorrhea and dysmenorrhea; Abdominal pain due to deficiency and cold, rheumatic arthralgia, falling injury, carbuncle ulcer; Intestinal dryness and constipation	煎服，6～12g Decoction, 6-12g
熟地黄 Rehmannia glutinosa	甘，微温。归肝、肾经 Sweet, slightly warm. Return to liver and kidney meridians	补血滋阴，益精填髓 Enriching blood and nourishing yin, replenishing essence and filling marrow	血虚萎黄，心悸怔忡，月经不调，崩漏下血；肝肾阴虚，腰膝酸软，骨蒸潮热，盗汗遗精，内热消渴；肝肾亏虚，精血不足，眩晕耳鸣，须发早白 Blood deficiency and chlorosis, palpitations, irregular menstruation, metrorrhagia and bleeding; Liver and kidney yin deficiency, soreness and weakness of waist and knees, bone steaming and tidal fever, night sweats and spermatorrhea, internal heat to quench thirst; Deficiency of liver and kidney, insufficient essence and blood, dizziness and tinnitus, premature graying of beard and hair	煎服，9～15g Decoction, 9-15g
阿胶 Donkey-hide gelatin	甘，平。归肺、肝、肾经 Gan, Ping. Return to lung, liver and kidney meridians	补血滋阴，润燥止血 Enriching blood and nourishing yin, moistening dryness and stopping bleeding	血虚萎黄，眩晕心悸，肌痿无力；热病阴伤，心烦不眠，虚风内动，手足瘛疭；肺燥咳嗽，劳嗽咯血；吐血衄血，尿血便血，崩漏下血，妊娠胎漏 Blood deficiency and chlorosis, dizziness and palpitations, muscle weakness; Fever, yin injury, upset and sleeplessness, internal movement of deficiency wind, and hands and feet; Lung dryness and cough, fatigue cough and hemoptysis; Hematemesis and epistaxis, hematuria and hematochezia, hemorrhagia, pregnancy and fetal leakage	3～9g，烊化兑服 3-9g, closed and taken

续表

药名 Drug name	药性 Medicinal properties	功效 Efficacy	主治 Indications	用法用量 Usage and Dosage
何首乌 Polygonum multiflorum	苦、甘、涩，微温。归肝、心、肾经 Bitter, sweet, astringent, slightly warm. Returns to the liver, heart and kidney meridians.	制何首乌：补肝肾，益精血，乌须发，强筋骨，化浊降脂。生何首乌：解毒，消痈，截疟，润肠通便 Preparation of Polygonum multiflorum: tonifying liver and kidney, replenishing essence and blood, blackening beard and hair, strengthening muscles and bones, resolving turbidity and lowering lipids. Raw Polygonum multiflorum: detoxification, elimination of carbuncle, interception of malaria, moistening intestines and laxative	血虚萎黄，眩晕耳鸣，须发早白，腰膝酸软，肢体麻木，崩漏带下；疮痈、瘰疬、风疹瘙痒；久疟体虚；肠燥便秘 Blood deficiency and chlorosis, dizziness and tinnitus, premature graying of beard and hair, soreness and weakness of waist and knees, numbness of limbs, and metrorrhagia; Sore carbuncle, scrofula, rubella itching; Chronic malaria and physical weakness; Intestinal dryness and constipation	制何首乌：煎服，6～12g；生何首乌：煎服，3～6g Preparation of Polygonum multiflorum: Decoction, 6-12g; Raw Polygonum multiflorum: Decoction, 3-6g
白芍 Radix paeoniae alba	苦、酸，微寒。归肝、脾经 Bitter, sour, slightly cold. Return to liver and spleen meridians	养血调经，敛阴止汗，柔肝止痛，平抑肝阳 Nourish blood and regulate menstruation, restrain yin and stop perspiration, soften liver and relieve pain, and calm liver yang	血虚萎黄，月经不调，崩漏下血；自汗、盗汗；胁痛、腹痛、四肢挛痛；肝阳上亢，头痛眩晕 Blood deficiency and chlorosis, irregular menstruation, metrorrhagia and bleeding; Spontaneous sweating, night sweats; Hypochondriac pain, abdominal pain, limb cramps; Hyperactivity of liver yang, headache and dizziness	煎服，6～15g Decoction, 6-15g

（三）补阴药

17.3 Yin-tonifying drugs

本类药物性味多甘寒（凉），主归肺、胃、肝、肾经，有滋补阴液、清热润燥功效，主治肺、胃、肝、肾等脏腑阴虚证，见皮肤、咽喉、口鼻、眼目干燥或肠燥便秘等阴液不足或午后潮热、盗汗、五心烦热、两颧发红等阴虚内热症状。常见补阴药包括北沙参、麦冬、龟甲、鳖甲等（表10–26）。

This kind of medicine is sweet and cold (cool) in nature and taste, mainly belongs to the lung, stomach, liver and kidney meridians, and has the effects of nourishing yin liquid, clearing away heat and moistening dryness. It is mainly used to treat yin deficiency syndrome of lung, stomach, liver and kidney and other internal heat symptoms of yin deficiency such as skin, throat, nose and mouth, dry eyes or intestinal dryness and constipation, or tidal fever in the afternoon, night sweats, dysphoria with feverish sensation in chest, palms and soles, and redness of both zygomatic bones. Common yin-tonifying drugs include Adenophora ginseng, Ophiopogon japonicus, tortoise shell, turtle shell, etc. (Table 10-26).

表 10-26 常见补阴药

Table 10-26 Common yin-tonifying drugs

药名 **Drug name**	药性 **Medicinal properties**	功效 **Efficacy**	主治 **Indications**	用法用量 **Usage and Dosage**
北沙参 Adenophora northern	甘、微苦，微寒。归肺、胃经 Sweet, slightly bitter, slightly cold. Return to lung and stomach meridians	养阴清肺，益胃生津 Nourishing yin and clearing lung, benefiting stomach and promoting fluid production	肺阴虚证；胃阴虚证 Lung yin deficiency syndrome; Syndrome of stomach yin deficiency	煎服，5～12g Decoction, 5-12g
麦冬 Ophiopogon japonicus	甘、微苦，微寒。归心、肺、胃经 Sweet, slightly bitter, slightly cold. Return to the heart, lung and stomach meridians	养阴生津，润肺清心 Nourishing yin and promoting fluid production, moistening lung and clearing heart	胃阴虚证；肺阴虚证；心阴虚证 Stomach yin deficiency syndrome; Lung yin deficiency syndrome; Heart yin deficiency syndrome	煎服，6～12g Decoction, 6-12g
龟甲 tortoise shell	咸、甘，微寒。归肝、肾、心经 Salty, sweet and slightly cold. Return to liver, kidney and heart meridians	滋阴潜阳，益肾强骨，养血补心，固经止崩 Nourishing yin and hiding yang, nourishing kidney and strengthening bones, nourishing blood and nourishing heart, strengthening meridian and stopping collapse	肝肾阴虚证；肾虚筋骨痿弱；阴血亏虚之惊悸、失眠、健忘；月经量多 Liver and kidney yin deficiency syndrome; Kidney deficiency and weakness of muscles and bones; Palpitations, insomnia and forgetfulness caused by yin and blood deficiency; Heavy menstrual flow	煎服，9～24g，宜打碎先煎 Decoction, 9-24g, it is advisable to break and decoct first
鳖甲 Turtle shell	咸，微寒。归肝、肾经 Salty, slightly cold. Return to liver and kidney meridians	滋阴潜阳，退热除蒸，软坚散结 Nourishing yin and hiding yang, reducing fever and removing steam, softening hardness and dispersing stagnation	肝肾阴虚证；癥瘕积聚，久疟疟母 Liver and kidney yin deficiency syndrome; Accumulation of symptoms, chronic malaria	煎服，9～24g，宜先煎 Decoction, 9-24g, it is advisable to decoct first

（四）补阳药

17.4 Yang tonic medicine

本类药物味多甘辛咸，性温热，主归肾经。以温补肾阳为主要功效，主治肾阳虚证，症见形寒肢冷、腰膝酸软、性欲淡漠、阳痿早泄、遗精滑精、尿频遗尿、宫寒不孕。常见补阳药包括鹿茸、淫羊藿、杜仲、续断、菟丝子等（表 10–27）。

This kind of medicine is sweet, pungent and salty in taste, warm and hot in nature, and mainly belongs to the kidney meridian. With the main effect of warming and tonifying kidney yang, it is mainly used to treat kidney yang deficiency syndrome, with symptoms such as cold body and limbs, soreness and weakness of waist and knees, apathy of sexual desire, impotence and premature ejaculation, spermatorrhea and slippery spermatorrhea, frequent urination and enuresis, and infertility due to uterine cold. Common yang–tonifying drugs include velvet antler, epimedium, eucommia ulmoides, Dipscaci radix, dodder, etc. (Table 10–27).

表 10–27　常见补阳药

Table 10–27　Common Yang–tonifying drugs

药名 Drug name	药性 Medicinal properties	功效 Efficacy	主治 Indications	用法用量 Usage and Dosage
鹿茸 Velvet antler	甘、咸，温。归肾、肝经 Sweet, salty, warm. Return to kidney and liver meridians	壮肾阳，益精血，强筋骨，调冲任，托疮毒 Strengthening kidney yang, replenishing essence and blood, strengthening muscles and bones, regulating Chong Ren, and supporting sore poison	肾阳不足，精血亏虚，阳痿滑精，宫冷不孕；腰脊冷痛，筋骨痿软；冲任虚寒，崩漏带下；阴疽不敛 Insufficient kidney yang, essence and blood deficiency, impotence and slippery sperm, uterine cold infertility; Cold pain in the lumbar spine, weak muscles and bones; Chong Ren deficiency cold, metrorrhagia belt; Yin gangrene does not converge	研末冲服，1～2g Grind into powder and take, 1-2g
淫羊藿 Epimedium	辛、甘，温。归肝、肾经 Pungent, sweet, warm. Return to liver and kidney meridians	补肾阳，强筋骨，祛风湿 Tonify kidney yang, strengthen muscles and bones, and dispel rheumatism	肾阳虚衰，阳痿遗精，筋骨痿软；风湿痹痛，麻木拘挛 Kidney yang deficiency, impotence and spermatorrhea, muscle and bone weakness; Rheumatic arthralgia, numbness and convulsion	煎服，6～10g Decoction, 6-10g
杜仲 Eucommia ulmoides	甘、温。归肝、肾经 Sweet, warm. Return to liver and kidney meridians	补肝肾，强筋骨，安胎 Tonify liver and kidney, strengthen muscles and bones, and prevent fetus	肝肾不足，腰膝酸痛，筋骨无力，头晕目眩；肝肾亏虚，妊娠漏血，胎动不安 Liver and kidney deficiency, soreness of waist and knees, weakness of muscles and bones, dizziness; Liver and kidney deficiency, blood leakage during pregnancy, fetal movement restlessness	煎服，6～10g Decoction, 6-10g

续表

药名 Drug name	药性 Medicinal properties	功效 Efficacy	主治 Indications	用法用量 Usage and Dosage
续断 Dipscaci radix	苦、辛，微温。归肝、肾经 Bitter, pungent, slightly warm. Return to liver and kidney meridians	补肝肾，强筋骨，续折伤，止崩漏 Tonify liver and kidney, strengthen muscles and bones, continue fracture and injury, and stop metrorrhagia	肝肾不足，腰膝酸软，风湿痹痛；跌仆损伤，筋伤骨折；肝肾亏虚，崩漏，胎漏，胎动不安 Liver and kidney deficiency, soreness and weakness of waist and knees, rheumatism and arthralgia; Fall injury, tendon injury and fracture; Liver and kidney deficiency, metrorrhagia, fetal leakage, fetal restlessness	煎服，9～15g Decoction, 9-15g
菟丝子 Dodder	辛、甘，平，趋向升浮。归肝、肾、脾经 Xin, sweet, flat, tend to rise and float. Return to liver, kidney and spleen meridians	补益肝肾，固精缩尿，安胎，明目，止泻；外用消风祛斑 Tonify liver and kidney, strengthen essence and reduce urine, prevent fetus, improve eyesight, and stop diarrhea; External use to eliminate wind and remove freckles	肝肾不足，腰膝酸软，阳痿遗精，遗尿尿频；肾虚胎漏，胎动不安；肝肾不足，目暗耳鸣；脾肾虚泻；白癜风 Liver and kidney deficiency, soreness and weakness of waist and knees, impotence and spermatorrhea, enuresis and frequent urination; Kidney deficiency and fetal leakage, fetal movement restlessness; Liver and kidney deficiency, dark eyes and tinnitus; Spleen and kidney deficiency diarrhea; Vitiligo	煎服，6～12g Decoction, 6-12g

十八、收涩药
18 Astringent medicines

凡以收敛固涩为主要功效，主要用于各种滑脱病证的药物，称为收涩药。

All drugs whose main effect is astringent and astringent and are mainly used for various types of spondylolisthesis diseases are called astringent medicines.

本类药物大多味酸涩，性温或平，主归肺、脾、肾、大肠经，具有固表止汗、敛肺止咳、涩肠止泻、固精缩尿、固崩止带等作用。

Most of these drugs are sour and astringent in taste, warm or flat in nature, mainly belong to the lung, spleen, kidney and large intestine meridians, and have the functions of consolidating the surface and stopping perspiration, constraining the lung and relieving cough, astringent intestines and stopping diarrhea, consolidating essence and urination, and consolidating collapse and stopping belt.

收涩药治疗久病体虚、正气不固、脏腑功能衰退所致的自汗盗汗、久咳虚喘、久泻久痢、遗精滑精、遗尿尿频、崩带不止等滑脱不禁的病证。常见收涩药包括五味子、山茱萸、桑螵蛸、乌梅等（表 10–28）。

The astringent medicine can treat spontaneous sweating and night sweats, chronic cough and asthma, chronic diarrhea and chronic dysentery, spermatorrhea and slippery spermatorrhea, frequent enuresis and frequent collapse caused by chronic illness and physical weakness, weakness of healthy qi, and decline of viscera function. Common astringent drugs include Schisandra chinensis, cornus officinalis, mulberry cuttlebone, ebony plum, etc. (Table 10–28).

表 10–28　常见收涩药

Table 10–28　Common astringent drugs

药名 **Drug name**	药性 **Medicinal properties**	功效 **Efficacy**	主治 **Indications**	用法用量 **Usage and Dosage**
五味子 Schisandra chinensis	酸、甘，温。归肺、心、肾经 Sour, sweet, warm. Return to lung, heart and kidney meridians	收敛固涩，益气生津，补肾宁心 Astringent and solidified astringent, replenishing qi and promoting fluid production, tonifying kidney and calming heart	久咳虚喘；自汗盗汗；遗精滑精；久泻不止；津伤口渴，消渴；心悸，失眠，多梦 Chronic cough and asthma; spontaneous night sweats; Spermatorrhea and spermatorrhea; Prolonged diarrhea; Fluid injury thirst, quenching thirst; Palpitations, insomnia, dreaminess	煎服，2～6g Decoction, 2-6g
山茱萸 Cornus officinalis	酸、涩，微温。归肝、肾经 Sour, astringent, slightly warm. Return to liver and kidney meridians	补益肝肾，收涩固脱 Tonify liver and kidney, reduce astringency and solidify detoxification	肝肾不足证；遗精滑精；崩漏带下；大汗不止，体虚欲脱 Liver and kidney deficiency syndrome; Spermatorrhea and spermatorrhea; Under the metrorrhagic zone; Sweating profusely, weakness and desire to wear off	煎服，6～12g；急救固脱，20～30g Decoction, 6-12g; First aid solidification, 20-30g
桑螵蛸 Mulberry cuttlebone	甘、咸，平。归肝、肾经 Sweet, salty, flat. Return to liver and kidney meridians	固精缩尿，补肾助阳 Consolidate essence and reduce urine, tonify kidney and aid yang	遗精滑精，遗尿尿频，白浊；阳痿 Spermatorrhea and slippery spermatorrhea, enuresis, frequent urination, white turbidity; Impotence	煎服，5～10g Decoction, 5-10g
乌梅 ebony plum	酸、涩，平。归肝、脾、肺、大肠经 Sour, astringent, flat. Returns to liver, spleen, lung and large intestine meridians	敛肺涩肠，生津安蛔 Constrain the lungs and astringent intestines, promote fluid production and calm roundworms	肺虚久咳；久泻久痢；蛔厥腹痛，呕吐；虚热消渴；炒炭后能固冲止漏；外敷能消疮毒 Chronic cough due to lung deficiency; Chronic chronic diarrhea and chronic dysentery; Ascaris abdominal pain, vomiting; Deficiency of heat to quench thirst; After frying the charcoal, it can solidify the flushing and stop leakage; External application can eliminate sores	煎服，6～12g，大剂量可用至30g；外用适量 Decoction, 6-12g, large doses can be up to 30g; Appropriate amount for external use

十九、涌吐药
19 Vomiting drugs

凡以促使呕吐为主要功效，主要用于毒物、宿食、痰涎等停滞于胃脘或胸膈以上所致病证的药物，称为涌吐药。

Drugs with the main effect of promoting vomiting are mainly used for poisons, accommodation, phlegm and saliva, etc., which stagnate in the epigastric or above the chest and diaphragm, are called vomiting drugs.

涌吐药味多酸苦辛，性偏寒凉，主归胃经，功效升散涌泄。可用于误食毒物，停留胃中，尚未被吸收，或食积不化，堵塞胃脘，胀满疼痛，或痰涎壅盛，咽喉堵塞，呼吸急促，或痰浊上涌，清窍闭塞，癫痫发狂等证。

Vomiting drugs tastes sour, bitter and pungent, and is cold and cold in nature. It mainly returns to the stomach meridian, and its efficacy rises and disperses. It can be used for ingesting poisons by mistake, staying in the stomach, not being absorbed, or food accumulation, blockage of the epigastric cavity, fullness and pain, or excessive phlegm and salivary, throat blockage, shortness of breath, or turbid phlegm upwelling, obstruction of orifices, epilepsy and madness, etc.

本类药物药力峻猛，刺激性强，且多具毒性，为确保临床用药的安全，宜从小量开始，逐渐增加剂量，中病即止。服药后宜多饮温开水或辅以探吐之法，以助药力。常见涌吐药包括常山、胆矾等（表 10–29）。

This class of drugs is powerful, irritating, and toxic. In order to ensure the safety of clinical medication, it is advisable to start with a small amount and gradually increase the dosage, so as to stop the disease. After taking the medicine, it is advisable to drink more warm boiled water or supplement it with the method of exploring vomiting to help the medicine. Common vomiting drugs include Anti febrile dichroa, bile alum, etc. (Table 10–29).

表 10–29 常见涌吐药

Table 10–29 Common vomiting drugs

药名 **Drug name**	药性 **Medicinal properties**	功效 **Efficacy**	主治 **Indications**	用法用量 **Usage and Dosage**
常山 Anti febrile dichroa	苦、辛，寒，趋向升浮；有毒。归肺、肝、心经 Bitter, pungent, cold, tend to rise and float; Toxic. Return to lung, liver and heart meridians	涌吐痰涎，截疟 Spitting and salivation, cutting off malaria	痰饮停聚，胸膈痞塞；疟疾 Phlegm stops gathering, chest and diaphragm are blocked; malaria	煎服，5～9g；或入丸散。涌吐宜生用，截疟宜酒炒用 Decoction, 5-9g; Or enter the pill powder. It is suitable for raw use for vomiting, and it is suitable for stir-frying with wine for malaria interception

续表

药名 Drug name	药性 Medicinal properties	功效 Efficacy	主治 Indications	用法用量 Usage and Dosage
胆矾 Bile alum	酸、辛，寒；有毒。归肝、胆经 Sour, pungent, cold; Toxic. Return to liver and gallbladder meridians	涌吐，解毒化湿，蚀疮去腐 Vomiting, detoxifying and removing dampness, eroding sores and removing rot	风痰壅盛，误食毒物；口疮，牙疳，风眼赤烂；胬肉，肿毒不溃 Wind and phlegm are congested, and poison is ingested by mistake; Aphthous sores, chancre, red eyes; Pterygium, swollen and poisonous	温汤化服，0.1 ~ 0.3g。外用适量，研末撒或调敷，或水化外洗 Take warm soup and take it, 0.1-0.3g. Appropriate amount for external use, grind into powder, sprinkle or adjust application, or hydrate and wash externally

二十、攻毒杀虫去腐敛疮药

20 Drugs for attacking poisons, killing insecticides, removing rot and sores

凡以攻毒杀虫、去腐敛疮为主要功效，主要用于湿疹、疥癣、痈疽疮疡等病证的药物，称为攻毒杀虫去腐敛疮药。

All drugs that have the main effects of attacking poison, killing insects, and removing decay and sores, and are mainly used for eczema, mange, carbuncle and other diseases, are called drugs that attack poison, killing insects, removing decay and sores.

本类药物具有攻毒杀虫、去腐敛疮等功效。

This kind of medicine has the effects of attacking poison, killing insects, removing decay and sores, etc.

攻毒杀虫去腐敛疮药主要适用于湿疹、疥癣、痈疽疮疡证等。

Poison–attacking, insecticidal, decay–removing and sore drugs are mainly suitable for eczema, mange, carbuncle and ulcer syndrome, etc.

本类药物用药途径以外用为主。个别有毒药物需要内服时，宜作丸、散剂使用，以利于药物缓慢溶解吸收。本类药物多具有不同程度的毒性，无论外用与内服均应严格控制剂量和疗程，不宜过量或持续使用，以防发生毒性反应。常见攻毒杀虫去腐敛疮药包括硫黄、升药、硼砂等（表 10–30）。

The route of administration of this class of drugs is mainly for external use. When individual toxic drugs need to be taken orally, they should be used as pills and powders to facilitate the slow dissolution and absorption of drugs. Most of these drugs have varying degrees of toxicity. The dosage and course of treatment should be strictly controlled regardless of external and oral use, and should not be used excessively or continuously to prevent toxic reactions. Common drugs for attacking poisons, killing insecticides, removing decay and astringing sore include sulfur, hydrargyrum oxydatum crudum, borax, etc. (Table 10–30).

表 10–30　常见攻毒杀虫去腐敛疮药

Table 10–30　Common drugs for attacking poisons, kiuing insecticides removing decay and astringing sores

药名 Drug name	药性 Medicinal properties	功效 Efficacy	主治 Indications	用法用量 Usage and Dosage
硫黄 sulfur yellow	酸，温；有毒。归肾、大肠经 Sour, warm; Toxic. Return to kidney and large intestine meridian	外用解毒杀虫疗疮；内服补火助阳通便 External detoxification and insecticidal treatment of sores; Oral administration to tonify fire, help yang and laxate constipation	疥癣，湿疹，阴疽疮疡；阳痿，虚喘冷哮，虚寒便秘 Mange, eczema, vaginal gangrene ulcers; Impotence, deficiency asthma and cold wheezing, deficiency cold constipation	内服，1.5～3g，炮制后入丸、散服；外用适量 Oral administration, 1.5-3g, concocted into pills or powder; Appropriate amount for external use
升药 hydrargyrum oxydatum crudum	辛，热；有大毒。归肺、脾经 Xin, Re; It's poisonous. Return to lung and spleen meridians	拔毒，去腐 Remove poison, remove rot	痈疽溃后，脓出不畅，或腐肉不去，新肉难生；湿疹，黄水疮，顽癣，阴蚀，发际疮，粉刺 After the carbuncle ulcerates, the pus is not smooth, or the carrion does not go away, and new meat is difficult to produce; Eczema, yellow water sore, stubborn ringworm, negative erosion, hairline sore, acne	外用适量。本品只供外用，不能内服 Appropriate amount for external use. This product is for external use only, cannot be taken internally
硼砂 borax	甘、咸，凉。归肺、胃经 Sweet, salty and cool. Return to lung and stomach meridians	外用清热解毒，内服清肺化痰 External use to clear away heat and toxic materials, oral use to clear lung and resolve phlegm	咽喉肿痛，口舌生疮，目赤翳障；痰热咳嗽；痔疮肿痛 Sore throat, sores in the mouth and tongue, red eyes; Phlegm-heat cough; hemorrhoids swelling and pain	外用适量，研极细末干撒或调敷患处；或化水漱口，或入丸散含化内服，每次1.5～3g Appropriate amount for external use, grind extremely fine powder and dry sprinkle or adjust to the affected area; Or dissolve water and gargle your mouth, or put it into pills and powder and take it orally, 1.5-3g each time

第十一章　方剂基本知识
Chapter 11　Basic Knowledge of Prescriptions

第一节　方剂与治法
Section 1　Prescriptions and Treatments

一、方剂与治法的关系
1 The relationship between prescriptions and treatment methods

方剂，是在辨证论治确定治法之后，在治法的指导下，选择合适的药物，酌定用量，按照组方原则的要求妥善配伍而成，是临床辨证论治的主要工具之一。

Prescription is one of the main tools for clinical syndrome differentiation and treatment after the treatment method is determined based on syndrome differentiation, under the guidance of the treatment method, the appropriate drug is selected, the dosage is determined, and the prescription is properly compatible according to the requirements of the prescription principle.

二、常用治法
2 Commonly used treatments

1. 汗法　是通过开泄腠理、调畅营卫、宣肺散邪等作用，使在表的外感六淫之邪随汗而解的一类治法。

Sweating method　It is a kind of treatment method that relieves the six exogenous evil on the surface with sweat through the functions of opening and releasing the interstitial organs, regulating the camp and wei, and ventilating lung qi and dispersing the evil, so that the six exogenous evil on the surface can be relieved with sweat.

2. 吐法　是通过涌吐的方法，使停留在咽喉、胸膈、胃脘的痰涎、宿食或毒物从口中吐出的一类治法。

Emesis method　It is a kind of treatment method that makes the phlegm, food or poison that stays in the throat, chest diaphragm and stomach cavity spit out from the mouth through the method of spit.

3. 下法　是通过荡涤肠胃，泻出肠中积滞或积水、瘀血，使停留于胃肠的宿食、燥屎、冷积、瘀血、结痰、停水等从下窍谷道而出，以祛邪除病的一类治法。

Purgation method　It is to purge the stomach and intestines and discharge the stagnation or water and blood stasis in the intestines, so that the stagnant food, dry excrement, cold accumulation, blood stasis, phlegm accumulation, water stopping, etc. that stay in the stomach and intestines can come out from the lower orifices and valleys. It is a kind of treatment method to eliminate evil and diseases.

4. 和法　是通过和解与调和的方法，使半表半里之邪，或脏腑、阴阳、表里失和之证得以解除的一类治法。

Harmony method　It is a kind of treatment method that relieves the evil of half exterior and half interior, or the evidence of disharmony between viscera, yin and yang, and exterior and interior through reconciliation and reconciliation.

5. 温法　是通过温里祛寒，治疗里寒证的一类治法。

Warming method　It is a kind of treatment method that treats the inner cold syndrome by warming the inner and dispelling the cold.

6. 清法　是通过清热、泻火、凉血，解除里热之邪，治疗里热证的一类治法。

Clearing method　It is a kind of treatment method that treats internal heat syndrome by clearing away heat, purging fire, and cooling blood, relieving the evil of internal heat, and treating internal heat syndrome.

7. 消法　是通过消食导滞、行气活血、化痰利水，以及驱虫的方法，使气、血、痰、食、水、虫等所结聚而成的有形之邪渐消缓散的一类治法。

Digestive method　It is a kind of treatment method that gradually disappears and disperses the tangible evil formed by qi, blood, phlegm, food, water, insects, etc. through the methods of digesting food and guiding stagnation, promoting qi and blood circulation, resolving phlegm and diuresis, and repelling insects.

8. 补法　是通过补益人体气血阴阳不足或衰退的脏腑功能，治疗各种虚弱证候的一类治法。

Tonic method　It is a kind of treatment method that treats various weakness syndromes by replenishing the internal organs functions of insufficient or declining qi, blood, yin and yang of the human body.

第二节　方剂的组成
Section 2　Composition of Prescriptions

一、组成原则
1 Composition principles

方剂的组成原则，首先必须根据病情，辨证立法，然后依法组方。组方要符合“君、臣、佐、使”的基本形式。

The principle of composition of prescriptions must first be based on the illness, syndrome differentiation and legislation, and then formulate prescriptions according to law. The formula should conform to the basic form of “monarch, minister, assistant and envoy”.

1. 君药　即针对主病或主症起主要治疗作用的药物。

Monarch medicine　It is a drug that plays a major therapeutic role in the main disease or main symptom.

2. 臣药　有两种意义：一是指辅助君药加强治疗主病或主症的药物；二是指针对重要的兼病或兼症起主要治疗作用的药物。

Ministerial medicine　It has two meanings: one refers to the medicine that assists monarch medicine to strengthen the treatment of main diseases or main symptoms; The other refers to drugs that play a major therapeutic role for important concurrent diseases or concurrent diseases.

3. 佐药　有 3 种意义：①佐助药，是配合君、臣药以加强治疗作用，或直接治疗次要兼症的药物。②佐制药，是用以消除或减弱君、臣药的毒性，或能制约君、臣药峻烈之性的药物。③反佐药，即病重邪甚，可能拒药时，配用与君药性味相反而又能在治疗中起相成作用的药物，以防止药物格拒。

Adjuvant medicine　It has three meanings: ① Adjuvant drugs are combined with monarch and minister drugs to strengthen the therapeutic effect, or drugs that directly treat secondary concurrent diseases. ② Drugs used to eliminate or weaken the toxicity of monarch and ministerial drugs, or can restrict the severity of monarch and ministerial drugs. ③ Anti–adjuvant means that when the disease is serious and the evil is serious, and the drug may be rejected, use drugs that are opposite to the taste of the monarch’s medicine and can play a complementary role in the treatment to prevent drug rejection.

4. 使药　有两种意义：①引经药，是能引方中诸药至特定病所的药物。②调和药，是具有调和方中诸药作用的药物。

Making medicine　It has two meanings: ① Medicine for introducing menstruation can introduce various medicines in the prescription to medicines for specific diseases.

②Harmonizing drugs are drugs that have the effects of various drugs in the harmonizing prescription.

二、组成变化

2 Composition changes

方剂的组成变化主要有以下 3 种形式：

The composition changes of prescriptions mainly take the following three forms:

1. 药味加减　在主病、主症、基本病机及君药不变的前提下，改变方中的次要药物，以适应病情需要，即常说的“随证加减”。

Addition and subtraction of medicine flavor　On the premise that the main disease, main symptom, basic pathogenesis and monarch medicine remain unchanged, change the secondary drugs in the prescription to meet the needs of the disease, which is often referred to as “adding and subtracting according to the syndrome”.

2. 药量加减　药物的用量直接决定药力的大小，但在某些方剂中用量比例的变化还会改变方剂的配伍关系，从而可能改变该方功用。

Adding or subtracting the dosage of the drug　It directly determines the power of the drug, but the change of the dosage ratio in some prescriptions will also change the compatibility relationship of the prescription, which may change the function of the prescription.

3. 剂型更换　由于剂型不同，其功用和主治也有区别。如九味羌活汤是治疗外感风寒湿邪兼有里热所致感冒的常用方，倘若易汤为丸，则药力缓而疗效持久，可治疗内伤杂病。

Dosage form replacement　Due to different dosage forms, their functions and indications are also different. For example, Jiuwei Qianghuo Decoction is a commonly used prescription to treat colds caused by exogenous wind, cold, dampness and internal heat. If Yi Decoction is a pill, the medicine will be slow and the curative effect will be lasting, and it can treat internal injuries and miscellaneous diseases.

第三节　方剂的用法

Section 3　Usage of Prescriptions

一、方剂的剂型

1 Dosage form of prescription

方剂组成之后，根据病情需要与药物的特点制成一定的形态，称为剂型。方剂的剂型历史悠久，早在《黄帝内经》中就有汤、丸、散、膏、酒、丹等剂型，随着制药工业的发展，又研制了栓剂、糖浆剂、露剂、锭剂、条剂、线剂、搽剂、胶囊剂、灸剂、熨剂、灌肠剂、气雾剂、片剂、冲剂、注射剂等新的剂型。

After the prescription is composed, it is made into a certain form according to the needs of the disease and the characteristics of the drug, which is called the dosage form. The dosage forms of prescriptions have a long history. As early as the "*Huangdi Neijing*", there were decoction, pill, powder, ointment, wine, pill and other dosage forms. With the development of the pharmaceutical industry, new dosage forms such as suppositories, syrups, lotions, lozenges, strips, threads, liniments, capsules, moxibustion, ironing, enemas, aerosols, tablets, granules, and injections have been developed.

二、方剂的煎服法

2 The decoction method of the prescription

1. 煎药法 煎药用具一般以陶瓷器皿、砂锅为好。现代亦有使用不锈钢器皿，忌用铁器、铜器。

Decoction method Generally, ceramic utensils and casseroles are better for decoction utensils. In modern times, stainless steel utensils are also used, and iron and bronze utensils are avoided.

煎药用水以洁净、新鲜、无杂质为原则，自来水、蒸馏水均可，亦有用酒或水酒合煎者。

The water for decoction is clean, fresh and free of impurities. Tap water and distilled water can be used, and wine or water and wine can also be used for decoction.

加水量一般以高于饮片平面 3 ～ 5cm 为宜。每剂药一般煎煮 2 次。每次煎煮所得药量以 150mL 左右为宜。

Generally, the amount of water added should be 3–5cm higher than the plane of the decoction pieces. Each dose of medicine is usually decocted twice. The amount of medicine obtained by each decoction is about 150mL.

煎药火候常规先用武火，沸腾后即改用文火。同时，应根据药物性味及所需煎煮时间的要求，酌定火候。解表和泻下剂，煎煮时间宜短，其火宜急，水量宜少；补益之剂，煎煮时间宜长，其火宜慢，水量略多。

The decoction heat is conventionally used with strong fire first, and then slow fire is used after boiling. At the same time, the heat should be determined according to the requirements of the drug's nature and taste and the required decoction time. For exterior relief and purgative, the decoction time should be short, the fire should be urgent, and the water should be small; For tonic agents, the decoction time should be long, the fire should be slow, and the amount of water should be slightly more.

应先将药物浸泡 20 ～ 30 分钟之后再行煎煮。特殊煎药方法包括先煎、后下、包煎、单煎、烊化、冲服等。

The medicine should be soaked for 20–30 minutes before decoction. Special decoction methods include decoction first, then decoction, wrapped decoction, single decoction, closing and taking, etc.

2. 服药法 Take medicine

（1）服药时间 一般而言，病在上焦宜食后服，病在下焦宜食前服，补益药和泻下药宜空腹服，安神药宜临卧服，对胃肠有刺激的药应食后服。

medication time Generally speaking, the time of taking medicine should be taken after eating in the upper burner, before eating in the lower burner, tonic drugs and laxative drugs should be taken on an empty stomach, tranquilizing drugs should be taken while lying down, and drugs that irritate the gastrointestinal tract should be taken after eating.

（2）服药方法 服用汤剂，一般 1 日 1 剂，分 2 ～ 3 次温服。散剂和丸剂一般根据病情和具体药物定量，1 日服 2 ～ 3 次。

Medication method Take decoction, usually one dose a day, divided into 2–3 warm doses. Powders and pills are generally taken 2–3 times a day according to the condition and specific drug quantification.

第四节 常用方剂
Section 4 Commonly Used Prescriptions

一、解表剂
1 Exterior-relieving formulae

1. 概述 Overview

（1）概念 以解表药为主组成，具有发汗、解肌、透疹等作用，主治表证的方剂。

Concept Exterior-relieving formulae is mainly composed of exterior-relieving drugs, which have the functions of sweating, muscle-relieving, rash penetration, etc., and are mainly used to treat exterior syndromes.

（2）功效 发汗解表，体现“八法”中的“汗”法。

Efficacy Sweating and relieving exterior, reflecting the “sweating” method in the “eight methods”.

（3）应用 表证及麻疹、疮疡、水肿、痢疾等病初起见有表证者。

Application Superficial syndromes and measles, sores, edema, dysentery and other diseases with superficial syndromes at the beginning.

2. 常用方剂 麻黄汤、桂枝汤、小青龙汤、银翘散、麻黄杏仁甘草石膏汤、败毒散、九味羌活汤、桑菊饮等。

Commonly used prescriptions Mahuang Decoction, Guizhi Decoction, Xiaoqinglong Decoction, Yinqiao Powder, Mahuang Almond Licorice Gypsum Decoction, Baidu Powder, Jiuwei Qianghuo Decoction, Sangju Drink, etc.

3. 代表方剂 Representative prescriptions

（1）麻黄汤（《伤寒论》）Mahuang Decoction of *Treatise on Febrile Diseases*

组成：麻黄 9g，桂枝 6g，杏仁 6g，炙甘草 3g。

Composition: 9g of ephedra, 6g of cinnamon twig, 6g of almond and 3g of roasted licorice.

用法：水煎服，温覆取微汗。

Usage: Decoction in water, cover warm to remove slight sweat.

功效：发汗解表，宣肺平喘。

Efficacy: sweating and relieving exterior symptoms, ventilating lung qi and relieving asthma.

主治：外感风寒表实证。症见恶寒发热，头疼身痛，无汗而喘，舌苔薄白，脉浮紧。

Indications: Exogenous wind-cold symptoms. Symptoms include aversion to cold and fever, headache and body pain, wheezing without sweating, thin and white tongue coating, and tight pulse.

使用注意：发汗峻剂，宜暂用，不可久服。

Note for use: The sweating agent should be used temporarily, not for a long time.

组方原理：方中麻黄发汗解表，驱肌表之风寒，宣肺平喘，为君药。臣以桂枝，解肌发表，温通血脉，助麻黄加强发汗解表。佐以杏仁，降利肺气，与麻黄相伍，一宣一降，增强宣肺平喘之力，为宣降肺气的常用组合。炙甘草调和诸药，益气和中，为佐使药。四药合用，表寒得散，肺气得宣，则诸症可愈。

Principle of the prescription: Ephedra in the prescription causes sweating and relieves the exterior, repels the wind and cold on the exterior of the muscles, ventilates lung qi and relieves asthma, and is a monarch medicine. I use cinnamon twigs to relieve muscles, warm blood vessels, and help ephedra strengthen sweating and relieve exterior symptoms. Accompanied with almonds, it can lower lung qi, and combined with ephedra, one announcement and one lowering, and enhance the power of announcing lung and relieving asthma. It is a commonly used combination for announcing lung qi. Roasted licorice is an adjuvant medicine to harmonize various medicines, replenish qi and harmonize the middle. When the four medicines are used together, the cold on the surface can be dissipated and the lung qi can be released, and all symptoms can be cured.

（2）桂枝汤（《伤寒论》）Guizhi Decoction in *Treatise on Febrile Diseases*

组成：桂枝 9g，芍药 9g，炙甘草 6g，生姜 9g，大枣 3g。

Compositions: 9g of cassia twig, 9g of peony, 6g of roasted licorice, 9g of ginger and 3g of jujube.

用法：水煎服，温覆取微汗。药后啜热稀粥一碗，以助药力。

Usage: Decoction in water, cover warm to remove slight sweat. After the medicine, sip a bowl of hot gruel to help the medicine.

功效：解肌发表，调和营卫。

Efficacy: relieving muscles and publishing, harmonizing camp and guard.

主治：外感风寒表虚证。症见恶风发热，汗出，头痛，鼻鸣干呕，苔白不渴，脉浮缓或浮弱。

Indications: Exogenous wind–cold superficial deficiency syndrome. Symptoms include aversion to wind, fever, sweating, headache, nasal sounds and retching, white fur without thirst, and slow or weak pulse.

使用注意：外感风寒表实无汗者禁用。

Note for use: It is forbidden for those with exogenous wind–cold and no sweat.

组方原理：方中桂枝为君，解肌发表而祛在表之风邪。芍药为臣，益阴敛营，既可补营阴之不足，又可敛固营阴以防营阴外泄。生姜辛温，既助桂枝辛散表邪，又兼和胃止呕；大枣甘平，意在益气补中，且可滋脾生津。姜、枣相配，是补脾和胃、调和营卫的常用组合，共为佐药。炙甘草调和药性，合桂枝辛甘化阳以实卫，合芍药酸甘化阴以和营，兼佐使之用。

Principle of the prescription: Guizhi is the king in the prescription, which relieves the muscles and dispels the wind evil on the surface. Paeonia lactiflora is a minister, which can benefit yin and restrain camp, which can not only supplement the deficiency of camp yin, but also restrain and consolidate camp yin to prevent camp yin from leaking out. Ginger is pungent and warm, which not only helps guizhi pungent to disperse exterior pathogens, but also harmonizes the stomach and stops vomiting; Jujube is sweet and smooth, which is intended to replenish qi and tonify the middle, and can nourish the spleen and promote fluid production. The combination of ginger and jujube is a common combination of tonifying the spleen and stomach, harmonizing the camp and health, and is an adjuvant. Roasted licorice is used to harmonize the medicinal properties, combined with cinnamon branch pungent and sweet to dissolve yang to strengthen health, combined with paeonic acid sweet to dissolve yin to harmonize camp, and also used as an auxiliary.

（3）银翘散（《温病条辨》）Yinqiao San of *Differentiation of Febrile Diseases*

组成：连翘 30g，金银花 30g，苦桔梗 18g，薄荷 18g，竹叶 12g，生甘草 15g，荆芥穗 12g，淡豆豉 15g，牛蒡子 18g。

Comprises 30g of forsythia suspensa, 30g of honeysuckle, 18g of bitter platycodon grandiflorum, 18g of peppermint, 12g of bamboo leaf, 15g of raw licorice, 12g of schizonepeta spike, 15g of light tempeh and 18g of burdock.

用法：上为散。每服六钱（18g），鲜芦根汤煎，香气大出，即取服，勿过煮。亦可作汤剂，水煎服，用量按原方比例酌减。

Usage: The upper is powder. Each serving is six qian (18g), decocted in fresh reed root soup, and the aroma is strong. Take it immediately and do not overcook it. It can also be used as a decoction, decoction in water, and the dosage is reduced according to the proportion of the original prescription.

功效：辛凉透表，清热解毒。

Efficacy: pungent and cool, penetrating the surface, clearing away heat and detoxifying.

主治：温病初起。症见发热，微恶风寒，无汗或有汗不畅，头痛口渴，咳嗽咽痛，舌尖红，苔薄白或薄黄，脉浮数。

Indications: Initial onset of febrile disease. Symptoms include fever, slight aversion to wind and cold, no sweating or poor sweating, headache and thirst, cough and sore throat, red tongue tip, thin white or thin yellow coating, and floating pulse.

使用注意：外感风寒及湿热病初起者禁用。不宜久煎。

Note for use: It is forbidden for patients with exogenous wind-cold and damp-heat disease at the beginning. It should not be frying for a long time.

组方原理：方中金银花、连翘气味芳香，既能疏散风热，清热解毒，又可辟秽化浊，在透散卫分表邪的同时，兼顾了温热病邪易蕴成毒及多夹秽浊之气的特点，故重用为君药。薄荷、牛蒡子疏散风热，清利头目，且可解毒利咽。荆芥穗、淡豆豉辛而微温，解表散邪，二者虽属辛温，但辛而不烈、温而不燥，配入辛凉解表方中，增强辛散透表之力，是为去性取用之法。以上四药俱为臣药。芦根、竹叶清热生津，桔梗开宣肺气而止咳利咽，同为佐药。甘草既可调和药性，护胃安中，又合桔梗利咽止咳，是属佐使之用。

Prescription principle: The smell of honeysuckle and forsythia suspensa in the prescription is fragrant, which can not only evacuate wind and heat, clear away heat and detoxify, but also eliminate filth and turbidity. While dispersing external pathogens, it also takes into account the characteristics of warm and heat pathogens that are easy to accumulate into poison and more filthy and turbid, so it is reused as a monarch medicine. Peppermint and burdock evacuate wind and heat, clear the head, and can detoxify and soothe the throat. Schizonepeta spike and light tempeh are pungent and slightly warm, which can relieve the exterior and dispel pathogenic factors. Although they are pungent and warm, they are pungent but not strong, warm but not dry. They are combined with the pungent and cool exterior recipe to enhance the power of pungent and dispersing the exterior. It is a method to use it for sex. The above four medicines are all ministerial medicines. Reed root and bamboo leaf clear away heat and promote fluid production, and Platycodon grandiflorum opens lung qi and relieves cough and relieves throat. They are both adjuvants. Licorice can not only reconcile the medicinal properties, protect the stomach and calm the middle, but also combine with Platycodon grandiflorum to relieve the throat and relieve cough. It is an adjuvant.

4. 经典条文选读 Selected readings of classic articles

（1）麻黄汤　太阳病，头痛发热，身疼腰痛，骨节疼痛，恶风，无汗而喘者，麻黄汤主之。(《伤寒论》第 35 条）

Ephedra Decoction is the main treatment for patients with Taiyang disease, headache and fever, body pain and low back pain, joint pain, aversion to wind, and wheezing without sweating. (Article 35 of *Treatise on Febrile Diseases*)

（2）桂枝汤　太阳中风，阳浮而阴弱，阳浮者，热自发，阴弱者，汗自出。啬啬恶寒，淅淅恶风，翕翕发热，鼻鸣干呕者，桂枝汤主之。(《伤寒论》第 12 条）

Guizhi Decoction has a stroke in the sun, with floating yang and weak yin. If the yang is floating, the heat is spontaneous, and if the yin is weak, the sweat is spontaneous. Guizhi Decoction is the main treatment for those who are stingy with aversion to cold, wind, fever, nasal ringing and retching. (Article 12 of *Treatise on Febrile Diseases*)

（3）银翘散　太阴风温、温热、温疫、冬温，初起恶风寒者，桂枝汤主之；但热不恶寒而渴者，辛凉平剂银翘散主之。(《温病条辨》上焦篇第 4 条）

Yinqiao San is too yin wind warm, warm heat, warm epidemic, and winter warm, and Guizhi Decoction is the main treatment for those who have initial aversion to wind and cold; However, for those who are thirsty without aversion to cold due to heat, Yinqiao San, a pungent and cooling calming agent, is the main treatment. (Article 4 of the Shangjiao Chapter in *Differentiation of Febrile Diseases*)

二、泻下剂
2 Purgative formulae

1. 概述 Overview

（1）概念　以泻下药为主组成，具有通导大便或攻逐水饮等作用，治疗里实证的方剂。

Concept　Purgative formulae is mainly composed of laxative drugs, which have the functions of circulating stool or attacking water and drinking, etc., and is a demonstrated prescription in treatment.

（2）功效　泻下通便、攻积逐水，体现“八法”中的“下”法。

Efficacy　purging and laxative, attacking accumulation and expelling water, reflecting the “lower” method in the “eight methods”.

（3）应用　里实证，包括热结、寒结、燥结、水结等。

Application　Evidence in application, including hot knot, cold knot, dry knot, water knot, etc.

2. 常用方剂　大承气汤、小承气汤、调胃承气汤、温脾汤、麻子仁丸、济川煎、十枣汤等。

Commonly used prescriptions　Dachengqi Decoction, Xiaochengqi Decoction, Tiaowei

Chengqi Decoction, Wenpi Decoction, Maziren Pills, Jichuan Decoction, Shizao Decoction, etc.

3. 代表方剂 Representative prescriptions

（1）大承气汤（《伤寒论》）Dachengqi Decoction in *Treatise on Febrile Diseases*

组成：大黄 12g，厚朴 15g，枳实 12g，芒硝 9g。

Consists of 12g of rhubarb, 15g of magnolia officinalis, 12g of bitter aurantium and 9g of mirabilite.

用法：水煎服，先煎厚朴、枳实，后下大黄，芒硝溶服。

Usage: Decoction in water, first decoct Magnolia officinalis and Citrus aurantii, then add rhubarb and dissolve Glauber's salt.

功效：峻下热结。

Efficacy: Junxia heat knot.

主治：①阳明腑实证。症见大便不通，频转矢气，腹痛拒按、按之则硬，脉沉实。②热结旁流证。症见下利清水、色纯清，脐腹疼痛、按之坚硬有块，脉滑实。

Indications: ① Evidence of Yangming fu organs. The symptoms include obstructed stool, frequent turning to sagittal qi, abdominal pain refusing to press, hardness when pressed, and heavy and solid pulse. ② Syndrome of thermal junction flow. The symptoms include clear water, pure color, pain in the umbilicus and abdomen, hard and lumpy when pressed, and slippery and solid pulse.

使用注意：气血亏虚或肠胃无热结者禁用。

Note for use: It is forbidden for patients with qi and blood deficiency or no heat knot in the stomach and intestines.

组方原理：方中大黄苦寒降泄，泄热通便，荡涤胃肠实热积滞，为君药。芒硝咸寒润降，软坚润燥，助大黄泄热通便，为臣药。厚朴下气除满，枳实行气消痞，既能消痞除满，又助硝、黄荡涤积滞，为佐药。

Principle of the prescription: Rhubarb in the prescription is a monarch medicine to reduce the bitter cold and relieve discharge, release heat and laxative constipation, and clean up the excess heat and stagnation in the gastrointestinal tract. Glauber's salt is salty, cold and moistening, soft and firm, and moistens dryness. It helps rhubarb relieve heat and relieve constipation. It is a ministerial medicine. Magnolia officinalis can eliminate fullness, and trifoliate orange can eliminate fullness, which can not only eliminate fullness, but also help nitrate and yellow remove stagnation, and is an adjuvant.

（2）大黄附子汤（《金匮要略》）Dahuang Fuzi Decoction in *Synopsis of the Golden Chamber*

组成：大黄 9g，附子 9g，细辛 3g。

Composition: 9g of rhubarb, 9g of aconite and 3g of asarum.

用法：水煎服。

Usage: Decoction in water.

功效：温里散寒，泻结行滞。

Efficacy: Warming the interior and dispelling cold, purging stagnation.

主治：寒积里实证。症见腹痛便秘，发热，手足厥冷，舌苔白腻，脉弦紧。

Indications: Symptoms of cold accumulation. Symptoms include abdominal pain, constipation, fever, cold hands and feet, white and greasy tongue coating, and tight pulse.

使用注意：大黄用量一般不超过附子。

Note: The dosage of rhubarb generally does not exceed that of aconite.

组方原理：方中重用大辛大热之附子，温阳散寒，为君药。以苦寒之大黄，泻下通便，荡涤积滞，为臣药。佐以细辛温通散寒止痛，并助附子温阳散寒之力。大黄性味虽苦寒，但配伍附子、细辛等大辛大热之品，相反相成，寒性被制而泻下之功存。

Prescription principle: The prescription reuses aconite with great pungent and great heat to warm yang and dispel cold, which is the monarch medicine. Bitter and cold rhubarb is used as a minister's medicine to purge constipation and purge stagnation. It is supplemented with asarum to warm, dispel cold and relieve pain, and helps aconite to warm yang and dispel cold. Although the nature and taste of rhubarb are bitter and cold, it is compatible with aconite, asarum and other pungent and hot medicinals, which are opposite and complementary, and the cold nature is controlled and the effect of purging remains.

（3）麻子仁丸（《伤寒论》）Maziren Pill in *Treatise on Febrile Diseases*

组成：麻子仁 500g，芍药 250g，枳实 250g，大黄 500g，厚朴 250g（炙去皮），杏仁 250g。

Comprises 500g of hemp seed seed, 250g of peony lactiflora, 250g of bitter aurantium, 500g of rhubarb, 250g of magnolia officinalis (roasted and peeled) and 250g of almond.

用法：蜜丸，每服 9g，每日 2 ～ 3 次；亦可按原方用量比例改用汤剂煎服。

Usage: Honey pills, 9g each, 2 to 3 times a day; It can also be decocted with decoction according to the proportion of the original prescription.

主治：肠胃燥热，津液不足。

Indications: stomach dryness and heat, insufficient body fluid.

使用注意：津亏血少者不宜久服。孕妇慎用。

Note for use: People with fluid deficiency and blood deficiency should not take it for a long time. Use with caution in pregnant women.

组方原理：方中麻子仁性味甘平，功善润肠通便，重用为君药。大黄泄热通便；杏仁润燥通便，且善降肺气，因肺与大肠相表里，肺气降则肠气通；芍药养阴敛津，和里缓急，共为臣药。枳实下气破结，厚朴行气除满，为佐药。蜂蜜润肠通便，调和诸药，为使药。

Principle of the prescription: The pockmark kernel in the prescription is sweet and flat in nature, good in moistening the intestines and relaxing constipation, and can be reused as a monarch medicine. Rhubarb relieves heat and laxative; Almonds moisten dryness and relieve constipation, and are good at lowering lung qi. Because the lungs and the large intestine are external and internal, when the lung qi is lowered, the intestinal qi is circulated; Paeonia lactiflora nourishes yin and converges fluid, and is a minister's medicine together. Citrus aurantii breaks the knot under qi, and Magnolia officinalis promotes qi and removes fullness, which is an adjuvant. Honey moistens the intestines and relieves constipation, reconciles various medicines, and is a medicine.

4. 经典条文选读 Selected readings of classic articles

（1）大承气汤　阳明病，脉迟，虽汗出不恶寒者，其身必重，短气，腹满而喘，有潮热者，此外欲解，可攻里也。手足濈然汗出者，此大便已硬也，大承气汤主之；若汗多，微发热恶寒者，外未解也，其热不潮，未可与承气汤；若腹大满不通者，可与小承气汤，微和胃气，勿令至大泄下。(《伤寒论》第 208 条）

Dachengqi Decoction Yangming disease, late pulse, although sweating and not aversion to cold, the body will be heavy, short of breath, full abdomen and wheezing, and tidal fever. In addition, if you want to solve it, you can attack the inside. If the hands and feet are sweating, the stool is already hard, and Dachengqi Decoction is the main factor; If you have excessive sweating, slight fever and aversion to cold, the external situation is not solved, and the heat is not damp, so it cannot be used with Chengqi Decoction; If the abdomen is full and blocked, it can be used with Xiaochengqi Decoction to slightly harmonize the stomach qi, so as not to cause a large discharge. (Article 208 of *Treatise on Febrile Diseases*)

（2）大黄附子汤　胁下偏痛，发热，其脉紧弦，此寒也，以温药下之，宜大黄附子汤。(《金匮要略・腹满寒疝宿食病脉证治》)

Dahuang Aconite Decoction has pain and fever under the hypochondriac side, and its pulse is tight and stringy. This cold is also used to treat it with warm medicine. Dahuang Aconite Decoction is suitable. (*Synopsis of the Golden Chamber・Syndrome and Treatment of Abdominal Fullness, Cold Hernia, Food Disease and Pulse Disease*)

（3）麻子仁丸　趺阳脉浮而涩，浮则胃气强，涩则小便数，浮涩相搏，大便则硬，其脾为约，麻子仁丸主之。(《伤寒论》第 247 条）

The Yang pulse of Maziren Pill is floating and astringent. If it is floating, the stomach qi is strong, and if it is astringent, the number of urination is counted. If it is floating and astringent, the stool is hard, and the spleen is about, which is dominated by Maziren Pill. (Article 247 of *Treatise on Febrile Diseases*)

三、和解剂
3 Harmonizing-releasing formulae

1. 概述 Overview

（1）概念　具有和解少阳、调和肝脾、调和肠胃等作用，治疗邪在少阳、肝脾不和、肠胃不和等证的方剂，统称和解剂。

Concept It has the functions of reconciling Shaoyang, harmonizing liver and spleen, and harmonizing stomach and intestines, and is a prescription for treating pathogens in Shaoyang, disharmony between liver and spleen, and disharmony between stomach and intestines, collectively referred to as harmonizing–releasing formulae.

（2）功效 和解少阳，病位属半表半里，属"八法"中的"和"法。

Efficacy Reconciliation of Shaoyang, the disease position belongs to half exterior and half internal, which belongs to the "harmony" method in the "eight methods".

（3）应用 少阳证，或肝郁脾虚、肝脾不和证，寒热互结、肠胃不和证等。

Application Shaoyang syndrome, or liver stagnation and spleen deficiency, liver–spleen disharmony syndrome, cold–heat combination, intestinal and gastrointestinal disharmony syndrome, etc.

2. 常用方剂 小柴胡汤、大柴胡汤、逍遥散、半夏泻心汤、蒿芩清胆汤、四逆散、痛泻要方。

Commonly used prescriptions Xiaochaihu Decoction, Dachaihu Decoction, Xiaoyao Powder, Banxia Xiexin Decoction, Haoqin Qingdan Decoction, Sini Powder, and Tongxie Yaofang.

3. 代表方剂 Representative prescriptions

（1）小柴胡汤（《伤寒论》）Xiaochaihu Decoction in *Treatise on Febrile Diseases*

组成：柴胡 24g，黄芩 9g，人参 9g，炙甘草 9g，半夏 9g，生姜 9g，大枣 4 枚。

Composition: 24g of bupleurum, 9g of scutellaria baicalensis, 9g of ginseng, 9g of roasted licorice, 9g of pinellia ternata, 9g of ginger and 4 jujube.

用法：水煎服。

Usage: Decoction in water.

功效：和解少阳。

Efficacy: Reconciles Shaoyang.

主治：①伤寒少阳证。症见往来寒热，胸胁苦满，默默不欲饮食，心烦喜呕，口苦，咽干，目眩，舌苔薄白，脉弦者。②热入血室证。症见妇人中风，经水适断，寒热发作有时。③疟疾、黄疸等病而见少阳证者。

Indications: ① Typhoid fever and Shaoyang syndrome. Symptoms include cold and heat, bitterness and fullness in the chest and hypochondrium, silent reluctance to eat and drink, upset and vomiting, bitter mouth, dry throat, dizziness, thin and white tongue coating, and stringy pulse. ② Syndrome of heat entering the blood chamber. The symptoms are that the woman has a stroke, menstrual water is suitably interrupted, and cold and heat attacks occur sometimes. ③ Patients with Shaoyang syndrome due to malaria, jaundice and other diseases.

使用注意：阴虚血少者禁用。

Note for use: It is forbidden for patients with yin deficiency and blood deficiency.

组方原理：方中柴胡透泄少阳之邪，并能疏泄气机之郁滞，使少阳半表之邪得以疏散，为君药。黄芩清泄少阳半里之热，为臣药。君臣配伍，一透一清，和解少阳。胆气犯胃，胃失和降，佐以半夏、生姜和胃降逆止呕；邪从太阳传入少阳，缘于正气本虚，又佐以人参、大枣益气健脾，一方面扶正以助祛邪，另一方面益气以御邪内传。炙甘草助参、枣扶正，且能调和诸药，为使药。

Principle of the prescription: Bupleurum in the prescription can relieve the evil of Shaoyang, and can relieve the stagnation of qi, so that the evil of half-surface Shaoyang can be evacuated. It is a monarch medicine. Scutellaria baicalensis is a ministerial medicine for clearing away the heat of half a mile in Shaoyang. The monarch and minister are compatible, one transparent and one clear, and Shaoyang is reconciled. Gall qi invades the stomach, and the stomach loses harmony and lowers, supplemented with Pinellia ternata, ginger and stomach to reduce the reverse and stop vomiting; Evil is introduced into Shaoyang from the sun, due to the deficiency of righteous qi, and it is supplemented with ginseng and jujube to replenish qi and strengthen the spleen. On the one hand, it strengthens the body resistance to help eliminate evil, and on the other hand, it replenishes qi to prevent the internal transmission of evil. Roasted licorice helps ginseng and jujube strengthen body resistance, and can reconcile various medicines, which is a medicine.

（2）半夏泻心汤（《伤寒论》）Banxia Xiexin Decoction in *Treatise on Febrile Diseases*

组成：半夏 12g，黄芩 9g，干姜 9g，人参 9g，黄连 3g，大枣 4 枚，炙甘草 9g。

Composition: 12g of pinellia ternata, 9g of scutellaria baicalensis, 9g of dried ginger, 9g of ginseng, 3g of coptis chinensis, 4 pieces of jujube and 9g of roasted licorice.

用法：水煎服。

Usage: Decoction in water.

功效：寒热平调，消痞散结。

Efficacy: leveling cold and heat, eliminating ruffians and dispersing stagnation.

主治：寒热互结之痞证。症见心下痞，但满而不痛，或呕吐，肠鸣下利，舌苔腻而微黄。

Indications: Syndrome of cold and heat combination. The symptoms include heart ruff, but full but not painful, or vomiting, intestinal sounds, and greasy and yellowish tongue coating.

使用注意：气滞或食积所致的心下痞满，不宜用。

Note for use: It is not suitable for fullness under the heart caused by qi stagnation or food accumulation.

组方原理：方中以半夏为君，散结除痞，又善降逆止呕。臣以干姜温中散寒，黄芩、黄连泄热开痞。以上四味相伍，具有寒热平调、辛开苦降之用。然寒热互结，又缘于中虚失运，故方中又以人参、大枣甘温益气，以补脾虚，为佐药。使以甘草补脾和中而调诸药。

Principle of the prescription: Pinellia ternata is used as the king in the prescription, which can dissipate stagnation and eliminate ruffians, and is also good at reducing adverse reactions and stopping vomiting. I used dried ginger to warm the middle and dispel cold, while Scutellaria baicalensis and Coptis chinensis released heat and opened ruffians. The above four flavors are combined with each other, which has the functions of leveling cold and heat, opening pungent and reducing bitterness. However, the interaction of cold and heat is due to middle deficiency and loss of transportation. Therefore, ginseng and jujube are used in the prescription to warm and replenish qi to tonify spleen deficiency as adjuvants. Use licorice to tonify the spleen and harmonize the middle and adjust various medicines.

4. 经典条文选读 Selected readings of classic articles

（1）小柴胡汤　伤寒五六日，中风，往来寒热，胸胁苦满，嘿嘿不欲饮食，心烦喜呕，或胸中烦而不呕，或渴，或腹中痛，或胁下痞硬，或心下悸，小便不利，或不渴，身有微热，或咳者，小柴胡汤主之。(《伤寒论》第 96 条）

Xiaochaihu Decoction typhoid fever on the 5th or 6th day, stroke, cold and heat, bitterness and fullness in the chest and hypochondrium, silently, no desire to eat and drink, upset and vomiting, or irritation in the chest but not vomiting, or thirst, or abdominal pain, or hardness in the hypochondrium, or palpitations under the heart, difficulty urinating, or lack of thirst, slight heat in the body, or cough, Xiaochaihu Decoction is the main treatment. (Article 96 of *Treatise on Febrile Diseases*)

（2）半夏泻心汤　伤寒五六日，呕而发热者，柴胡汤证具，而以他药下之，柴胡汤证仍在者，复与柴胡汤，此虽已下之，不为逆，必蒸蒸而振，却发热汗出而解。若心下满而硬痛者，此为结胸也，大陷胸汤主之；但满而不痛者，此为痞，柴胡不中与之，宜半夏泻心汤。(《伤寒论》第 149 条）

Banxia Xiexin Decoction typhoid fever for five or six days, vomiting and fever, Bupleurum Decoction evidence, but with other medicines, Bupleurum Decoction evidence still exists, reuse Bupleurum Decoction, although this has been prescribed, it is not reverse, it will steam and vibrate, but the fever and sweat will solve. If the heart is full and hard and painful, this is chest knot, and Daxianxiong Decoction is the main factor; However, if it is full but not painful, this is a ruffian, and if Bupleurum is not neutral, it is suitable for Banxia Xiexin Decoction. (Article 149 of *Treatise on Febrile Diseases*)

四、清热剂

4 Heat clearing formulae

1. 概述 Overview

（1）概念　以清热药为主组成，具有清热、泻火、凉血、解毒、滋阴透热等作用的方剂。

Concept Heat clearing formulae is a prescription mainly composed of heat-clearing medicine, which has the functions of clearing away heat, purging fire, cooling blood, detoxifying, nourishing yin and permeating heat, etc.

（2）功效 清热、泻火、凉血、解毒、滋阴透热等，体现“八法”中的“清”法。

Efficacy Clearing away heat, purging fire, cooling blood, detoxifying, nourishing yin and permeating heat, etc., reflecting the “clearing” method in the “eight methods”.

（3）应用 表证已解，里热正盛，或热虽盛尚未结实。

Application Superficies-syndrome has been solved, the internal heat is full, or the heat is not yet strong although it is full.

2. 常用方剂 白虎汤、清营汤、黄连解毒汤、凉膈散、普济消毒饮、导赤散、龙胆泻肝汤、清胃散、芍药汤、青蒿鳖甲汤、仙方活命饮、六一散、犀角地黄汤、清瘟败毒饮、左金丸、玉女煎、白头翁汤。

Commonly used prescriptions Baihu Decoction, Qingying Decoction, Huanglian Jiedu Decoction, Liangge Powder, Puji Disinfection Decoction, Daochi Powder, Longdan Xiegan Decoction, Qingwei Powder, Shaoyao Decoction, Qinghao Biejia Decoction, Xianfang Huoming Decoction, Liuyi Powder, Rhinoceros Horn Dihuang Decoction, Qingwen Baidu Decoction, Zuojin Pill, Yu Nu Decoction, Pulsatilla Decoction.

3. 代表方剂 Representative prescription

白虎汤（《伤寒论》） Baihu Decoction in *Treatise on Febrile Diseases*

组成：石膏 30g，知母 9g，炙甘草 6g，粳米 9g。

Composition: 30g of gypsum, 9g of anemarrhena, 6g of roasted licorice and 9g of japonica rice.

用法：水煎至米熟汤成，去滓温服。

Usage: Decoction in water until the rice is cooked and the soup is made, remove the dregs and take warm.

功效：清热生津。

Efficacy: clearing away heat and promoting fluid production.

主治：气分热盛证。症见壮热面赤，汗出恶热，烦渴引饮，脉洪大有力，脉滑数。

Indications: Syndrome of qi separation and excessive heat. The symptoms include strong heat and red face, sweating and aversion to heat, polydipsia and drinking, strong and strong pulse, and slippery pulse.

使用注意：无汗、口不渴、脉浮弦细或沉者，禁用。

Note for use: It is forbidden for those who have no sweat, no thirst in the mouth, and thin or heavy pulse.

组方原理：方中石膏清热泻火，解肌透热，为清泻气分实热之要药，为君药。知母苦寒质润，清热生津，与石膏相须为用，为臣药。粳米、炙甘草益胃生津，并防大寒之剂损伤胃气，为佐药。炙甘草兼能调和诸药，为使药。

Prescription principle: Gypsum in the prescription clears away heat and purges fire, relieves muscles and permeates heat. It is an important medicine for clearing away qi and separating excess heat, and it is a monarch medicine. Anemarrhena is bitter, cold and moist, clears away heat and produces fluid production, and is used in conjunction with gypsum as a minister's medicine. Japonica rice and roasted licorice can benefit the stomach and promote fluid production, and prevent cold from damaging stomach qi. They are adjuvants. Roasted licorice can also reconcile various medicines, which is a medicine.

4. 经典条文选读 Selected readings of classic articles

白虎汤　三阳合病，腹满身重，难以转侧，口不仁面垢，谵语遗尿。发汗则谵语。下之则额上生汗，手足逆冷。若自汗出者，白虎汤主之。(《伤寒论》第 219 条)

Baihu Decoction is a combination of three yang diseases, with heavy abdomen and body, difficulty in turning sides, insensitive mouth and facial dirt, delirium and enuresis. Sweating leads to delirium. If you go down, you will sweat on your forehead, and your hands and feet will be cold. If you sweat spontaneously, Baihu Decoction is the main treatment. (Article 219 of *Treatise on Febrile Diseases*)

五、温里剂

5 Interior-warming formulae

1. 概述 Overview

(1) 概念　以温热药为主组成，具有温里助阳、散寒通脉的作用，用于治疗里寒证的方剂。

Concept　Interior-warming formulae is mainly composed of warming medicine, which has the functions of warming the internal and helping yang, dispelling cold and dredging the veins. It is a prescription used to treat internal cold syndrome.

(2) 功效　温中祛寒、回阳救逆、温经散寒等，体现“八法”中的“温”法。

Efficacy　warming the middle and dispelling cold, returning yang and saving adverse effects, warming meridians and dispelling cold, etc., reflecting the “warming” method in the “eight methods”.

(3) 应用　里寒证。

Application　Internal cold syndrome.

2. 常用方剂　理中丸、小建中汤、四逆汤、当归四逆汤、阳和汤、吴茱萸汤。

Commonly used prescriptions　Lizhong Pill, Xiaojianzhong Decoction, Sini Decoction, Danggui Sini Decoction, Yanghe Decoction, and Evodia Decoction.

3. 代表方剂 Representative prescriptions

(1) 理中丸(《伤寒论》) Lizhong Pill in *Treatise on Febrile Diseases*

组成：人参 6g，干姜 5g，炙甘草 6g，白术 9g。

Composition: 6g of ginseng, 5g of dried ginger, 6g of roasted licorice and 9g of atractylodes macrocephala.

用法：蜜丸，1 次 9g，1 日 2 次，小儿酌减；或水煎服。

Usage: Honey pills, 9g once, 2 times a day, reduce in children; Or decoction in water.

功效：温中祛寒，补气健脾。

Efficacy: Warm the middle and dispel cold, invigorate qi and strengthen spleen.

主治：①中焦虚寒证。症见呕吐下利，脘腹疼痛，喜温喜按，不欲饮食，畏寒肢冷，舌淡苔白，脉沉细。②阳虚失血证。③小儿慢惊，病后喜唾涎沫，以及胸痹等由中焦虚寒所致者。

Indications: ① Zhongjiao deficiency and cold syndrome. The symptoms include vomiting, abdominal pain, warmth and pressing, no desire to eat and drink, cold limbs, pale tongue with white coating, and deep and thin pulse. ② Yang deficiency and blood loss syndrome. ③Children with slow alarm, salivation after illness, and chest paralysis caused by deficiency and cold in the middle jiao.

组方原理：干姜味辛性热，温阳散寒，为扶阳抑阴之要药，为君药。人参味甘性温，补中气，培后天，以助运化，为臣药。君臣相配，复中阳，益脾气。佐以白术，燥湿健脾。佐使炙甘草，益气和中，调和诸药。

Prescription principle: Dried ginger is pungent in taste and hot in nature, warms yang and dispels cold. It is an important medicine for supporting yang and suppressing yin, and it is a monarch medicine. Ginseng is sweet in taste and warm in nature, tonifying the middle qi, cultivating the day after tomorrow, and helping transportation and transformation. It is a ministerial medicine. The match of monarch and minister can restore the middle yang and benefit the temper. Accompanied by Atractylodes macrocephala, drying dampness and strengthening spleen. Adjuvant roasted licorice, replenishing qi and harmonizing the middle, and harmonizing various medicines.

（2）四逆汤（《伤寒论》）Sini Decoction in *Treatise on Febrile Diseases*

组成：炙甘草 6g，干姜 9g，生附子 10g。

Compositions: 6g of roasted licorice root, 9g of dried ginger and 10g of raw aconite root.

用法：水煎服，附子先煎 1 小时，再加余药同煎。

Usage: Decoction in water, decoct aconite for 1 hour first, and then add the remaining medicine to decoct together.

功效：回阳救逆。

Efficacy: Returning Yang and saving rebellion.

主治：①心肾阳衰之寒厥证。症见四肢厥逆，神衰欲寐，面色苍白，恶寒蜷卧，腹痛下利，呕吐不渴，甚或冷汗淋漓，舌淡，苔白滑，脉微欲绝。②误汗亡阳者。

Indications: ① Cold syndrome of heart and kidney yang failure. The symptoms include convulsion of the limbs, sleepiness, pale complexion, aversion to cold and lying curled up, abdominal pain, vomiting and not thirsty, or even dripping cold sweat, pale tongue, white and slippery coating, and slightly exhausted pulse. ② Those who sweat and die Yang by mistake.

使用注意：生附子宜先煎 1 小时，再加余药同煎。药后出现呕吐格拒者，可凉服。

Note for use: Raw aconite should be decocted for 1 hour first, and then the remaining medicine should be added to decoct together. If vomiting occurs after the medicine, it can be taken cold.

组方原理：本方以大辛大热之生附子为君药，温壮元阳，破散阴寒，以救助心肾衰竭之阳气。以辛热之干姜为臣药，温中焦，散阴寒，以固守后天之本。生附子与干姜相须为用，是回阳救逆的基本配伍。佐使炙甘草，一则甘温补气，使生附子、干姜回阳救逆之中兼有益气补虚之效；二则缓解君臣药物的峻烈之性，使生附子、干姜无暴散虚阳之虞；三则调和药性，并能使药力作用持久。

Principle of prescription: This prescription takes aconite, a raw material of great pungent and great heat, as the monarch medicine to warm and strengthen Yuanyang, break and disperse yin and cold, and help the yang qi of heart and kidney failure. Take pungent and hot dried ginger as ministerial medicine, warm the middle jiao, disperse yin and cold, and stick to the acquired foundation. Raw aconite and dried ginger are used together, which is the basic compatibility of returning yang and saving adverse disease. Adjuvant to roasted licorice, one is sweet and warm to invigorate qi, so that raw aconite and dried ginger can return yang and save adverse effects, and it has the effect of benefiting qi and invigorating deficiency; The second is to alleviate the severity of the drugs of monarch and minister, so that raw aconite and dried ginger are not in danger of violently dispersing deficiency yang; Third, it can harmonize the medicinal properties and make the effect of the medicine last.

4. 经典条文选读 Selected readings of classic articles

（1）理中丸　大病差后，喜唾，久不了了，胸上有寒，当以丸药温之，宜理中丸。（伤寒论》第 396 条）

After the serious illness of Lizhong Pill, the patient like to spit, and it won't last for a long time. If there is a cold on the chest, I should use pills to warm it. Lizhong Pill is advisable. (Article 396 of *Treatise on Febrile Diseases*)

（2）四逆汤　少阴病，脉沉者，急温之，宜四逆汤。（《伤寒论》第 323 条）

Sini Decoction is suitable for those with Shaoyin disease and heavy pulse. Sini Decoction is suitable for urgent warmth. (Article 323 of *Treatise on Febrile Diseases*)

六、补益剂

6 Tonic formulae

1. 概述 Overview

（1）概念　以补益药为主组成，具有补益人体气、血、阴、阳等作用，治疗各种虚证的方剂。

Concept　Tonic formulae is mainly composed of tonic drugs, which have the functions of tonifying qi, blood, yin and yang of the human body, and are a prescription for treating various deficiency syndromes.

（2）功效　补气、补血、补阴、补阳，体现“八法”中的“补”法。

Efficacy　Tonifying qi, blood, yin and yang, embodying the “tonifying” method in the “eight methods”.

（3）应用　气虚、血虚、阴虚、阳虚等。

Application　Qi deficiency, blood deficiency, yin deficiency, yang deficiency, etc.

2. 常用方剂　四君子汤、参苓白术散、补中益气汤、生脉散、玉屏风散、四物汤、归脾汤、六味地黄丸、一贯煎、百合固金汤、肾气丸、炙甘草汤、当归补血汤、大补阴丸、左归丸、右归丸、地黄饮子。

Commonly used prescriptions　Sijunzi Decoction, Shenling Baizhu Powder, Buzhong Yiqi Decoction, Shengmai Powder, Yupingfeng Powder, Siwu Decoction, Guipi Decoction, Liuwei Dihuang Pill, Yiguanjian, Baihe Gujin Decoction, Shenqi Pill, Zhigancao Decoction, Danggui Buxue Decoction, Dabuyin Pill, Zuogui Pill, Yougui Pill, Dihuang Yinzi.

3. 代表方剂 Representative prescriptions

（1）四君子汤（《太平惠民和剂局方》）Sijunzi Decoction in *Taiping Huimin and Medicine Bureau Prescription*

组成：人参 9g，白术 9g，茯苓 9g，炙甘草 6g。

Composition: 9g of ginseng, 9g of atractylodes macrocephala, 9g of poria cocos and 6g of roasted licorice.

用法：水煎服。

Usage: Decoction in water.

功效：益气健脾。

Efficacy: replenishing qi and invigorating spleen.

主治：脾胃气虚证。症见面色萎白，语声低微，气短乏力，食少便溏，舌淡苔白，脉虚缓。

Indications: Spleen and stomach qi deficiency syndrome. The symptoms include withering and white color, low voice, shortness of breath and fatigue, poor appetite and loose stool, pale tongue with white coating, and weak and slow pulse.

组方原理：方中人参健脾养胃，为君药。白术健脾燥湿，助君药之力，为臣药。茯苓渗湿健脾，为佐药。苓、术合用，健脾祛湿之功益著。炙甘草益气和中，调和诸药，为使药。

Prescription principle: Ginseng in the prescription strengthens the spleen and nourishes the stomach, and is a monarch medicine. Atractylodes macrocephala invigorates the spleen and dries dampness, helps the power of the monarch’s medicine, and is a minister’s medicine. Poria cocos infiltrates dampness and strengthens the spleen, and is an adjuvant. The combination of Ling and Shu has the effect of strengthening the spleen and removing dampness. Roasted licorice replenishes qi and harmonizes the middle, harmonizes various medicines, and is shi medicine.

（2）四物汤（《仙授理伤续断秘方》）Siwu Decoction in *The Secret Recipe for Immortal Teaching and Continuing Injuries*

组成：当归 9g，川芎 6g，白芍 9g，熟地黄 15g。

Composition: 9g of Chinese angelica, 6g of Chuanxiong, 9g of white peony root and 15g of prepared rehmannia glutinosa.

用法：水煎服。

Usage: Decoction in water.

功效：补血和血。

Efficacy: Tonic and blood.

主治：营血虚滞证。症见心悸失眠，头晕目眩，面色无华，形瘦乏力，妇人月经不调、量少或经闭不行，脐腹作痛，舌淡，脉细弦或细涩。

Indications: Syndrome of deficiency and stagnation of blood. Symptoms include palpitations, insomnia, dizziness, dull complexion, thinness and weakness, irregular menstruation, low volume or amenorrhea, umbilical and abdominal pain, pale tongue, thin or astringent pulse.

使用注意：阴虚发热及血崩气脱之证不宜用。

Note for use: It is not suitable for symptoms of yin deficiency, fever and blood collapse and qi depletion.

组方原理：方中熟地黄补血滋阴，为君药。当归养血补肝，和血调经，为臣药。白芍养血敛阴，缓急止痛；川芎活血行气，祛瘀止痛，共为佐药。

Prescription principle: Rehmannia glutinosa in the prescription nourishes blood and nourishes yin, and is a monarch medicine. Angelica sinensis nourishes blood and nourishes liver, harmonizes blood and regulates menstruation, and is a ministerial medicine. Paeony lactiflora nourishes blood and converges yin, relieves urgency and relieves pain; Ligusticum chuanxiong is used as an adjuvant for promoting blood circulation and promoting qi, removing blood stasis and relieving pain.

（3）肾气丸（《金匮要略》）Shenqi Pill in *Synopsis of the Golden Chamber*

组成：干地黄 24g，薯蓣 12g，山茱萸 12g，泽泻 9g，茯苓 9g，牡丹皮 9g，桂枝 3g，附子 3g。

Comprises 24g of dried rehmannia glutinosa, 12g of dioscorea zingiberensis, 12g of cornus officinalis, 9g of alisma orientalis, 9g of poria cocos, 9g of peony bark, 3g of cinnamon twig and 3g of aconite.

用法：炼蜜和丸；亦可为汤剂，水煎服。

Usage: Refining honey and pills; It can also be taken as a decoction, decocted in water.

功效：补肾助阳，化生肾气。

Efficacy: Tonifying kidney and helping yang, transforming kidney qi.

主治：肾阳不足证。症见腰痛脚软，身半以下常有冷感，少腹拘急，小便不利，或小便反多，入夜尤甚，阳痿早泄，舌淡而胖，脉虚弱，尺部沉细；以及痰饮、水肿、消渴、脚气、转胞等。

Indications: Syndrome of kidney yang deficiency. Symptoms include low back pain and soft feet, often cold feeling below half of the body, less abdominal tightness, difficult urination, or excessive urination, especially at night, impotence and premature ejaculation, pale and fat tongue, weak pulse, and heavy and thin ulnar; As well as phlegm drinking, edema, thirst quenching, athlete's foot, transcytosis, etc.

使用注意：肾阴不足、虚火上炎者，不宜用。

Note for use: It is not suitable for patients with insufficient kidney yin and inflammation due to deficiency fire.

组方原理：方中用干地黄为君，滋补肾阴，益精填髓。臣以山茱萸补肝肾，涩精气；薯蓣健脾气，固肾精。二药与地黄相配，补肾填精之功益著。臣以附子、桂枝温肾助阳，鼓舞肾气。佐以茯苓健脾益肾，泽泻、牡丹皮降相火而制虚阳浮动，且茯苓、泽泻均有渗湿泄浊、通调水道之功。

Prescription principle: In the prescription, dried rehmannia glutinosa is used as the king, which nourishes kidney yin, replenishes essence and fills marrow. I use dogwood to nourish the liver and kidney and astringent essence; Dioscorea zingiberensis strengthens temper and strengthens kidney essence. The two medicines are matched with Rehmannia glutinosa, which is beneficial to tonify the kidney and fill essence. I use aconite and cinnamon twigs to warm the kidney and help yang, and inspire kidney qi. It is supplemented with Poria cocos to invigorate the spleen and kidney, Alisma and Peony Bark to reduce phase fire and control deficiency yang floating, and both Poria cocos and Alisma have the functions of seeping dampness and turbidity, and regulating waterways.

4. 经典条文选读 Selected readings of classic articles

肾气丸　男子消渴，小便反多，以饮一斗，小便一斗，肾气丸主之。(《金匮要略·消渴小便不利淋病脉证并治》)

Kidney Qi Pills are used to quench thirst and urinate too much. Drink a bucket and urinate a bucket. Kidney Qi Pills are the main treatment. (*Synopsis of the Golden Chamber · Combined Treatment of Gonorrhea Pulse Syndrome with Diabetes and Diabetes Urination*)

七、安神剂
7 Tranquilizing formulae

1. 概述 Overview

（1）概念　以安神药为主组成，具有安神定志作用，治疗神志不安病证的方剂。

Concept　Tranquilizing formulae is mainly composed of tranquilizing drugs, which have the effect of tranquilizing the mind and calming the mind, and are a prescription for treating uneasy diseases and syndromes.

（2）功效　重镇安神、滋养安神。

Efficacy　Tranquilization with heavy material, nourish and calm the nerves.

（3）应用　心悸健忘、虚烦失眠的虚证失眠或惊狂易怒、烦躁不安的实证失眠。

Application　Deficiency syndrome insomnia with palpitations, amnesia, deficiency and insomnia, or empirical insomnia with panic, irritability and restlessness.

2. 常用方剂　天王补心丹、酸枣仁汤、朱砂安神丸、柏子养心丸。

Commonly used prescriptions　Tianwang Buxin Dan, Suanzaoren Decoction, Zhusha Anshen Pill, and Baizi Yangxin Pill.

3. 代表方剂 Representative prescription

酸枣仁汤（《金匮要略》）Suanzaoren Decoction in *Synopsis of the Golden Chamber*

组成：酸枣仁 15g(炒)，甘草 3g，知母 6g，茯苓 6g，川芎 6g。

Composition: 15g of ziziphus jujube kernel (stir–fried), 3g of licorice, 6g of anemarrhena, 6g of poria cocos and 6g of chuanxiong.

用法：水煎，分 3 次温服。

Usage: Decoction in water and take warm in 3 times.

功效：养血安神，清热除烦。

Efficacy: nourishing blood and tranquilizing the nerves, clearing away heat and removing annoyance.

主治：肝血不足，虚热内扰证。症见虚烦失眠，心悸不安，头目眩晕，咽干口燥，舌红，脉弦细。

Indications: Insufficient liver blood, internal disturbance of deficiency heat. Symptoms include deficiency, insomnia, palpitations, dizziness, dry throat and dry mouth, red tongue, and thin pulse.

组方原理：方中重用酸枣仁，养血补肝，宁心安神，为君药。茯苓宁心安神；知母滋阴润燥，清热除烦，共为臣药。佐以川芎之辛散，调肝血而疏肝气，与大量酸枣仁相伍，辛散与酸收并用，补血与行血结合，具有养血调肝之妙。甘草和中缓急，调和诸药，为使。

Prescription principle: Ziziphus jujube kernels are reused in the prescription to nourish blood and liver, calm the heart and calm the nerves, and are the monarch medicine. Poria cocos calms the heart and calms the nerves; Anemarrhena nourishes yin and moistens dryness, clears away heat and removes annoyance, and is a minister’s medicine. Accompanied by the pungent powder of Ligusticum chuanxiong, it can regulate liver blood and soothe liver qi. It is combined with a large amount of jujube kernels. The pungent powder and sour–shrink are used together, and the combination of nourishing blood and promoting blood, which has the wonderful effect of nourishing blood and regulating the liver and medium and urgent, and reconcile various medicines for the purpose of making.

4. 经典条文选读 Selected readings of classic articles

酸枣仁汤　虚劳虚烦不得眠，酸枣仁汤主之。(《金匮要略·血痹虚劳病脉证并治》)

Suanzaoren Decoction is the main reason for fatigue, fatigue and annoyance, and you can't sleep, and Suanzaoren Decoction is the main reason. (*Synopsis of the Golden Chamber · Combined Treatment of Blood Paralysis, Deficiency, Fatigue, Disease and Pulse Syndrome*)

八、开窍剂
8 Resuscitation formulae

1. 概述 Overview

（1）概念　开窍剂是以芳香开窍药为主组成，具有开窍醒神作用，治疗窍闭神昏证的方剂。

Concept　Resuscitation formulae is mainly composed of chinese materia medica that resuscitate with aromatics, which has the function of inducing resuscitation and awakening mind, and is a formula for treating the unconsciousness caused by orifice closure.

（2）功效　开窍醒神。

Efficacy　Inducing resuscitation and mind-awakening .

（3）应用　邪热内闭或寒痰闭阻之闭证。

Appliance　The pattern of pathogenic heat internal block or block syndrome of cold-phlegm obstruction .

2. 常用方剂　安宫牛黄丸、紫雪、至宝丹、苏合香丸。

Commonly used formulas　Peaceful Palace Bovine Bezoar Pill（安宫牛黄丸）, Purple Snow Elixir（紫雪）, Supreme Jewel Elixir（至宝丹）and Storax Pill（苏合香丸）.

3. 代表方剂 Representative formula

安宫牛黄丸（《温病条辨》）　Peaceful Palace Bovine Bezoar Pill in *Differentiation of Febrile Diseases*

组成：牛黄 30g，郁金 30g，水牛角浓缩粉（原为犀角）30g，黄连 30g，朱砂 30g，冰片 7.5g，麝香 7.5g，珍珠 15g，山栀 30g，雄黄 30g，黄芩 30g。

Composition: Calculus Bovis（牛黄）30g, Radix Curcumae（郁金）30g, Cornu Bubali concentrated powder（水牛角浓缩粉）(formerly Cornu Rhinocerotis) 30g, Rhizoma Coptidis（黄连）30g, Cinnabaris（朱砂）30g, Borneolum Syntheticum（冰片）7.5 g, Moschus（麝香）7.5g, Margarita（珍珠）15g, Fructus Gardeniae（山栀）30g, Realgar（雄黄）30g and Radix Scutellariae（黄芩）30g.

用法：以水牛角浓缩粉 30g 替代犀角。以上 11 味，珍珠水飞或粉碎成极细粉，朱砂、雄黄分别水飞成极细粉；黄连、黄芩、栀子、郁金粉碎成细粉；将牛黄、水牛角浓缩粉、麝香、冰片研细，与上述粉末配研，过筛，混匀，加适量炼蜜制成大蜜丸。每服1丸，1日1次；小儿3岁以内1次1/4丸，4～6岁1次1/2丸，1日1次；或遵医嘱。

Usage: Replace Cornu Rhinocerotis（犀角）with 30g Cornu Bubali concentrated powder（水牛角浓缩粉）. The above 11 medicinals, Margarita（珍珠）grind with water or crushed into extremely fine powder, Cinnabaris（朱砂）and Realgar（雄黄）grind with water into extremely fine powder respectively; Rhizoma Coptidis（黄连）, Radix Scutellariae（黄芩）, Fructus Gardeniae（山栀）,Radix Curcumae（郁金）crushed into fine powder, Calculus Bovis（牛黄）, Cornu Bubali concentrated powder（水牛角浓缩粉）, Moschus（麝香）, Borneolum Syntheticum（冰片）grind into fine powder, mix with the above powders, sieve, mix evenly, and add proper amount of simmered honey to make big honey pills. Take 1 pill each time, once a day; 1/4 pill once for children under 3 years old, 1/2 pill once for children aged 4–6 years old, once a day; Or follow the doctor's advice.

亦作散剂：按上法制得，每瓶装1.6g。每服1.6g，1日1次；小儿3岁以内1次0.4g，4～6岁1次0.8g，1日1次；或遵医嘱。

Also used as powder: 1.6g per bottle according to the above method. Take 1.6g each time once a day; Children under 3 years old once 0.4g, 4–6 years old once 0.8g, once a day; or follow the doctor's advice.

功效：清热解毒，开窍醒神。

Efficacy: Clearing heat and resolving toxins, inducing resuscitation and awakening mind.

主治：①邪热内陷心包证。症见高热烦躁，神昏谵语，舌蹇肢厥，舌红或绛，脉数有力。②中风昏迷，小儿惊厥属邪热内闭者。

Indications: ① Pathogenic heat entering the pericardium. Symptoms include high fever, unconsciousness, delirious speech, inflexible tongue, reversal counterflow cold of the four limbs, red or crimson tongue, and powerful and rapid pulse. ② Wind–stroke fainting and pediatric convulsion belong to pathogenic heat internal block.

使用注意：孕妇忌用。

Note: Avoid using for pregnant women.

组方原理：方中牛黄清心解毒，辟秽开窍；水牛角清心凉血解毒；麝香芳香开窍醒神。三药相配，是清心开窍、凉血解毒的常用组合，共为君药。臣以黄连、黄芩、山栀清热泻火解毒，合牛黄、水牛角则清解心包热毒之力颇强；冰片、郁金芳香辟秽，化浊通窍，以增麝香开窍醒神之功。佐以雄黄，助牛黄辟秽解毒；朱砂、珍珠镇心安神，以除烦躁不安。炼蜜为丸，和胃调中，为使药。原方以金箔为衣，取其重镇安神之效。

Principle of formula: Niuhuang in the prescription clears heart and detoxifies, eliminates filth and induces resuscitation; Buffalo horn clears heart, cools blood and detoxifies; Musk fragrance awakens mind. The combination of the three drugs is a common combination of clearing heart fire, inducing resuscitation, cooling blood and detoxifying, and they are all monarch drugs. Use Coptis chinensis, Scutellaria baicalensis Georgi and Gardenia gardenia to clear away heat, purge fire and detoxify, and combine bezoar and buffalo horn to clear away pericardial heat and toxin; Borneol and Curcuma aromatis are fragrant to eliminate filth, turn turbidity and dredge orifices, so as to increase musk's ability to induce resuscitation and wake up. Accompanied by realgar, it helps bezoar to eliminate filth and detoxify; Cinnabar and pearl calm the nerves to eliminate irritability. Refining honey is a pill, harmonizing the stomach and regulating the middle, in order to make medicine. The original prescription takes gold foil as clothing, and takes the effect of calming the nerves in its important town.

4. 经典条文选读 Selected readings of classic articles

安宫牛黄丸　阳明温病，斑疹温痘，温疮，温毒，发黄，神昏谵语者，安宫牛黄丸主之。(《温病条辨》中焦篇第 9 条）

Angong Niuhuang Pill is the main one for Yangming febrile disease, macula, warm acne, warm sore, warm toxin, yellowing, faint delirium. (Article 9 of Middle Jiao Pian in Tiaobian of *Epidemic Febrile Diseases*)

九、理气剂
9 Qi-regulating formulae

1. 概述 Overview

（1）概念　理气剂是以理气药为主组成，具有行气或降气作用，治疗气滞或气逆证的方剂，统称理气剂。

Concept　Qi-regulating formulae is mainly composed of qi-regulating drugs, which have the function of promoting qi circulation or lowering qi, and are collectively referred to as qi-regulating drugs for treating qi stagnation or qi inversion syndrome.

（2）功效　行气、降气。

Efficacy　Promoting qi circulation and lowering qi.

（3）应用　气滞或气逆证。

Application　Qi stagnation or Qi inversion syndrome.

2. 常用方剂　越鞠丸、半夏泻心汤、苏子降气汤、定喘汤、旋覆代赭汤、柴胡疏肝散、瓜蒌薤白白酒汤、天台乌药散。

Commonly used prescriptions　Yueju Pill, Banxia Xiexin Decoction, Suzi Jiangqi Decoction, Dingchuan Decoction, Xuanfu Daizhe Decoction, Chaihu Shugan Powder, Gualou Xiebai Liquor Decoction and Tiantai Wuyao Powder.

3. 代表方剂 Representative prescription

（1）半夏厚朴汤（《金匮要略》）Banxia Houpo Decoction in *Synopsis of Golden Chamber*

组成：半夏 12g，厚朴 9g，茯苓 12g，生姜 12g，苏叶 6g。

Composition: Pinellia ternata 12g, Magnolia officinalis 9g, Poria cocos 12g, Ginger 12g and Perilla leaves 6g.

用法：水煎服。

Usage: Decoct with water.

功效：行气散结，降逆化痰。

Efficacy: Promoting qi circulation, resolving stagnation, lowering adverse effects and eliminating phlegm.

主治：梅核气。症见咽中如有物阻，咯吐不出，吞咽不下，胸膈满闷，或咳或呕，苔白润或滑腻，脉弦缓或弦滑。

Indications:Globus hysteriocus. Symptoms include obstruction in pharynx, inability to vomit, inability to swallow, stuffy chest diaphragm, cough or vomiting, white or greasy fur, and slow or slippery pulse.

组方原理：方中半夏化痰散结，降逆和胃；厚朴行气化湿，下气除满。两药相伍，痰气并治，共为君药。茯苓渗湿健脾，与半夏相合，一治“生痰之源”，一治“贮痰之器”，使痰无由生，为臣药。生姜降逆消痰，和胃止呕，助君药化痰降逆之力，并制半夏毒，为佐药。苏叶入肝肺经，既可疏肝理气、宣散郁结，又能宣肺利咽，引药力上达于咽喉；且与君药相配，降逆之中寓升散之性，使气机升降有调，为佐使药。

Principle of prescription: Pinellia ternata in the prescription can eliminate phlegm and dissipate stagnation, reduce adverse effects and harmonize stomach; Magnolia officinalis can be vaporized and damp, and can be filled The two drugs are combined, phlegm and qi are treated together, and they are monarch drugs. Poria cocos permeates dampness and strengthens spleen, which is combined with Pinellia ternata. It is a minister medicine for treating “the source of phlegm” and “the device of storing phlegm”. Ginger can reduce adverse effects and eliminate phlegm, harmonize stomach and stop vomiting, and help monarch to eliminate phlegm and reduce adverse effects, and make Pinellia ternata poison as an adjuvant medicine. The perilla leaves enter the liver and lung meridians, which can not only soothe the liver and regulate qi, dispel stagnation, but also disperse the lung and relieve sore throat, and the drug attraction reaches the throat; And it is matched with monarch medicine, and it contains the nature of ascending and dispersing in descending inverse, which makes the qi activity rise and fall in tune, and is an auxiliary medicine.

（2）旋覆代赭汤（《伤寒论》）Xuanfu Daizhe Decoction in *Treatise on Febrile Diseases*

组成：旋覆花 9g，人参 6g，代赭石 3g，炙甘草 9g，半夏 9g，生姜 15g，大枣 4 枚。

Composition: Inula 9g, ginseng 6g, ochre 3g, Radix Glycyrrhizae Preparata 9g, Pinellia ternata 9g, ginger 15g and jujube 4.

用法：水煎服。

Usage: Decoct with water.

功效：降逆化痰，益气和胃。

Efficacy: Reducing adverse effects, eliminating phlegm, invigorating qi and harmonizing stomach.

主治：胃虚痰气逆阻证。症见心下痞硬，噫气不除，或反胃呃逆，吐涎沫，舌苔白腻，脉缓或滑。

Indications: Stomach deficiency and phlegm–qi reverse obstruction syndrome. Symptoms include hard heart, stagnation of qi, nausea, hiccup, salivation, white and greasy tongue coating, slow or slippery pulse.

使用注意：方中代赭石用量不可过重。

Note: The dosage of ochre in the prescription should not be too large.

组方原理：方中旋覆花下气消痰，降逆止噫，为君药。代赭石善镇冲逆，助旋覆花降逆止呕，为臣药。半夏燥湿祛痰，降逆和胃；生姜用量独重，和胃降逆止呕；人参、炙甘草、大枣健脾益气，调胃和中，为佐药。炙甘草又可调和药性，用为使药。

Principle of prescription: Inula flowers in the prescription lower qi to eliminate phlegm, lower adverse effects and stop alas, which is the monarch medicine. Instead of ochre, it is a minister medicine, which is good at relieving adverse effects and helping inula flowers to reduce adverse effects and stop vomiting. Pinellia ternata, eliminating dampness and expectorant, lowering adverse effects and harmonizing The dosage of ginger is heavy alone, which harmonizes the stomach, reduces adverse effects and stops vomiting; Ginseng, Radix Glycyrrhizae Preparata and Jujube are adjuvant medicines for invigorating spleen and qi, regulating stomach and harmonizing middle warmer. Radix Glycyrrhizae Preparata can also harmonize its medicinal properties and be used as a medicine.

4. 经典条文选读 Selected readings of classic articles

（1）半夏厚朴汤　妇人咽中如有炙脔，半夏厚朴汤主之。(《金匮要略·妇人杂病脉证并治》)

Banxia Houpo Decoction is the main body of Banxia Houpo Decoction if there is a roasted preserve in the woman's throat. (*Synopsis of Golden Chamber*, *Combined Treatment of Women's Miscellaneous Diseases and Pulse Syndromes*)

（2）旋覆代赭汤　伤寒发汗，若吐若下，解后心下痞硬，噫气不除者，旋覆代赭汤主之。(《伤寒论》第 161 条)

Xuan Fu Daizhe Decoction is the master of typhoid fever and sweating. If you vomit, your heart will be hard and hard after solution, and your breath will not be removed. (Article 161 of *Treatise on Febrile Diseases*)

十、理血剂

10 Blood-regulating formulae

1. 概述 Overview

（1）概念　理血剂是以理血药为主组成，具有活血祛瘀或止血作用，主治瘀血证或出血病证的方剂。

Concept Blood-regulating formulae is mainly composed of blood-regulating drugs, which has the functions of promoting blood circulation, removing blood stasis or stopping bleeding, and is mainly a prescription for treating blood stasis syndrome or hemorrhagic disease syndrome.

（2）功效 活血化瘀、止血。

Efficacy Promoting blood circulation, removing blood stasis and stopping bleeding.

（3）应用 瘀血证或出血证。

Application Blood stasis syndrome or bleeding syndrome.

2. 常用方剂 桃核承气汤、血府逐瘀汤、补阳还五汤、复元活血汤、小蓟饮子、温经汤、十灰散、咳血方、桂枝茯苓丸。

Commonly used prescriptions Taoren Chengqi Decoction, Xuefu Zhuyu Decoction, Buyang Huanwu Decoction, Fuyuan Huoxue Decoction, Xiaoji Yinzi, Wenjing Decoction, Shihui Powder, Kexue Prescription and Guizhi Fuling Pill.

3. 代表方剂 Representative prescription

血府逐瘀汤（《医林改错》） Xuefu Zhuyu Decoction in *Correcting Mistakes in Medical Forest*

组成：桃仁 12g，红花 9g，当归 9g，生地黄 9g，川芎 4.5g，赤芍 6g，牛膝 9g，桔梗 4.5g，柴胡 3g，枳壳 6g，甘草 6g。

Composition: Peach kernel 12g, safflower 9g, Angelica sinensis 9g, Rehmannia glutinosa 9g, Chuanxiong 4.5 g, Radix Paeoniae Rubra 6g, Achyranthes bidentata 9g, Platycodon grandiflorum 4.5 g, Bupleurum root 3g, Fructus Aurantii 6g and Glycyrrhiza uralensis Fisch 6g.

用法：水煎服。

Usage: Decoct with water.

功效：活血化瘀，行气止痛。

Efficacy: Promoting blood circulation, removing blood stasis, promoting qi circulation and relieving pain.

主治：胸中血瘀证。症见胸痛，头痛，日久不愈，痛如针刺而有定处，或呃逆日久不止，或饮水即呛，干呕，或内热瞀闷，或心悸怔忡，失眠多梦，急躁易怒，入暮潮热，唇暗或两目暗黑，舌质暗红，或舌有瘀斑、瘀点，脉涩或弦紧。

Indications: Blood stasis syndrome in chest. Symptoms include chest pain, headache, persistent pain like acupuncture, hiccup for a long time, choking and retching after drinking water, or stuffy internal heat, palpitation, insomnia, dreaminess, irritability, hot flashes at dusk, dark lips or dark eyes, dark red tongue, or ecchymosis, petechia, astringent pulse or string-tight pulse.

使用注意：孕妇忌用。

Note: Avoid using for pregnant women.

组方原理：方中桃仁破血行滞而润燥，红花活血祛瘀以止痛，共为君药。赤芍、川芎助君药活血祛瘀；牛膝入血分，性善下行，能祛瘀血，通血脉，并引血下行，使血不瘀于胸中，瘀热不上扰，共为臣药。生地黄清热凉血，滋阴养血；合当归养血，使祛瘀而不伤正；合赤芍清热凉血，以清瘀热。三者养血益阴，清热活血为佐药。桔梗、枳壳，一升一降，宽胸行气，桔梗并能载药上行；柴胡疏肝解郁，升达清阳，与桔梗、枳壳同用，尤善理气行滞，使气行则血行，亦为佐药。甘草调和诸药，为使药。

Principle of prescription: Peach kernel breaks blood stagnation and moistens dryness, while safflower promotes blood circulation and removes blood stasis to relieve pain, which are all monarch drugs. Radix Paeoniae Rubra and Ligusticum Chuanxiong help the monarch to promote blood Achyranthes bidentata enters the blood, which is good at going down, can remove blood stasis, dredge blood vessels, and induce blood to go down, so that blood stasis is not in the chest, and blood stasis and heat are not disturbed. Rehmannia glutinosa clears heat and cools blood, nourishes yin and nourishes blood; Combine Angelica sinensis to nourish blood, so as to remove blood stasis without hurting positive; Combined with Radix Paeoniae Rubra to clear away heat and cool blood. The three are adjuvant drugs for nourishing blood and benefiting yin, clearing heat and promoting blood circulation. Platycodon grandiflorum, Fructus Aurantii, one liter and one drop, wide chest and qi circulation, Platycodon grandiflorum and can carry medicine upward; Bupleurum soothes liver and relieves depression, and rises to clear yang. It is used together with Platycodon grandiflorum and Fructus Aurantii. It is especially good at regulating qi and stagnation, making qi flow lead to blood flow, and it is also an adjuvant medicine. Licorice blends various medicines to make medicines.

十一、祛湿剂
11 Dampness-dispelling formulae

1. 概述 Overview

（1）概念　祛湿剂是以祛湿药为主组成，具有化湿利水、通淋泄浊等作用，用以治疗水湿病证的方剂。

Concept　Dampness-dispelling formulae is mainly composed of dampness-eliminating drugs, which have the functions of eliminating dampness and promoting diuresis, dredging stranguria and removing turbidity, and are used to treat water-dampness diseases.

（2）功效　燥湿和胃，清热祛湿，利水渗湿，温化寒湿，祛湿化浊，祛风胜湿。

Efficacy　Eliminating dampness and harmonizing stomach, clearing away heat and dampness, promoting diuresis and eliminating dampness, warming cold and dampness, eliminating dampness and turbidity, and dispelling wind and eliminating dampness.

（3）应用　内湿和外湿。

Application　Internal dampness and external dampness.

2. 常用方剂　平胃散、藿香正气散、茵陈蒿汤、三仁汤、八正散、五苓散、真武汤、独活寄生汤、甘露消毒丹、连朴饮、猪苓汤、防己黄芪汤、苓桂术甘汤、实脾散、萆薢分清饮。

Commonly used prescriptions Pingwei Powder, Huoxiang Zhengqi Powder, Yinchenhao Decoction, Sanren Decoction, Bazheng Powder, Wuling Powder, Zhenwu Decoction, Duhuo Jisheng Decoction, Ganlu Disinfection Dan, Lianpu Decoction, Zhuling Decoction, Fangji Huangqi Decoction, Linggui Shugan Decoction, Shipi Powder and Bixie Fenqing Decoction.

3. 代表方剂 Representative prescription

（1）三仁汤（《温病条辨》）Sanren Decoction in *Differentiation of Febrile Diseases*

组成：杏仁 15g，滑石 18g，通草、白蔻仁、竹叶、厚朴各 6g，生薏苡仁 18g，半夏 15g。

Composition: Almond 15g, Talc 18g, Tongcao, Coco kernel, Bamboo leaf, Magnolia officinalis 6g each, Coix seed 18g, Pinellia ternata 15g.

用法：水煎服。

Usage: Decoct with water.

功效：宣畅气机，清利湿热。

Efficacy: Disseminate qi activity, clear away damp heat.

主治：湿温初起或暑温夹湿之湿重于热证。头痛恶寒，身重疼痛，肢体倦怠，面色淡黄，胸闷不饥，午后身热，苔白不渴，脉弦细而濡。

Indications: Dampness at the beginning of dampness and temperature or dampness mixed with summer heat and temperature is heavier than heat syndrome. Headache, aversion to cold, heavy body pain, limb burnout, pale yellow complexion, chest tightness and no hunger, hot body in the afternoon, white fur and no thirst, and thin and moist pulse.

使用注意：热重于湿者，不宜使用。

Attention to use: If heat is heavier than wet, it should not be used.

组方原理：方中以滑石为君，清热利湿而解暑。以薏苡仁、杏仁、白蔻仁“三仁”为臣，其中薏苡仁淡渗利湿以健脾，使湿热从下焦而去；白蔻仁芳香化湿，利气宽胸，畅中焦之脾气以助祛湿；杏仁宣利上焦肺气，盖肺主一身之气，气化则湿亦化。佐以通草、竹叶甘寒淡渗，助君药利湿清热之效；半夏、厚朴行气除满，化湿和胃，以助君臣理气除湿之功。

Principle of prescription: Talc is the king in the prescription, clearing heat and promoting diuresis to relieve summer heat. The “three kernels” of coix seed, almond and white coix seed are the ministers, in which coix seed permeates lightly and promotes diuresis to strengthen the spleen and make damp heat go away from the lower energizer; White cardamom is fragrant and damp-eliminating, promoting qi and broadening chest, and smoothing the temper of middle energizer to help eliminate dampness; Almonds promote the upper energizing lung qi, cover the lung and control the whole body qi, and when gasification occurs, dampness also changes. With the effect of dredging grass, sweet, cold and light infiltration of bamboo leaves, and helping monarch to promote diuresis and clear away heat; Pinellia ternata and Magnolia officinalis promote qi circulation, eliminate dampness and harmonize stomach, so as to help monarch and minister regulate qi and remove dampness.

（2）五苓散（《伤寒论》）Wuling Powder in *Treatise on Febrile Diseases*

组成：猪苓 9g，泽泻 15g，白术 9g，茯苓 9g，桂枝 6g。

Composition: Polyporus umbellatus 9g, Alisma orientalis 15g, Atractylodes macrocephala 9g, Poria cocos 9g and Cassia twig 6g.

用法：散剂，每服 6 ～ 10g，多饮热水，取微汗；亦可作汤剂，水煎服，温服取其微汗。

Usage: Powder, take 6–10g each, drink more hot water and take slight sweat; It can also be used as decoction, decocted with water, and taken warmly to take its slight sweat.

功效：利水渗湿，温阳化气。

Efficacy: Promoting diuresis and dampness, warming yang and transforming qi.

主治：①蓄水证。症见小便不利，头痛微热，烦渴欲饮，甚则水入即吐，舌苔白，脉浮。②痰饮。症见脐下动悸，吐涎沫而头目眩晕，或短气而咳者。③水湿内停证。症见水肿，泄泻，小便不利，以及霍乱吐泻等。

Indications: ① Water storage syndrome. Symptoms include dysuria, headache, slight heat, polydipsia, vomiting when water enters, white tongue coating and floating pulse. ② Phlegm retention. Symptoms include palpitation under umbilicus, spitting and foaming, and dizziness of the leader, or short breath and cough. ③ Syndrome of internal stop due to water dampness. Symptoms include edema, diarrhea, dysuria, and cholera vomiting and diarrhea.

组方原理：方中重用泽泻为君，利水渗湿。臣以茯苓、猪苓助君药利水渗湿。佐以白术补气健脾以运化水湿，合茯苓既可彰健脾制水之效，又可奏输津四布之功。膀胱的气化有赖于阳气的蒸腾，故又佐以桂枝温阳化气以助利水，并可辛温发散以祛表邪，一药而表里兼治。

Principle of prescription: Alisma orientalis is reused in the prescription to promote diuresis and dampness. I used Poria cocos and Polyporus umbellatus to help the monarch with diuresis and dampness With Atractylodes macrocephala Koidz invigorating qi and spleen to transport water and dampness, combined with Poria cocos can not only strengthen spleen and make water, but also play the role of delivering fluid and four cloth. The gasification of bladder depends on the transpiration of yang–qi, so it is accompanied by cassia twig to warm yang and transform qi to help diuresis, and it can be pungent and warm to dispel exterior evil, and one medicine can treat both exterior and interior.

（3）真武汤（《伤寒论》）Zhenwu Decoction in *Treatise on Febrile Diseases*

组成：茯苓 9g，芍药 9g，白术 6g，生姜 9g，炮附子 9g。

Composition: Poria cocos 9g, Paeonia lactiflora 9g, Atractylodes macrocephala 6g,

Ginger 9g and Aconitum carmichaeli 9g.

用法：水煎服。

Usage: Decoct with water.

功效：温阳利水。

Efficacy: Warming yang and promoting diuresis.

主治：①阳虚水泛证。症见小便不利，四肢沉重疼痛，浮肿，腰以下为甚，畏寒肢冷，腹痛，下利，或咳，或呕，舌淡胖，苔白滑，脉沉细。②太阳病发汗太过，阳虚水泛证。症见汗出不解，其人仍发热，心下悸，头眩，身瞤动，振振欲擗地。

Indications: ① Syndrome of yang deficiency and flooding of water. Symptoms include dysuria, heavy pain and edema of limbs, especially below the waist, chills, cold limbs, abdominal pain, lower diuresis, cough or vomiting, pale and fat tongue, white and smooth fur, and heavy and thin pulse. ② Excessive sweating due to sun disease, yang deficiency and flooding of water. When the symptoms are puzzled by sweating, the person still has fever, palpitation, dizzy head, moving body, and wants to move to the ground.

组方原理：本方以大辛大热之附子为君，温肾助阳，化气行水。白术健脾燥湿，茯苓利水渗湿，二者合用，使脾气得复，湿从小便去，共为臣药。生姜既助附子温阳散寒，又合苓、术宣散水湿，兼能和胃降逆止呕，为佐药。配伍酸收之白芍，其义有四：一者利小便以行水气，二者柔肝缓急以止腹痛，三者敛阴舒筋以解筋肉瞤动，四者可防止附子燥热伤阴，亦为佐药。

Principle of prescription: This prescription takes Aconitum carmichaeli, which is hot and pungent, as the monarch, warming kidney and helping yang, transforming qi and moving water. Atractylodes macrocephala Koidz invigorates spleen and dries dampness, and Poria cocos promotes diuresis and seeps dampness. The two are used together to restore spleen temper and remove dampness from childhood Ginger not only helps Aconitum carmichaeli warm yang and dispel cold, but also combines cocos, disperses water and dampness, and can harmonize stomach, lower adverse effects and stop vomiting, which is an adjuvant medicine. The combination of sour–shrink white peony root has four meanings: one is to facilitate urination to promote moisture, the other is to soften the liver to relieve abdominal pain, the third is to astringe yin and relax muscles to relieve muscle movement, and the fourth is to prevent aconite from damaging yin due to dryness and heat, which is also an adjuvant medicine.

4. 经典条文选读 Selected readings of classic articles

（1）三仁汤　头痛恶寒，身重疼痛，舌白不渴，脉弦细而濡，面色淡黄，胸闷不饥，午后身热，状若阴虚，病难速已，名曰湿温。汗之，则神昏耳聋，甚则目瞑不欲言；下之，则洞泄；润之，则病深不解。长夏、深秋、冬日同法，三仁汤主之。（《温病条辨》上焦篇第 43 条）

Sanren Decoction has headache, aversion to cold, heavy body pain, white tongue without thirst, thin and moist pulse, pale yellow complexion, chest tightness without hunger, hot body in the afternoon, yin deficiency in shape, and difficult illness, so it is called damp temperature. If you sweat, you will be faint and deaf, and even your eyes will not speak; If you go down, the hole will leak; If you moisten it, you will be deeply puzzled. Long summer, late autumn and winter are the same, and Sanren Tang is the master. –Article 43 of Shangjiao Chapter in *Differentiation of Febrile Diseases*;

（2）五苓散　太阳病，发汗后，大汗出，胃中干，烦躁不得眠，欲得饮水者，少少与饮之，令胃气和则愈。若脉浮，小便不利，微热消渴者，五苓散主之。（《伤寒论》第71条）

Wuling Powder has sun disease. After sweating, it sweats out, the stomach is dry, and it is irritable and sleepless. If you want to drink water, you should drink it less, so that the stomach will be healed. If the pulse is floating, the urine is unfavorable, and the thirst is slightly hot, Wuling Powder is the main one. –Article 71 of *Treatise on Febrile Diseases*;

（3）真武汤　太阳病发汗，汗出不解，其人仍发热，心下悸，头眩，身瞤动，振振欲擗地者，真武汤主之。（《伤寒论》第82条）

Zhenwu Decoction sweats due to sun disease, and the sweat is puzzled. People still have fever, palpitation, dizziness, body movement, and vibration to get to the ground. Zhenwu Decoction is the master. –Article 82 of *Treatise on Febrile Diseases*.

十二、祛痰剂

12 Phlegm-resolving formulae

1. 概述 Overview

（1）概念　祛痰剂是以祛痰药为主组成，具有消除痰饮作用，治疗各种痰病的方剂。

Concept　Phlegm-resolving formulae is mainly composed of expectorants, which has the function of eliminating phlegm retention and treating various phlegm diseases.

（2）功效　燥湿化痰、清热化痰、润燥化痰、温化寒痰和治风化痰。

Efficacy　Eliminating dampness and eliminating phlegm, clearing heat and eliminating phlegm, moistening dryness and eliminating phlegm, warming cold phlegm and treating wind and eliminating phlegm.

（3）应用　痰证，包括湿痰、热痰、燥痰、寒痰和风痰等。

Application　Phlegm syndrome, including damp phlegm, hot phlegm, dry phlegm, cold phlegm and wind phlegm.

2. 常用方剂　二陈汤、温胆汤、半夏白术天麻汤、止嗽散、清气化痰丸、小陷胸汤。

Commonly used prescriptions　Erchen Decoction, Wendan Decoction, Banxia Baizhu Tianma Decoction, Zhisou Powder, Qingqi Huatan Pill and Xiaoxianxiong Decoction.

3. 代表方剂 Representative prescription

二陈汤（《太平惠民和剂局方》）Er Chen Decoction in *Taiping Huimin Heji Bureau Prescription*

组成：半夏 15g，橘红 15g，白茯苓 9g，炙甘草 4.5g。

Composition: Pinellia ternata 15g, Orange 15g, Poria cocos 9g, Radix Glycyrrhizae Preparata 4.5 g.

用法：加生姜 7 片，乌梅 1 个，水煎服。

Usage: Add 7 slices of ginger and 1 dark plum, and decoct them with water.

功效：燥湿化痰，理气和中。

Efficacy: Eliminating dampness and phlegm, regulating qi and harmonizing middle warmer.

主治：湿痰证。症见咳嗽痰多、色白易咳，胸膈痞闷，恶心呕吐，肢体困重，或头眩心悸，舌苔白滑或腻，脉滑。

Indications: Damp phlegm syndrome. Symptoms include cough with excessive phlegm, white color and easy cough, stuffy chest and diaphragm, nausea and vomiting, heavy limbs, dizziness and palpitation, white or greasy tongue coating and slippery pulse.

使用注意：燥痰者慎用。吐血、消渴、阴虚、血虚者忌用。

Attention: Use with caution for those with dry phlegm. Avoid vomiting blood, diabetes, yin deficiency and blood deficiency.

组方原理：方中半夏尤善燥湿化痰，且能和胃降逆，为君药。湿痰既成，每致气机阻遏，故以橘红为臣，既可理气行滞，又能燥湿化痰。痰由湿生，湿自脾来，故佐以茯苓健脾渗湿，以杜生痰之源。加生姜，既能制半夏之毒，又能助半夏化痰降逆、和胃止呕；复用少许乌梅，收敛肺气，与半夏、橘红相伍，散中兼收，使其祛痰不伤正气，且有“欲劫之而先聚之”之意，共为佐药。炙甘草为佐使，健脾和中，调和诸药。

Principle of prescription: Pinellia ternata in the prescription is especially good at eliminating dampness and phlegm, and can harmonize the stomach and lower adverse effects, so it is the monarch medicine. Damp phlegm is accomplished, which causes qi activity to be blocked. Therefore, orange is the minister, which can not only regulate qi and stagnation, but also eliminate dampness and phlegm. Phlegm comes from dampness, and dampness comes from spleen. Therefore, Poria cocos is used to strengthen spleen and permeate dampness, which is the source of phlegm. Adding ginger can not only control the poison of Pinellia ternata, but also help Pinellia ternata to eliminate phlegm and reduce adverse effects, harmonize the stomach and stop vomiting; Reuse a little dark plum, converge lung qi, combine it with Pinellia ternata and orange, and collect it in powder, so that it can eliminate phlegm without hurting healthy qi, and it has the meaning of “getting together first if you want to rob it”, which is an adjuvant medicine. Radix Glycyrrhizae Preparata is an adjuvant, which strengthens the spleen and harmonizes the middle.

十三、治风剂
13 Wind-eliminating formulae

1. 概述 Overview

（1）概念 治风剂是以辛散祛风或息风止痉的药物为主组成，具有疏散外风或平息内风作用，治疗风病的方剂。

Concept Wind-eliminating formulae is mainly composed of pungent powder for dispelling wind or relieving wind and spasm, which has the function of evacuating external wind or calming internal wind and treating wind diseases.

（2）功效 疏散外风，平息内风。

Efficacy Evacuate the external wind and calm the internal wind.

（3）应用 感受外风或内生风邪。

Application Feel external wind or endogenous wind evil.

2. 常用方剂 川芎茶调散、消风散、镇肝熄风汤、羚角钩藤汤、天麻钩藤饮。

Commonly used prescriptions Chuanxiong Tea Tiaosan, Xiaofeng Powder, Zhengan Xifeng Decoction, Lingjiao Gouteng Decoction and Tianma Gouteng Decoction.

3. 代表方剂 Representative prescription

（1）川芎茶调散（《太平惠民和剂局方》）Chuanxiong Tea Adjustment Powder in *Taiping Huimin Heji Bureau Prescription*

组成：川芎、荆芥各 120g，白芷、羌活、甘草各 60g，细辛 30g，防风 45g，薄荷 120g。

Composition: Ligusticum Chuanxiong and Schizonepeta tenuifolia 120g each, Angelica dahurica, Notopterygium root and Glycyrrhiza uralensis Fisch 60g each, Asarum 30g, Saposhnikovia.

用法：散剂，每服 6g，每日 2 次，清茶调下；水煎服。

Usage: Powder, 6g each time, twice a day, mixed with green tea; Decoct in water.

功效：疏风止痛。

Efficacy: Dispel wind and relieve pain.

主治：外感风邪头痛。症见偏正头痛或颠顶作痛，恶寒发热，目眩鼻塞，舌苔薄白，脉浮者。

Indications: Headache due to exogenous wind evil. Symptoms include headache or top pain, aversion to cold and fever, dizziness and stuffy nose, thin and white tongue coating and floating pulse.

使用注意：用量宜轻，不宜久煎。

Attention: The dosage should be light and should not be decocted for a long time.

组方原理：方中川芎辛香走窜，上达头目，善于祛风活血而止头痛，为“诸经头痛之要药"，长于治少阳、厥阴经头痛，为君药。薄荷轻清上行，疏散风邪，清利头目；羌活、白芷祛风止痛，其中羌活善治太阳经头痛，白芷善治阳明经头痛，细辛散寒止痛并长于治少阴经头痛，三药助川芎疏风止痛之力；荆芥、防风辛散上行，疏散风邪，共为臣药。用时以清茶调下，取茶叶的苦寒性味，既可上清头目，又能制约风药的过于温燥与升散，升中有降。甘草调和诸药，甘缓以防辛散耗气，为佐使药。

Principle of prescription: Ligusticum Chuanxiong is pungent and fragrant, reaching the leader, and is good at dispelling wind and promoting blood circulation to stop headache. It is the "key medicine for headache in various meridians", and is good at treating headache in Shaoyang and Jueyin meridians, and is the monarch medicine. Mint goes up lightly, evacuates wind evil, and clears the leader; Notopterygium root and Angelica dahurica can dispel wind and relieve pain, among which Notopterygium root is good at treating headache of Sun Meridian, Angelica dahurica is good at treating headache of Yangming Meridian, Asarum can dispel cold and relieve pain and is good at treating headache of Shaoyin Meridian, and the three drugs can help Chuanxiong dispel wind and relieve pain; Schizonepeta tenuifolia and Fangfeng Powder go up to evacuate wind evil, which are all ministerial medicines. When you use it, you can adjust it with green tea, and take the bitter and cold taste of tea, which can not only clear the leader, but also restrict the wind medicine from being too warm and dry, rising and scattering, and falling in rising. Glycyrrhiza uralensis Fisch blends various medicines, which is sweet and slow to prevent pungent powder from consuming qi.

（2）镇肝熄风汤（《医学衷中参西录》）Zhengan Xifeng Decoction in *Record of Chinese Medicine*

组成：怀牛膝 30g，生赭石 30g，生龙骨 15g，生牡蛎 15g，生龟甲 15g，生杭芍 15g，玄参 15g，天冬 15g，川楝子 6g，生麦芽 6g，茵陈 6g，甘草 4.5g。

Composition: Achyranthes bidentata 30g, raw ochre 30g, raw keel 15g, raw oyster 15g, raw tortoise shell 15g, raw Paeonia lactiflora 15g, Scrophularia ningpoensis 15g, asparagus 15g, toosendan 6g, raw malt 6g, wormwood 6g and licorice 4.5g.

用法：水煎服。

Usage: Decoct with water.

功效：镇肝息风，滋阴潜阳。

Efficacy: Calm liver and calm wind, nourish yin and submerge yang.

主治：类中风。症见头晕目眩，目胀耳鸣，脑部热痛，心中烦热，面色如醉，或时常噫气，或肢体渐觉不利，口角㖞斜，甚或眩晕颠仆，昏不知人，移时始醒，或醒后不得复原，精神短少，脉弦长有力者。

Indications: Stroke–like. Symptoms include dizziness, eye swelling and tinnitus, hot pain in the brain, vexation and heat in the heart, drunken complexion, or frequent breath, or gradual discomfort in limbs, oblique spat, or even dizziness, faintness, awakening when moving, or not recovering after waking up, lack of spirit, and long and strong pulse.

使用注意：气虚血瘀之中风不宜用。

Note: Apoplexy due to qi deficiency and blood stasis should not be used.

组方原理：方中重用怀牛膝引血下行，补益肝肾，为君药。代赭石镇潜肝阳，牛膝、代赭石相伍，则可使并走于上的气血下行；龙骨、牡蛎重镇潜阳，为臣药。君臣相合，降逆潜阳，镇肝息风以治标。龟甲、玄参、天冬、白芍滋养阴液，意在治本。肝性喜条达，故用茵陈、川楝子、生麦芽清肝热、舒肝气，三药配伍既可清泄肝阳之有余，又可顺肝木之性。甘草调和诸药，配麦芽和胃调中，防止金石类药物碍胃之弊，均为佐使药。

Principle of prescription: Achyranthes bidentata is reused in the prescription to induce blood to descend and tonify liver and kidney, which is the monarch medicine. On behalf of ochre town hidden liver yang, Achyranthes bidentata, on behalf of ochre, can make and go up the qi and blood downward; Keel, an important oyster town, is a minister medicine. The combination of monarch and minister, lowering the inverse and subduing yang, and calming the liver and stopping the wind to treat the symptoms. Tortoise shell, Scrophularia ningpoensis, Asparagus asparagus and Radix Paeoniae Alba nourish yin liquid, Liver is fond of strips, so Herba Artemisiae, Fructus Toosendan and raw malt are used to clear liver heat and soothe liver qi. The compatibility of the three drugs can not only clear away liver yang, but also follow the nature of liver wood. Glycyrrhiza uralensis Fisch blends various medicines, combines malt with stomach to regulate the middle, and prevents epigraphic drugs from obstructing the stomach, all of which are adjuvant medicines.

十四、消食剂

14 Digestive formulae

1. 概述 Overview

（1）概念　消食剂是以消食药为主组成，具有消食运脾、化积导滞等作用，主治各种食积证的方剂。

Concept　Digestive formulae is mainly composed of digestion-promoting drugs, which have the functions of digestion-promoting, spleen-transporting, stagnation-promoting, etc. It is a prescription for treating various food accumulation syndromes.

（2）功效　消食化滞、健脾消食。

Efficacy　Promoting digestion and stagnation, strengthening spleen and promoting digestion.

（3）应用　食积证。

Application　Food retention syndrome.

2. 常用方剂　保和丸、健脾丸、枳实导滞丸。

Commonly used prescriptions　Baohe Pill, Jianpi Pill and Zhishi Daozhi Pill.

3. 代表方剂 Representative prescription

保和丸（《丹溪心法》） Baohe Pill in *Danxi Heart Method*

组成：山楂 18g，神曲 6g，半夏、茯苓各 9g，陈皮、连翘、莱菔子各 3g。

Composition: Hawthorn 18g, Divine Composition 6g, Pinellia ternata, Poria cocos 9g each, dried tangerine peel, Forsythia suspensa, radish seed 3g each.

用法：上药共为末，水泛为丸，每服 6 ～ 9g，温开水送下；亦可作汤剂，水煎服。

Usage: The above medicine is the end, and the water is flooded into pills, each taking 6–9g, and sending it with warm boiled water; It can also be used as decoction and decocted with water.

功效：消食化滞，理气和胃。

Efficacy: Resolve digestion and stagnation, regulate qi and harmonize stomach.

主治：食积证。症见脘腹痞满胀痛，嗳腐吞酸，恶食呕逆，或大便泄泻，舌苔腻，脉滑。

Indications: Syndrome of food retention. Symptoms include abdominal fullness, swelling and pain, belly rot, acid swallowing, vomiting, or stool diarrhea, greasy tongue coating and slippery pulse.

使用注意：属攻伐之剂，不宜久服。

Attention to use: It is an attack agent and should not be taken for a long time.

组方原理：方中以山楂为君药，可消一切饮食积滞，尤善消肉食油腻之积。臣以神曲消食健胃，更长于化酒食陈腐之积；莱菔子消食下气，长于消麦面痰气之积。三药同用，可消各种饮食积滞。佐以半夏、陈皮行气化滞，和胃止呕；茯苓健脾利湿，和中止泻。食积易于化热，故又佐以苦而微寒之连翘，既可散结以助消积，又可清解食积所生之热。

Principle of prescription: Hawthorn is the monarch medicine in the prescription, which can eliminate all dietary stagnation, especially the greasy meat. Use Divine Comedy to promote digestion and strengthen the stomach, which is longer than the stale product of wine and food; Raphani seeds promote digestion and lower qi, which is longer than eliminating phlegm and qi in wheat noodles. Using the three drugs together can eliminate various dietary stagnation. Accompanied by Pinellia ternata and dried tangerine peel, qi stagnation, stomach harmony and vomiting; Poria cocos strengthens spleen, promotes diuresis, and stops diarrhea. Food accumulation is easy to turn heat, so it is accompanied by bitter and slightly cold Forsythia suspensa, which can not only disperse the accumulation to help eliminate the accumulation, but also clear the heat caused by food accumulation.

第十二章　针灸基本知识
Chapter 12　Basic Knowledge of Acupuncture and Moxibustion

针灸学因其操作方便、经济安全、疗效明显、适应证广等优点，逐步发展成为专门学科。本章主要介绍经络学、腧穴学的基础知识。

Acupuncture and moxibustion has gradually developed into a specialized subject because of its advantages of convenient operation, economic safety, obvious curative effect and wide indications. This chapter mainly introduces the basic knowledge of meridian science and acupoint science.

第一节　腧穴学总论
Section 1　General Introduction of Acupoint Science

腧穴是人体脏腑经络气血输注于体表的特殊部位，也是疾病的反应点和针灸施术的部位。

Acupoints are the special parts where qi and blood of viscera and meridians are infused into the body surface, and they are also the reaction points of diseases and the parts where acupuncture is performed.

一、腧穴的分类
1 Classification of Acupoints

人体腧穴通常分为十四经穴、奇穴、阿是穴三类。

Acupoints of human body are usually divided into three categories: fourteen meridian points, strange points and Ashi points.

凡归属于十二正经和任脉、督脉的腧穴，称为十四经穴，简称经穴。一些具有确定的名称和位置，但尚未归入或不便于归入十四经脉系统的腧穴，统称奇穴。阿是穴既无固定名称，又无固定位置，仅以疾病压痛点或其他反应点作为针灸施术部位的一类腧穴，因按压患者痛处，患者会发出“啊”声，故命名“阿是穴”。

All acupoints belonging to the twelve meridians, Ren meridians and Du meridians are called fourteen meridians, or meridians for short. Some acupoints with definite names and locations, but which have not been classified or are inconvenient to be classified into the fourteen meridians system, are collectively called strange acupoints. Ashi Point has neither a fixed name nor a fixed position. Only the tenderness points of diseases or other reaction points are used as a class of acupoints at the acupuncture site. Because the patient presses the pain points, the patient will make a "ah" sound, so it is named "Ashi Point".

二、腧穴的主治特点
2 The indications of acupoints

腧穴的主治特点主要体现在近治作用、远治作用和特殊作用三个方面。

The indications of acupoints are mainly reflected in three aspects: near treatment, remote treatment and special treatment.

1. 近治作用 腧穴具有治疗其所在部位的局部及其临近组织、器官病证的作用。

Near-treatment Acupoints have the function of treating diseases and syndromes of local parts and adjacent tissues and organs where they are located.

2. 远治作用 腧穴具有治疗本经脉循行所经过的远隔部位的脏腑、组织、器官病证的作用，即"经脉所过，主治所及"。腧穴的远治作用与经络的循行密切相关。

Remote treatment Acupoints have the function of treating the diseases and syndromes of viscera, tissues and organs in distant parts where the meridians pass, that is, "where the meridians pass, where the indications reach". The remote treatment of acupoints is closely related to the circulation of meridians.

3. 特殊作用 腧穴具有双向良性调节作用和相对特殊的治疗作用。如腹泻时针天枢可止泻，便秘时针天枢可通便。

Special treatment Acupoints have two-way benign regulation and relatively special therapeutic effect. Such as diarrhea hour hand Tian Shu can stop diarrhea, constipation hour hand Tian Shu can relieve constipation.

三、腧穴定位法
3 Acupoint positioning method

腧穴定位法是指确定腧穴位置的基本方法，又称取穴法。取穴法主要有体表标志定位法、骨度折量定位法、手指同身寸定位法和简便取穴法。

Acupoint positioning method refers to the basic method of determining the position of acupoints, also known as acupoint selection method. Point selection methods mainly include body surface mark positioning, bone degree and folding positioning, finger same body cun positioning and simple point selection.

1. 体表标志定位法 是以人体的体表标志为依据来确定腧穴位置的方法。体表标志分为固定标志和活动标志两类，前者如骨节和肌肉所形成的突起或凹陷、五官轮廓、发际、指（趾）甲、乳头、肚脐等，后者如关节、肌肉、肌腱、皮肤等随着活动而出现的空隙、凹陷、皱纹等。

The body surface mark positioning method It is a method to determine the position of acupoints based on the body surface mark of human body. Body surface signs can be divided into two types: fixed signs and active signs. The former is such as protrusions or depressions formed by joints and muscles, facial contours, hairline, nails, nipples, navel, etc., while the latter is such as gaps, depressions, wrinkles, etc. of joints, muscles, tendons, skin, etc.

2. 骨度折量定位法 又称“骨度法”（表 12–1）。

Bone fracture positioning method It is also called “bone fracture method” (Table 12–1).

表 12–1 骨度折量寸表

Table 12–1 Bone Fracture Cun Table

部位 Location	起止点 Starting and ending point	折量寸 Fold Cun	度量方法 Measurement method	说明 Description
头面部 Head and face	前发际正中至后发际正中 Median front hairline to median back hairline	12 寸 12 cun	直量 Straight quantity	确定头部腧穴的纵向距离 Determine the longitudinal distance of head acupoints
	眉间（印堂）至前发际正中 Eyebrow (Yintang) to the center of front hairline	3 寸 3 cun	直量 Straight quantity	确定前额部腧穴的纵向距离 Determine the longitudinal distance of forehead acupoints
	前额两发角（头维）之间 Between the two hair angles (head dimensions) of the forehead	9 寸 9 cun	横量 Transverse quantity	确定头前部腧穴的横向距离 Determine the transverse distance of acupoints in front of the head
	耳后两乳突（完骨）之间 Between the two hair angles (head dimensions) of the forehead	9 寸 9 cun	横量 Transverse quantity	确定头后部腧穴的横向距离 Determine the transverse distance of acupoints at the back of the head
	第 7 颈椎棘突下至后发际正中 The spinous process of the 7th cervical spine descends to the middle of the posterior hairline	3 寸 3 cun	直量 Straight quantity	确定后颈部腧穴的纵向距离 Determine the longitudinal distance of acupoints in the posterior neck
胸腹胁部 Thoracoabdominal hypochondrium	胸骨上窝（天突）至胸剑联合中点 Superior sternal fossa (celestial process) to the midpoint of chest-sword joint	9 寸 9 cun	直量 Straight quantity	确定胸部任脉穴的纵向距离 Determine the longitudinal distance of Ren meridian points in chest
	胸剑联合中点（歧骨）至脐中 From the midpoint of thoracic-sword joint (disambiguation bone) to the umbilicus	8 寸 8 cun	直量 Straight quantity	确定上腹部腧穴的纵向距离 Determine the longitudinal distance of acupoints in the upper abdomen

续表

部位 Location	起止点 Starting and ending point	折量寸 Fold Cun	度量方法 Measurement method	说明 Description
胸腹胁部 Thoracoabdominal hypochondrium	脐中至耻骨联合上缘（曲骨） From the middle umbilicus to the upper edge of pubic symphysis (curved bone)	5 寸 5 cun	直量 Straight quantity	确定下腹部腧穴的纵向距离 Determine the longitudinal distance of acupoints in lower abdomen
	两乳头之间 Between two nipples	8 寸 8 cun	横量 Transverse quantity	确定胸腹部腧穴的横向距离 Determine the transverse distance of thoracic and abdominal acupoints
	腋窝顶点至第 11 肋游离端 Axillary apex to free end of 11th rib	12 寸 12 cun	直量 Straight quantity	确定胁肋部腧穴的纵向距离 Determine the longitudinal distance of hypochondriac acupoints
背腰部 Back waist	第 7 颈椎棘突下（大椎）至尾骶 Subspinous process (greater vertebra) to caudal sacrum of the 7th cervical spine	21 椎 21 vertebrae	直量 Straight quantity	督脉腧穴定位依据 Location basis of Du meridian acupoints
	肩胛骨内缘至后正中线 From the inner edge of scapula to the posterior midline	3 寸 3 cun	横量 Transverse quantity	确定背腰部腧穴的横向距离 Determine the transverse distance of acupoints on the back and waist
	肩峰缘至后正中线 Acromion margin to posterior midline	8 寸 8 cun	横量 Transverse quantity	确定肩背部腧穴的横向距离 Determine the transverse distance of acupoints on shoulder and back
下肢部 Lower extremity	腋前、后纹头至肘横纹（平肘尖） Anterior and posterior axillary striation head to elbow transverse striation (flat elbow tip)	9 寸 9 cun	直量 Straight quantity	确定上臂部腧穴的纵向距离 Determine the longitudinal distance of acupoints on the upper arm
	肘横纹（平肘尖）至腕掌（背）侧横纹 Transverse striation of elbow (flat elbow tip) to transverse striation of carpometacarpal (dorsal) side	12 寸 12 cun	直量 Straight quantity	确定前臂部腧穴的纵向距离 Determine the longitudinal distance of forearm acupoints
	耻骨联合上缘至股骨内上髁上缘 Superior edge of pubic symphysis to superior edge of medial epicondyle of femur	18 寸 18 cun	直量 Straight quantity	确定大腿内侧腧穴的纵向距离 Determine the longitudinal distance of acupoints on the inner thigh
	胫骨内侧髁下方至内踝尖 From below the medial condyle of tibia to the tip of medial	13 寸 13 cun	直量 Straight quantity	确定小腿内侧腧穴的纵向距离 Determine the longitudinal distance of acupoints on the inner leg

续表

部位 Location	起止点 Starting and ending point	折量寸 Fold Cun	度量方法 Measurement method	说明 Description
下肢部 Lower extremity	股骨大转子至膝中（腘横纹） From greater trochanter of femur to middle knee (popliteal transverse striation)	19 寸 19 cun	直量 Straight quantity	确定大腿外后侧腧穴的纵向距离 Determine the longitudinal distance of acupoints on the outer back of thigh
	膝中（腘横纹）至外踝尖 Middle knee (popliteal transverse striation) to lateral malleolus tip	16 寸 16 cun	直量 Straight quantity	确定小腿外后侧腧穴的纵向距离 Determine the longitudinal distance of acupoints on the outer posterior side of the leg
	臀沟至腘横纹 Buttock sulcus to popliteal transverse striation	14 寸 14 cun	直量 Straight quantity	确定大腿后侧腧穴的纵向距离 Determine the longitudinal distance of acupoints on the back of thigh

3. 手指同身寸定位法 是以患者手指作为度量分寸来量取腧穴的定位方法，又称“指寸法”。手指同身寸包括中指同身寸、拇指同身寸和横指同身寸三种（图 12–1）。

Finger–in–body positioning method It is a positioning method that measures acupoints with patients' fingers as measurement discretion, also known as "finger–in–cun method". Finger body cun includes middle finger body cun, thumb body cun and horizontal finger body cun (Figure 12–1).

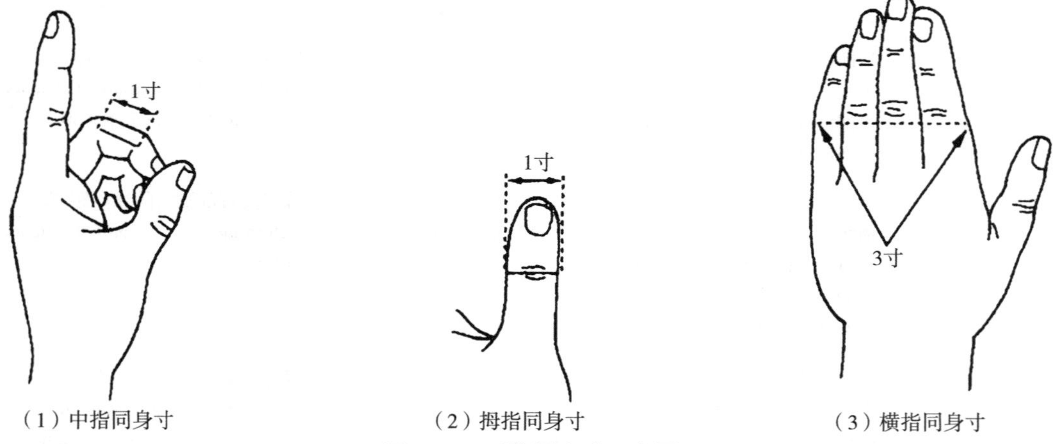

图 12–1 手指同身寸示意图

Figure 12–1 Schematic diagram of finger size

4. 简便取穴法 是临床总结出来的某些简单方便的取穴方法，是一种辅助取穴法。如患者立正姿势，双手自然下垂，其中指末端即为风市穴。

Simple acupoint selection method It is some simple and convenient acupoint selection methods summarized in clinic, and it is an auxiliary acupoint selection method. If the patient stands at attention, his hands droop naturally, and the end of the finger is Fengshi acupoint.

第二节 十二经脉及其常用腧穴
Section 2 Twelve Meridians and Their Common Acupoints

一、手太阴肺经
1 The hand Taiyin lung meridian

（一）经脉循行
1.1 Meridian circulation

手太阴肺经循行见图 12–2。
See Figure 12–2 for the lung meridian of hand Taiyin.

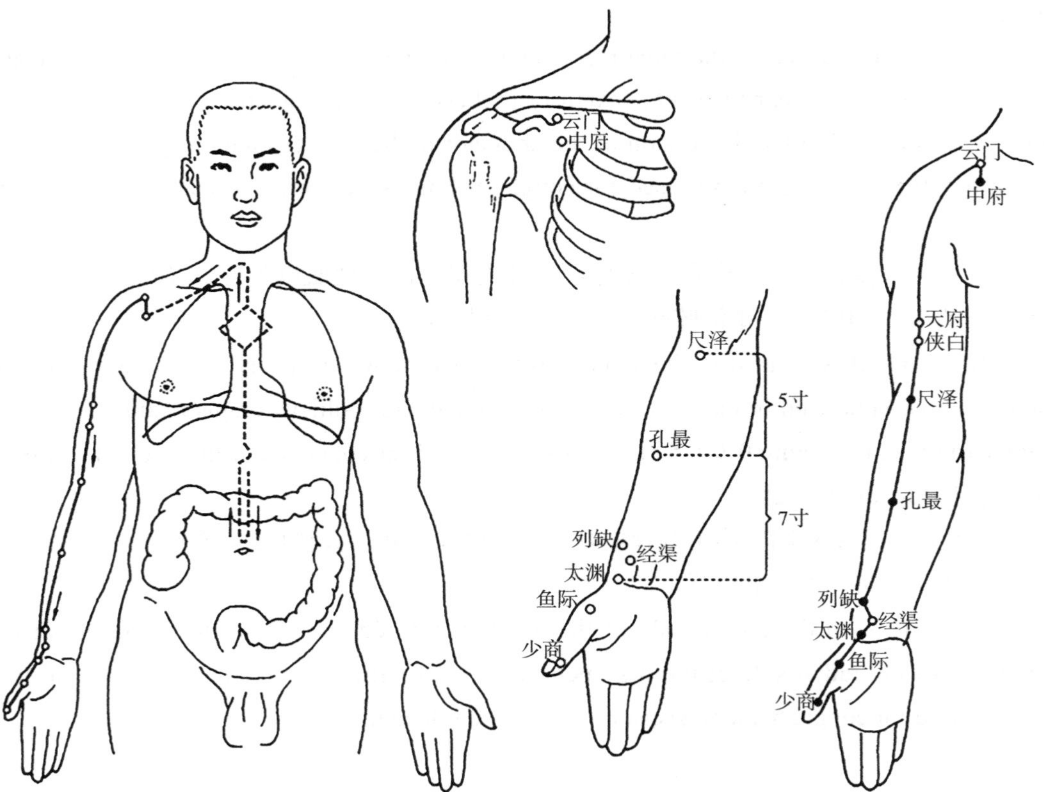

图 12–2 手太阴肺经循行及腧穴示意图
Figure 12–2 Schematic diagram of lung meridian circulation and acupoints of hand Taiyin

（二）常用腧穴

1.2 Common acupoints

手太阴肺经分布有 11 个腧穴：中府、云门、天府、侠白、尺泽、孔最、列缺、经渠、太渊、鱼际、少商。本经腧穴主要治疗喉、胸、肺及肺经循行部位的其他病症。

There are 11 acupoints distributed in the lung meridian of Hand Taiyin: Zhongfu, Yunmen, Tianfu, Xiabai, Chize, Kongzui, Lieque, Jingqu, Taiyuan, Yuji and Shaoshang. Acupoints of this meridian mainly treat other diseases of throat, chest, lung and lung meridian.

1. 尺泽 在肘区，肘横纹上，肱二头肌腱桡侧缘凹陷中。直刺 0.8 ～ 1.0 寸，或点刺放血。主治咳嗽、气喘、咽喉肿痛、肘臂挛痛等。

Chize It is located in the elbow area, on the transverse striation of elbow, and in the depression of the radial edge of biceps brachii tendon. Stab 0.8–1.0 cun straight, or prick and bleed. It is mainly used for cough, asthma, sore throat, elbow and arm twin pain, etc.

2. 列缺 在前臂，腕掌侧远端横纹上 1.5 寸，拇短伸肌腱与拇长展肌腱之间，拇长展肌腱沟的凹陷中。斜刺 0.3 ～ 0.5 寸。主治咳嗽、气喘、咽喉肿痛、头痛、项强等。

Lieque It is absent in the forearm, 1.5 cun above the transverse striation at the distal end of carpometacarpal side, between the extensor pollicis brevis tendon and the abductor pollicis longus tendon, and in the depression of the abductor pollicis longus tendon groove. Oblique prick 0.3–0.5 cun. It is mainly used for cough, asthma, sore throat, headache, strong neck, etc.

3. 太渊 在腕前区，桡骨茎突与舟状骨之间，拇长展肌腱尺侧凹陷中。避开桡动脉，直刺 0.3 ～ 0.5 寸。主治咳喘、胸背痛、无脉症等。

Taiyuan It is located in the anterior wrist area, between the styloid process of radius and scaphoid bone, and in the ulnar depression of abductor pollicis longus tendon. Avoid the radial artery and puncture 0.3–0.5 cun. It is mainly used for cough and asthma, chest and back pain, pulseless disease, etc.

4. 鱼际 在手外侧，第 1 掌骨桡侧中点赤白肉际处。直刺 0.5 ～ 0.8 寸。主治咳嗽、咯血、咽喉肿痛、小儿疳积等。

Yuji It is on the lateral side of the hand, at the red and white fleshy border at the midpoint of the radial side of the first metacarpal bone. Straight puncture 0.5–0.8 cun. It is mainly used for cough, hemoptysis, sore throat, infantile malnutrition, etc.

二、手阳明大肠经

2 The large intestine meridian of Hand Yangming

（一）经脉循行

2.1 Meridian circulation

手阳明大肠经循行见图 12–3。

The circulation of large intestine meridian in Hand Yangming is shown in Figure 12–3.

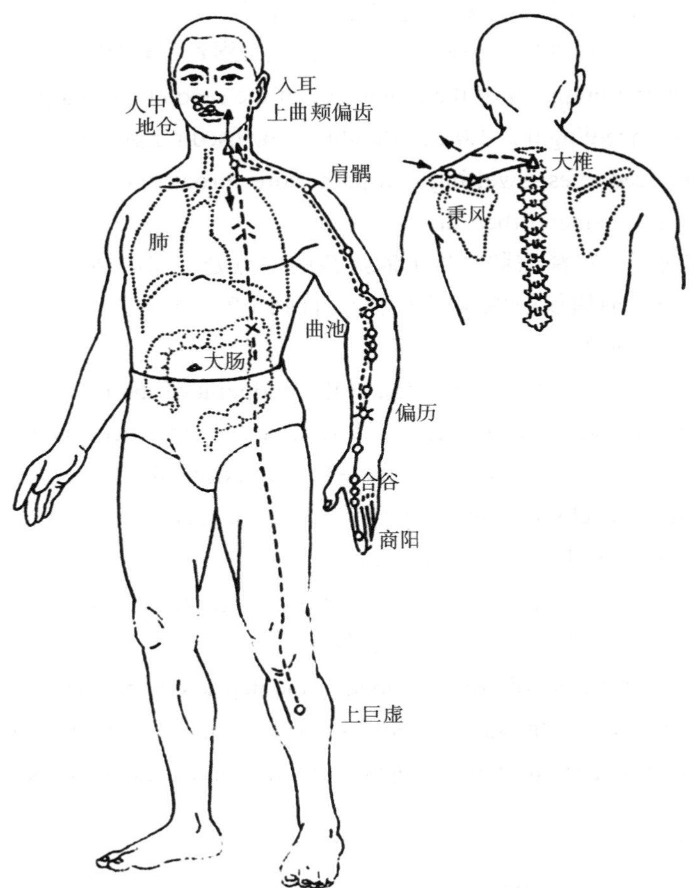

图 12–3　手阳明大肠经循行及腧穴示意图

Figure 12–3　Schematic diagram of large intestine meridian circulation and acupoints of hand Yangming

（二）常用腧穴

2.2 Common acupoints

手阳明大肠经分布有 20 个腧穴：商阳、二间、三间、合谷、阳溪、偏历、温溜、下廉、上廉、手三里、曲池、肘髎、手五里、臂臑、肩髃、巨骨、天鼎、扶突、口禾髎、迎香。本经腧穴主要治疗头面五官疾患、热病、皮肤病、肠胃病、神志病及大肠经循行部位的其他病症。

There are 20 acupoints distributed in the large intestine meridian of Shouyangming: Shangyang, Erjian, Sanjian, Hegu, Yangxi, Pianli, Wenliu, Xialian, Shanglian, Shousanli, Quchi, Elbow Liao, Shouwuli, Arm Yu, Shoulder Yu, Jugu, Tianding, Futu, Kouhe Liao and Yingxiang. Acupoints of this meridian mainly treat diseases of head, face and facial features, fever, skin diseases, gastrointestinal diseases, mental diseases and other diseases along the large intestine meridian.

1. 合谷 在手背，第 2 掌骨桡侧的中点处。直刺 0.5 ～ 1.0 寸，孕妇不宜针刺。主治头痛、目赤肿痛、咽喉肿痛、齿痛、耳聋、口㖞、滞产、经闭等。

Hegu It is at the midpoint of the radial side of the second metacarpal bone on the back of the hand. Straight needling 0.5–1.0 cun should not be used for pregnant women. It is mainly used for headache, red eyes, swelling and pain, sore throat, toothache, deafness,deviated mouth, prolonged labor, amenorrhea, etc.

2. 曲池 在肘区，尺泽与肱骨外上髁连线的中点处（屈肘 90°，肘横纹外侧端外凹陷中；极度屈肘时，肘横纹桡侧端凹陷中）。直刺 1.0 ～ 1.5 寸。主治咽喉肿痛、齿痛、目赤肿痛、头痛、热病等。

Quchi It is located in the elbow area, at the midpoint of the line connecting Chize and the lateral epicondyle of humerus (90 elbow flexion, in the outer depression of the lateral end of the transverse striation of elbow; When the elbow is extremely flexed, the radial end of the transverse striation of the elbow is sunken). Stab 1.0–1.5 cun straight. It is mainly used for sore throat, toothache, red eyes, headache, fever, etc.

3. 肩髃 在三角肌区，肩峰外侧缘前端与肱骨大结节两骨间凹陷中。直刺或向下斜刺 0.8 ～ 1.5 寸。主治上肢活动不利、肩痛不举等。

Jianyu It lies in the deltoid muscle area, in the depression between the front end of the lateral edge of acromion and the greater tubercle of humerus. Stab straight or obliquely down 0.8–1.5 cun. It is mainly used for adverse upper limb movement, shoulder pain and so on.

三、足阳明胃经

3 Foot Yangming Stomach Meridian

（一）经脉循行

3.1 Meridian circulation

足阳明胃经循行见图 12–4。

The stomach meridian of Foot Yangming is shown in Figure 12–4.

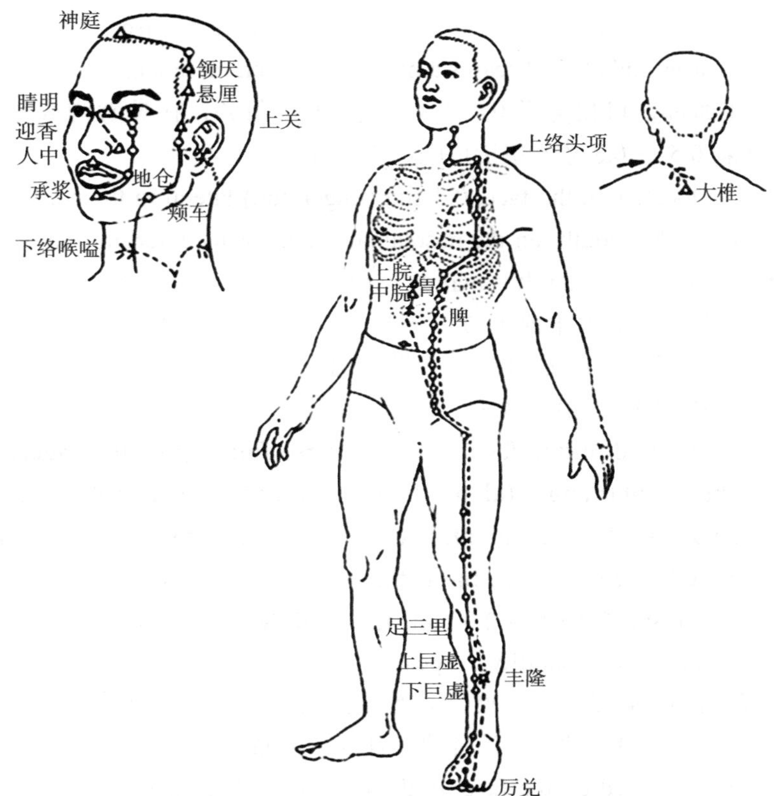

图 12-4 足阳明胃经循行及腧穴示意图

Figure 12-4 Schematic diagram of stomach meridian circulation and acupoints of Zuyangming

（二）常用腧穴

3.2 Common acupoints

足阳明胃经分布有 45 个腧穴：承泣、四白、巨髎、地仓、大迎、颊车、下关、头维、人迎、水突、气舍、缺盆、气户、库房、屋翳、膺窗、乳中、乳根、不容、承满、梁门、关门、太乙、滑肉门、天枢、外陵、大巨、水道、归来、气冲、髀关、伏兔、阴市、梁丘、犊鼻、足三里、上巨虚、条口、下巨虚、丰隆、解溪、冲阳、陷谷、内庭、厉兑。本经腧穴主治胃肠病、头面五官病、神志病、皮肤病、热病及胃经循行部位的其他病症。

There are 45 acupoints distributed in the stomach meridian of Zuyangming: Chengqi, Sibai, Juliao, Dicang, Daying, Buccal Car, Xiaguan, Touwei, Renying, Shuitu, Qishe, Quepen, Qihu, Warehouse, Wuyi, Yingchuang, Ruzhong, Rugen, Burong, Chengman, Liangmen, Guanmen, Taiyi, Sliding Meat Gate, Tian Shu, Wailing, Daju, Waterway, Return, Qichong, Tioguan, Futu, Yinshi, Liangqiu, Dubi, Zusanli, Upper Juxu, Tiaokou, Lower Juxu, Fenglong, Jiexi, Chongyang, Dagu, Inner Court and Lidui. Acupoints of this meridian are mainly used to treat gastrointestinal diseases, head, face and facial features diseases, mental diseases, skin diseases, fever diseases and other diseases along the stomach meridian.

1. 地仓　在面部，口角旁开 0.4 寸（指寸）（口角旁，在鼻唇沟或鼻唇沟延长线上）。平刺或斜刺 0.5 ～ 0.8 寸。主治口㖞、流涎等。

Dicang　It is located on the face, 0.4 cun (finger cun) lateral to the corner of the mouth (beside the corner of the mouth, on the nasolabial sulcus or its extension line). Horizontal or oblique insertion of 0.5 – 0.8 cun. It is mainly used to treat wry mouth and salivation, etc.

2. 颊车　在面部，下颌角前上方一横指（中指）（沿下颌角平分线上一横指，闭口咬紧牙关时咬肌隆起，放松时按之有凹陷处）。直刺 0.3 ～ 0.5 寸，或向地仓透刺 1.5 ～ 2.0 寸。主治口㖞、颊肿、齿痛、口噤不语等。

Jiache　It is located on the face, one transverse finger (middle finger) anterior and superior to the mandibular angle (along the midline of the mandibular angle, where the masseter muscle bulges when the mouth is closed and the teeth are clenched tightly and a depression can be felt when relaxed). Insert the needle perpendicularly for 0.3 – 0.5 cun, or perforate towards Dicang for 1.5 – 2.0 cun. It is mainly used to treat wry mouth, swollen cheek, toothache, trismus and inability to speak, etc.

3. 下关　在面部，颧弓下缘中央与下颌切迹之间凹陷中（闭口，上关直下，颧弓下缘凹陷中）。直刺 0.5 ～ 1.0 寸。主治耳鸣、耳聋、齿痛、口㖞、面痛等。

Xiaguan　It is located on the face, in the depression between the central lower margin of the zygomatic arch and the mandibular notch (with the mouth closed, directly below Shangguan, in the depression of the lower margin of the zygomatic arch). Insert the needle perpendicularly for 0.5 – 1.0 cun. It is mainly used to treat tinnitus, deafness, toothache, facial paralysis, facial pain, etc.

4. 天枢　在腹部，横平脐中，前正中线旁开 2 寸。直刺 1.0 ～ 1.5 寸。主治肠鸣腹胀、绕脐痛、便秘、泄泻、痢疾、癥瘕、月经不调、痛经等。

Tianshu　It is situated in the abdomen, at the same level as the umbilicus, 2 cun lateral to the anterior midline. The needle is inserted perpendicularly for 1.0 – 1.5 cun. It is mainly used to treat rumbling bowel sounds, abdominal distension, pain around the umbilicus, constipation, diarrhea, dysentery, abdominal masses, irregular menstruation, and dysmenorrhea, etc.

5. 足三里　在小腿外侧，犊鼻下 3 寸，犊鼻与解溪连线上（在胫骨前肌上取穴）。直刺 1.0 ～ 2.0 寸。主治胃痛、腹痛、呕吐、消化不良、泄泻、便秘、虚劳羸瘦、下肢痹痛、水肿等。

Zusanli　It is on the lateral side of the lower leg, 3 cun below Dubi, on the line connecting Dubi and Jiexi (the acupoint is located on the anterior tibialis muscle). The needle is inserted perpendicularly for 1.0 – 2.0 cun. It is mainly used to treat stomach pain, abdominal pain, vomiting, dyspepsia, diarrhea, constipation, asthenic fatigue and emaciation, pain and numbness of the lower extremities, edema, etc.

6. 丰隆 在小腿外侧，外踝尖上 8 寸，胫骨前肌外缘（犊鼻与解溪连线的中点，条口外侧一横指）。直刺 1.0 ～ 1.5 寸。主治下肢痿痹、癫、狂、痫、痰浊诸症等。

Fenglong It is on the lateral side of the lower leg, 8 cun above the tip of the lateral malleolus, on the outer edge of the anterior tibialis muscle (the midpoint of the line connecting Dubi and Jiexi, one transverse finger outside the lateral side of Tiáok ǒ u). The needle is inserted perpendicularly for 1.0 – 1.5 cun. It is mainly used to treat flaccidity and numbness of the lower extremities, epilepsy, mania, and other disorders caused by phlegm turbidity.

四、足太阴脾经

4 Foot Taiyin Spleen Meridian

（一）经脉循行

4.1 Meridian circulation

足太阴脾经循行见图 12–5。

The spleen meridian of Foot Taiyin is shown in Figure 12–5.

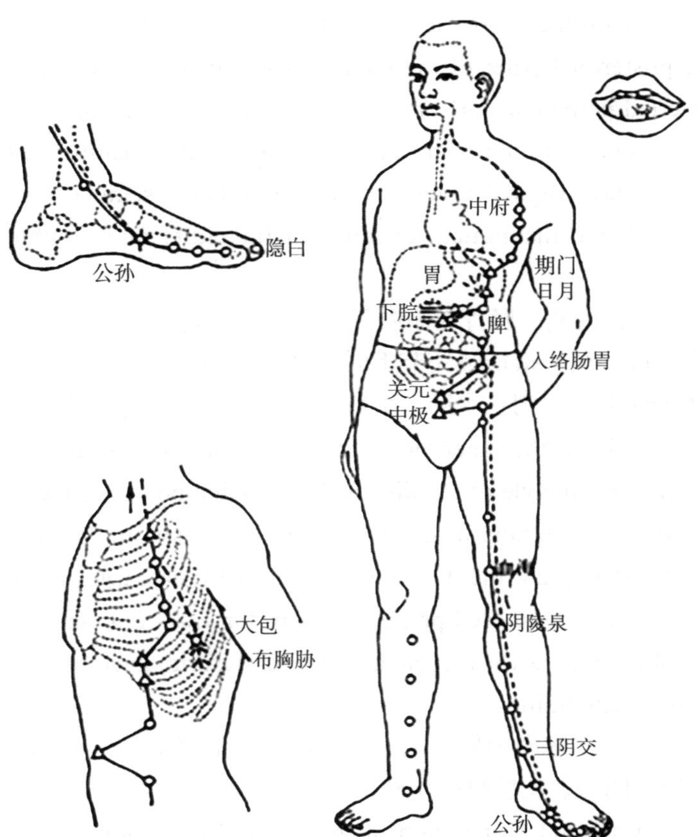

图 12–5 足太阴脾经循行及腧穴示意图

Figure 12–5 Schematic diagram of spleen meridian circulation and acupoints of Zutaiyin

（二）常用腧穴

4.2 Common acupoints

足太阴脾经分布有 21 个腧穴：隐白、大都、太白、公孙、商丘、三阴交、漏谷、地机、阴陵泉、血海、箕门、冲门、府舍、腹结、大横、腹哀、食窦、天溪、胸乡、周荣、大包。本经腧穴主治脾胃病、妇科病、前阴病，以及脾经循行部位的其他病症。

There are 21 acupoints distributed in the spleen meridian of Zutaiyin: Yinbai, Dadu, Taibai, Gongsun, Shangqiu, Sanyinjiao, Lougu, Diji, Yinlingquan, Xuehai, Jimen, Chongmen, Fushe, Fujie, Daheng, Fuai, Shidou, Tianxi, Xiongxiang, Zhourong, and Dabao. Acupoints of this meridian are mainly used to treat diseases of the spleen and stomach, gynecological diseases, anterior genital diseases, and other disorders in the areas along the meridian of the spleen.

1. 三阴交 在小腿内侧，内踝尖上 3 寸，胫骨内侧缘后际（交信上 1 寸）。直刺 1.0 ～ 1.5 寸，文献记载孕妇禁针。主治月经不调、经闭、带下、阴挺、遗精、阳痿、小便不利、遗尿、水肿、失眠、眩晕、下肢痿痹等。

Sanyinjiao It is on the inner side of the lower leg, 3 cun above the tip of the medial malleolus, at the posterior border of the medial aspect of the tibia (1 cun above Jiaoxin). The needle is inserted perpendicularly for 1.0 – 1.5 cun. It is recorded in the literature that acupuncture at this point is prohibited for pregnant women. It is mainly used to treat irregular menstruation, amenorrhea, vaginal discharge, uterine prolapse, seminal emission, impotence, dysuria, enuresis, edema, insomnia, vertigo, and flaccidity and numbness of the lower extremities, etc.

2. 阴陵泉 在小腿内侧，胫骨内侧髁下缘与胫骨内侧缘之间的凹陷中（用拇指沿胫骨内侧缘由下往上推，至拇指抵膝关节下时，胫骨向内上弯曲的凹陷中即本穴）。直刺 1.0 ～ 2.0 寸。主治腹胀、泄泻、水肿、黄疸、小便不利、膝痛、下肢痿痹等。

Yinlingquan It is on the inner side of the lower leg, in the depression between the lower edge of the medial condyle of the tibia and the medial border of the tibia (push upward along the medial border of the tibia with the thumb from the bottom. When the thumb reaches the lower part of the knee joint, the depression where the tibia curves inward and upward is this acupoint). The needle is inserted perpendicularly for 1.0 – 2.0 cun. It is mainly used to treat abdominal distension, diarrhea, edema, jaundice, dysuria, knee pain, and flaccidity and numbness of the lower extremities.

3. 血海 在股前区，髌底内侧端上 2 寸，股内侧肌隆起处。直刺 1.0 ～ 1.5 寸。主治月经不调、痛经、闭经、皮肤瘙痒、瘾疹、湿疹、丹毒等。

Xuehai It is in the anterior region of the thigh, 2 cun above the medial end of the patella, at the bulge of the vastus medialis muscle. The needle is inserted perpendicularly for 1.0 – 1.5 cun. It is mainly used to treat irregular menstruation, dysmenorrhea, amenorrhea, pruritus, urticaria, eczema, erysipelas, etc.

五、手少阴心经
5 Hand Shaoyin Heart Meridian

（一）经脉循行
5.1 Meridian circulation

手少阴心经循行见图 12–6。

The heart meridian of Hand Shaoyin is shown in Figure 12–6.

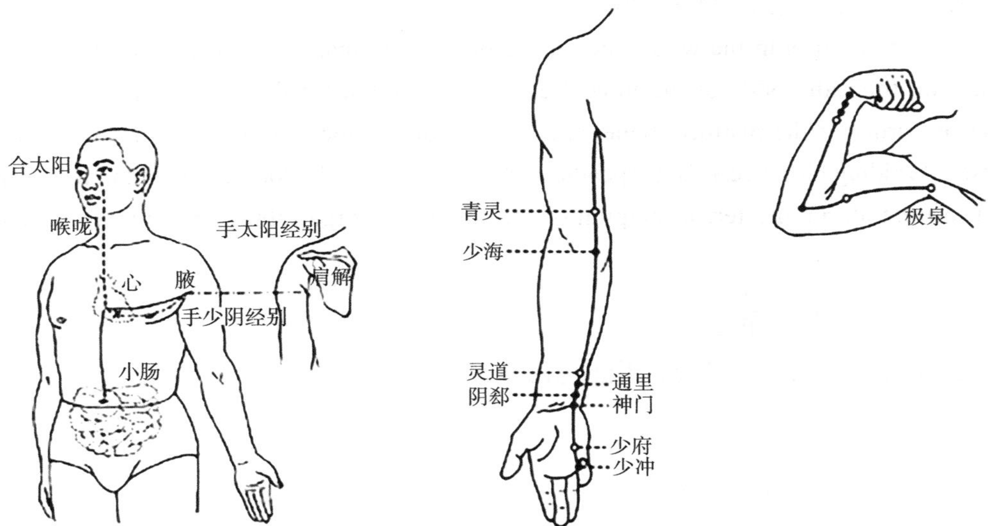

图 12–6 手少阴心经循行及腧穴示意图

Figure 12–6 Schematic diagram of heart meridian circulation and acupoints of Shoushaoyin

（二）常用腧穴
5.2 Common acupoints

本经分布有 9 个腧穴：极泉、青灵、少海、灵道、通里、阴郄、神门、少府、少冲。本经腧穴主要治疗心、胸、神志病，血证，肢痛痒疮，以及心经循行部位的其他病症。

There are 9 acupoints distributed in the heart meridian of Shoushaoyin: Jixuan, Qingling, Shaohai, Lingdao, Tongli, Yinxi, Shenmen, Shaofu and Shaochong. Acupoints of this meridian are mainly used to treat diseases of the heart, chest, and mind, bleeding disorders, limb pain, itching, and sores, as well as other disorders along the running path of the Heart Meridian of Hand Shaoyin.

1. 少海 在肘前区，横平肘横纹，肱骨内上髁前缘（屈肘，在肘横纹内侧端与肱骨内上髁连线的中点处）。直刺 0.5 ～ 1.0 寸。主治心痛、神志病、肘臂挛痛麻木等。

Shaohai It is in the anterior region of the elbow, at the same level as the transverse elbow crease, at the anterior margin of the medial epicondyle of the humerus (flex the elbow, and it is at the midpoint of the line connecting the medial end of the elbow crease and the medial epicondyle of the humerus). The needle is inserted perpendicularly for 0.5 – 1.0 cun. It is mainly used to treat heart pain, mental disorders, contracture and numbness of the elbow and arm, etc.

2. 神门 在腕前区，腕掌侧远端横纹尺侧端，尺侧屈腕肌腱的桡侧缘（在豌豆骨上缘桡侧凹陷中，于腕掌侧远端横纹上取穴）。避开血管直刺 0.3 ～ 0.5 寸。主治惊悸、怔忡、心烦、健忘、失眠、痴呆、癫、狂等。

Shenmen It is in the wrist anterior region, at the ulnar end of the distal wrist palmar crease, on the radial side of the ulnar flexor carpi tendon (in the radial depression of the superior border of the pisiform bone, and the acupoint is located on the distal wrist palmar crease). Avoiding blood vessels, perpendicularly insert the needle for 0.3 – 0.5 cun. It is mainly used to treat alarm and terror, palpitation, restlessness, forgetfulness, insomnia, dementia, epilepsy, mania, etc.

六、手太阳小肠经

6 Small Intestine Meridian of Hand Sun

（一）经脉循行

6.1 Meridian circulation

手太阳小肠经循行见图 12–7。

The circulation of small intestine meridian of hand sun is shown in Figure 12–7.

（二）常用腧穴

6.2 Common acupoints

手太阳小肠经分布有 19 个腧穴：少泽、前谷、后溪、腕骨、阳谷、养老、支正、小海、肩贞、臑俞、天宗、秉风、曲垣、肩外俞、肩中俞、天窗、天容、颧髎、听宫。本经腧穴主治头面五官病、热病、神志病，以及小肠经循行部位的其他病症。

There are 19 acupoints distributed in the small intestine meridian of Hand Sun: Shaoze, Qiangu, Houxi, Carpal Bone, Yanggu, Pension, Zhizheng, Xiaohai, Jianzhen, Yu Shu, Tianzong, Bingfeng, Quyuan, Jianwaishu, Jianzhongshu, Skylight, Tianrong, Quanliao and Tinggong. Acupoints of this meridian are mainly used to treat diseases of head, face and facial features, fever, mental diseases, and other diseases along the small intestine meridian.

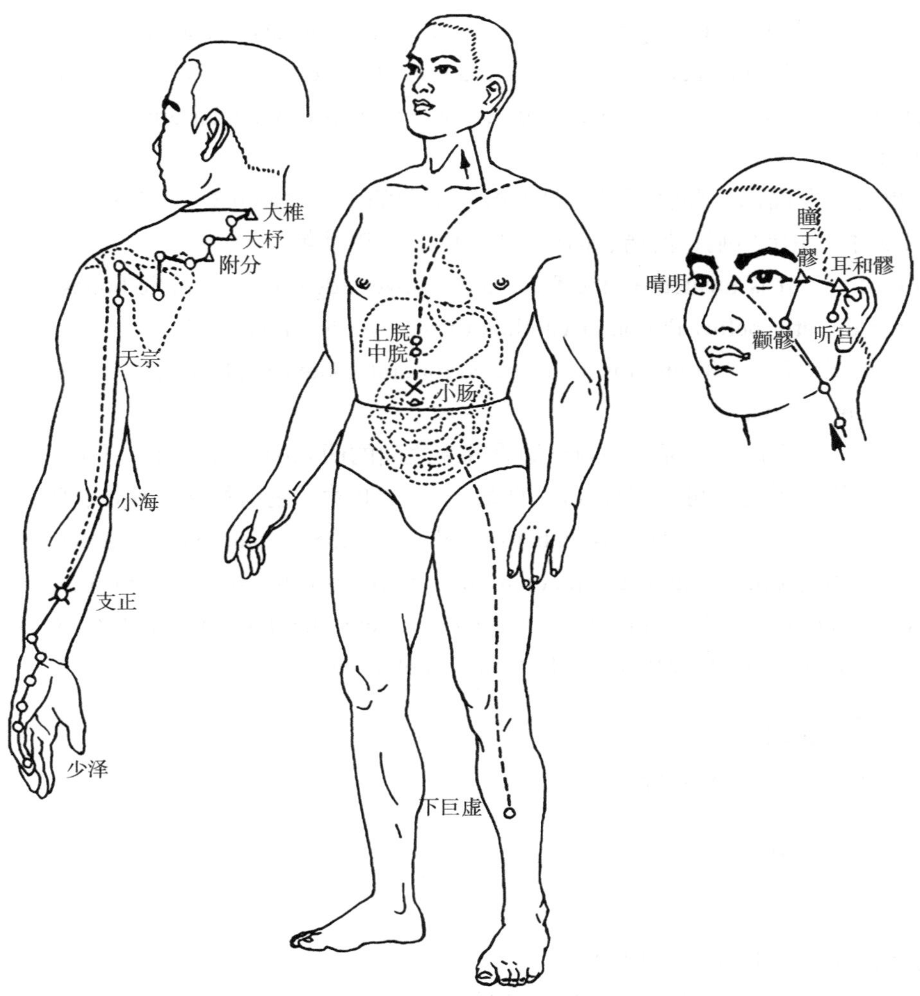

图 12–7 手太阳小肠经循行及腧穴示意图

Figure 12–7 Schematic diagram of small intestine meridian circulation and acupoints of hand sun

1. 小海　在肘后区，尺骨鹰嘴与肱骨内上髁之间凹陷处（微屈肘，在尺神经沟中，用手指弹敲此处时有触电麻感直达小指）。直刺 0.5 ～ 0.8 寸。主治肘臂疼痛、癫、狂、痫等。

Xiaohai It is located in the posterior elbow area, in the depression between the olecranon of ulna and the medial epicondyle of humerus (slightly flexing elbow, in the ulnar nerve groove, when you bounce here with your fingers, you will feel electric shock and numbness directly to your little finger). Straight puncture 0.5–0.8 cun. It is mainly used for elbow and arm pain, epilepsy, madness and epilepsy.

2. 天宗　在肩胛区，肩胛冈中点与肩胛骨下角连线的上 1/3 与下 2/3 交点凹陷中。直刺或斜刺 0.5 ～ 1.0 寸，遇到阻力不可强行进针。主治肩胛区疼痛、乳痈、气喘等。

Tianzong It is in the depression of the intersection point between the upper 1/3 and the lower 2/3 of the line connecting the midpoint of scapular spine and the lower corner of scapula. Straight stab or oblique stab 0.5–1.0 cun, and do not force the needle into the needle when encountering resistance. It is mainly used for treating pain in scapular area, breast carbuncle, asthma, etc.

3. 颧髎 在面部，颧骨下缘，目外眦直下凹陷中。直刺 0.3 ～ 0.5 寸，斜刺或平刺 0.5 ～ 1.0 寸。主治口㖞、齿痛、面痛、颊肿、眼睑瞤动等。

Quanliao It is located on the face, at the lower edge of zygomatic bones, and in the depression directly below the outer canthus of the eye. Straight prick 0.3–0.5 cun, oblique prick or flat prick 0.5–1.0 cun. It is mainly used for oral, toothache, facial pain, cheek swelling, eyelid movement, etc.

4. 听宫 在面部，耳屏正中与下颌骨髁突之间的凹陷中（微张口，耳屏正中前缘凹陷中，在耳门与听会之间）。微张口，直刺 0.5 ～ 1.0 寸。主治耳鸣、耳聋、聤耳等。

Tinggong It is in the depression between the face, the median tragus and the mandibular condyle (slightly open mouth, the median anterior edge of the tragus is in the depression, between the auricle and the auditory meeting). Open your mouth slightly and stab 0.5–1.0 cun straight. It is mainly used for tinnitus, deafness, tinnitus, etc.

七、足太阳膀胱经

7 Foot sun bladder meridian

（一）经脉循行

7.1 Meridian circulation

足太阳膀胱经循行见图 12–8。

The circulation of bladder meridian of foot sun is shown in Figure 12–8.

（二）常用腧穴

7.2 Common acupoints

足太阳膀胱经分布有 67 个腧穴：睛明、攒竹、眉冲、曲差、五处、承光、通天、络却、玉枕、天柱、大杼、风门、肺俞、厥阴俞、心俞、督俞、膈俞、肝俞、胆俞、脾俞、胃俞、三焦俞、肾俞、气海俞、大肠俞、关元俞、小肠俞、膀胱俞、中膂俞、白环俞、上髎、次髎、中髎、下髎、会阳、承扶、殷门、浮郄、委阳、委中、附分、魄户、膏肓、神堂、譩譆、膈关、魂门、阳纲、意舍、胃仓、肓门、志室、胞肓、秩边、合阳、承筋、承山、飞扬、跗阳、昆仑、仆参、申脉、金门、京骨、束骨、足通谷、至阴。本经腧穴主要治疗头、目、项、背、腰、下肢部病症及神志病，背部第一侧线的背俞穴及第二侧线相平的腧穴主治与其相关的脏腑、组织器官病症，第 1 ～ 6 胸椎两侧腧穴主治心、肺疾病，第 7 ～ 12 胸椎之间两侧腧穴主治肝、胆、脾、胃等疾病，第 1 腰椎～第 5 骶椎两侧腧穴主治肾、膀胱、大小肠、子宫等疾病。

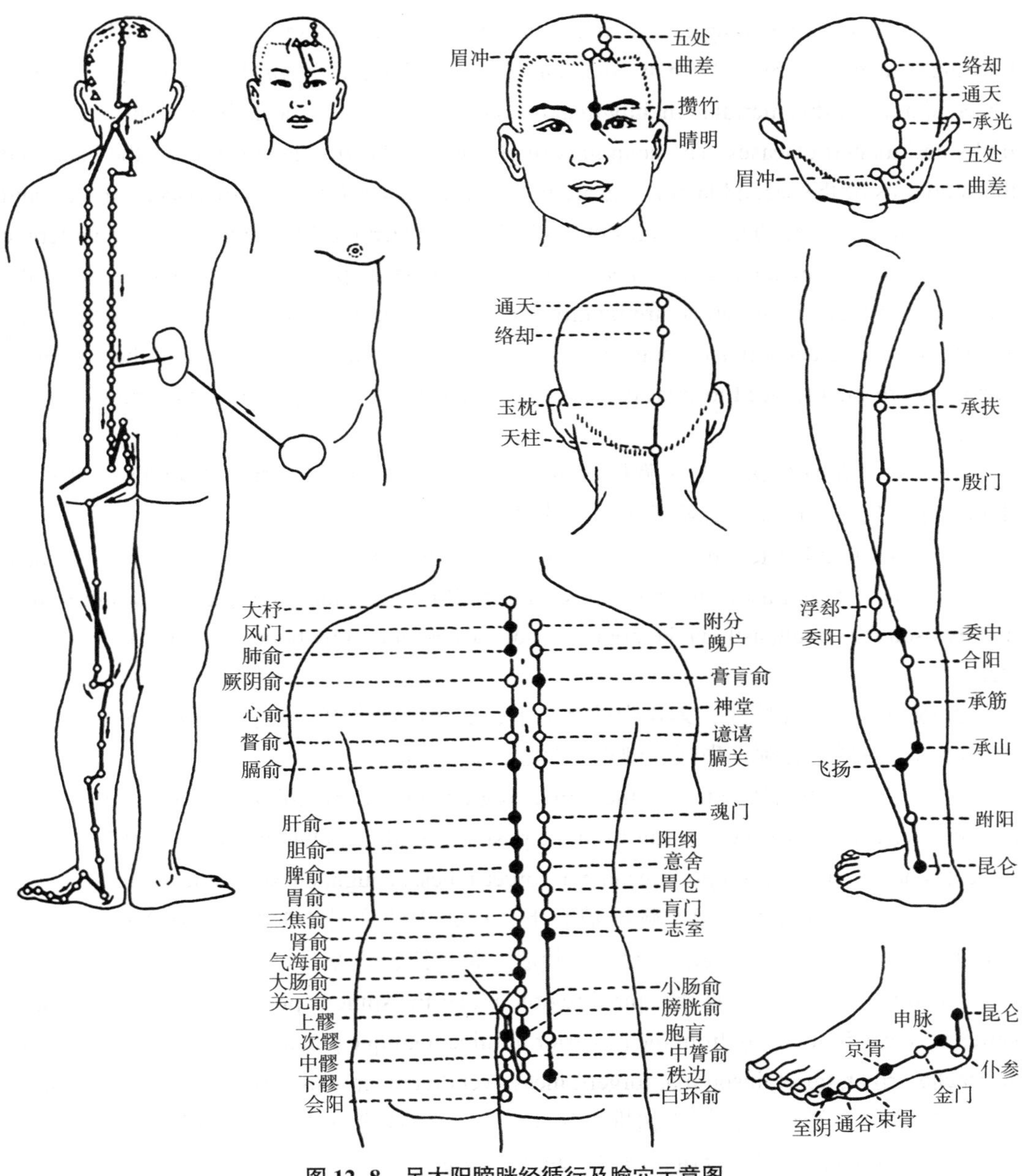

图 12–8 足太阳膀胱经循行及腧穴示意图

Figure 12–8 Schematic diagram of bladder meridian circulation and acupoints of foot sun

There are 67 acupoints distributed in the Bladder Meridian of Foot Sun: Jingming, Zanzhu, Meichong, Qucha, Wuchu, Chengguang, Tongtian, Luoque, Yuzhen, Tianzhu, Dazhu, Fengmen, Feishu, Jueyinshu, Xinshu, Dushu, Geshu, Ganshu, Danshu, Pishu, Weishu, Sanjiao Shu, Shenshu, Qihaishu, Dachangshu, Guanyuanshu, Xiaochangshu, Pangguangshu, Zhongyushu, Baihuanshu, Shangliao, Ciliao, Zhongliao, Xialiao, Huiyang, Chengfu, Yinmen, Fuqi, Weiyang, Weizhong, Fufen, Pohu, Gaohuang, Shentang, Yixi, Geguan, Hunmen,

Yanggang, Yishe, Weicang, Huangmen, Zhishi, Zhibian, Heyang, Chengjin, Chengshan, Feiyang, Fuyang, Kunlun, Pushen, Shenmai, Jinmen, Jinggu, Shugu, Foot Tonggu, and Yin. The acupoints of this meridian mainly treat diseases of head, eyes, neck, back, waist and lower limbs and mental diseases. The acupoints of Beishu on the first lateral line of the back and the acupoints of the second lateral line are mainly used to treat diseases of viscera, tissues and organs related to them. The acupoints on both sides between the 1st and 6th thoracic vertebrae are mainly used to treat diseases of heart and lung, and the acupoints on both sides between the 7th and 12th thoracic vertebrae are mainly used to treat diseases of liver, gallbladder, spleen and stomach. The acupoints on both sides between the 1st lumbar vertebrae and the 5th sacral vertebrae are mainly used to treat diseases of kidney, bladder, large and small intestines and uterus.

1. 肺俞 在脊柱区，第 3 胸椎棘突下，后正中线旁开 1.5 寸。斜刺 0.5 ～ 0.8 寸。主治咳嗽、气喘、咳血、骨蒸潮热、皮肤瘙痒等。

Feishu It is located in the spinal region, under the spinous process of the third thoracic vertebra, and 1.5 cun away from the posterior midline. Oblique puncture 0.5–0.8 cun. It is mainly used for cough, asthma, hemoptysis, hot flashes caused by bone steaming, itching skin, etc.

2. 厥阴俞 在脊柱区，第 4 胸椎棘突下，后正中线旁开 1.5 寸。斜刺 0.5 ～ 0.8 寸。主治心痛、惊悸、心烦、失眠、健忘、咳嗽、胸闷等。

Jueyinshu It is located in the spinal region, under the spinous process of the 4th thoracic vertebra, and 1.5 cun away from the posterior midline. Oblique puncture 0.5–0.8 cun. Indicates heartache, fright, upset, insomnia, forgetfulness, cough, chest tightness, etc.

3. 心俞 在脊柱区，第 5 胸椎棘突下，后正中线旁开 1.5 寸。斜刺 0.5 ～ 0.8 寸。主治心痛、惊悸、心烦、失眠、健忘、梦遗、癫、狂、痫等。

Xinshu It is located in the spinal region, under the spinous process of the fifth thoracic vertebra, and 1.5 cun away from the posterior midline. Oblique puncture 0.5–0.8 cun. Indicates heartache, fright, upset, insomnia, forgetfulness, wet dream, epilepsy, madness, epilepsy, etc.

4. 督俞 在脊柱区，第 6 胸椎棘突下，后正中线旁开 1.5 寸。斜刺 0.5 ～ 0.8 寸。主治心痛、胸闷、气喘、胃痛、腹痛、腹胀、呃逆等。

Dushu It is located in the spinal region, under the spinous process of the 6th thoracic vertebra, and 1.5 cun away from the posterior midline. Oblique puncture 0.5–0.8 cun. It is mainly used for heartache, chest tightness, asthma, stomachache, abdominal pain, abdominal distension, hiccup, etc.

5. 膈俞 在脊柱区，第 7 胸椎棘突下，后正中线旁开 1.5 寸。斜刺 0.5 ～ 0.8 寸。主治胃脘痛、呕吐、呃逆、噎膈、气喘、潮热、盗汗、皮肤瘙痒等。

Geshu It is in the spinal region, under the spinous process of the 7th thoracic vertebra, 1.5 cun away from the posterior midline. Oblique puncture 0.5–0.8 cun. It is mainly used for treating epigastric pain, vomiting, hiccup, choking diaphragm, asthma, hot flashes, night sweats, itching skin, etc.

6. 肝俞 在脊柱区，第 9 胸椎棘突下，后正中线旁开 1.5 寸。斜刺 0.5 ～ 0.8 寸。主治胁痛、黄疸、目疾、癫、狂、痫等。

Ganshu It is located in the spinal region, under the spinous process of the 9th thoracic vertebra, and 1.5 cun away from the posterior midline. Oblique puncture 0.5–0.8 cun. It is mainly used for hypochondriac pain, jaundice, eye disease, epilepsy, madness and epilepsy.

7. 胆俞 在脊柱区，第 10 胸椎棘突下，后正中线旁开 1.5 寸。斜刺 0.5 ～ 0.8 寸。主治胁痛、口苦、黄疸、呕吐、潮热等。

Danshu It is located in the spinal region, under the spinous process of the 10th thoracic vertebra, and 1.5 cun away from the posterior midline. Oblique puncture 0.5–0.8 cun. It is mainly used for hypochondriac pain, bitter taste, jaundice, vomiting, hot flashes, etc.

8. 脾俞 在脊柱区，第 11 胸椎棘突下，后正中线旁开 1.5 寸。斜刺 0.8 ～ 1.0 寸。主治腹胀、呕吐、泄泻、痢疾、便血、背痛等。

Pishu It is located in the spinal region, under the spinous process of the 11th thoracic vertebra, and 1.5 cun away from the posterior midline. Oblique prick 0.8–1.0 cun. It is mainly used for abdominal distension, vomiting, diarrhea, dysentery, hematochezia, back pain, etc.

9. 胃俞 在脊柱区，第 12 胸椎棘突下，后正中线旁开 1.5 寸。斜刺 0.8 ～ 1.0 寸。主治胃脘痛、呕吐、反胃、腹胀、肠鸣、完谷不化等。

Weishu It is located in the spinal region, under the spinous process of the 12th thoracic vertebra, and 1.5 cun away from the posterior midline. Oblique prick 0.8–1.0 cun. It is mainly used for treating epigastric pain, vomiting, nausea, abdominal distension, bowel sounds, etc.

10. 三焦俞 在脊柱区，第 1 腰椎棘突下，后正中线旁开 1.5 寸。直刺 0.8 ～ 1.0 寸。主治水肿、小便不利、腹胀、肠鸣、泄泻、痢疾等。

Sanjiaoshu It is 1.5 cun away from the spinal region, under the spinous process of the first lumbar spine and beside the posterior midline. Stab 0.8–1.0 cun straight. Indicates edema, dysuria, abdominal distension, bowel sounds, diarrhea, dysentery, etc.

11. 肾俞 在脊柱区，第 2 腰椎棘突下，后正中线旁开 1.5 寸。直刺 0.8 ～ 1.0 寸。主治头晕、耳鸣、耳聋、腰膝酸软、腰痛、遗精、阳痿、早泄、月经不调、带下、遗尿、水肿、小便不利等。

Shenshu It is located in the spinal region, under the spinous process of the second lumbar spine, and 1.5 cun away from the posterior midline. Stab 0.8–1.0 cun straight. It is mainly used for treating dizziness, tinnitus, deafness, soreness of waist and knees, lumbago, spermatorrhea, impotence, premature ejaculation, irregular menstruation, leukorrhagia, enuresis, edema, dysuria, etc.

12. 气海俞 在脊柱区，第 3 腰椎棘突下，后正中线旁开 1.5 寸。直刺 0.8 ～ 1.0 寸。

主治腰痛、腹痛、腹胀、肠鸣、泄泻、遗尿等。

Qihaishu It is 1.5 cun away from the spinal region, under the spinous process of the third lumbar spine and beside the posterior midline. Stab 0.8–1.0 cun straight. It is mainly used for treating low back pain, abdominal pain, abdominal distension, bowel sounds, diarrhea, enuresis, etc.

13. 大肠俞 在脊柱区，第 4 腰椎棘突下，后正中线旁开 1.5 寸。直刺 0.8 ～ 1.0 寸。主治腰痛、腹痛、腹胀、肠鸣、泄泻、便秘等。

Dachangshu It is located in the spinal region, under the spinous process of the 4th lumbar spine, and 1.5 cun away from the posterior midline. Stab 0.8–1.0 cun straight. It is mainly used for treating low back pain, abdominal pain, abdominal distension, bowel sounds, diarrhea, constipation, etc.

14. 关元俞 在脊柱区，第 5 腰椎棘突下，后正中线旁开 1.5 寸。直刺 0.8 ～ 1.0 寸。主治腰痛、腹痛、腹胀、肠鸣、泄泻、遗尿等。

Guanyuanshu It is 1.5 cun away from the spinal region, under the spinous process of the fifth lumbar spine and beside the posterior midline. Stab 0.8–1.0 cun straight. It is mainly used for treating low back pain, abdominal pain, abdominal distension, bowel sounds, diarrhea, enuresis, etc.

15. 小肠俞 在骶区，横平第 1 骶后孔，骶正中嵴旁开 1.5 寸（横平上髎）。直刺 0.8 ～ 1.0 寸。主治腹痛、泄泻、痢疾、遗精、遗尿、带下等。

Xiaochangshu It is located in the sacral region, horizontally flattening the first posterior sacral foramen, and opening 1.5 cun beside the median sacral crest. Stab 0.8–1.0 cun straight. It is mainly used for abdominal pain, diarrhea, dysentery, spermatorrhea, enuresis, leukorrhagia, etc.

16. 膀胱俞 在骶区，横平第 2 骶后孔，骶正中嵴旁开 1.5 寸（横平次髎）。直刺 0.8 ～ 1.0 寸。主治小便不利、尿频、遗尿、泄泻、便秘、腰骶痛等。

Pangguangshu It is located in the sacral region, horizontally flattening the second posterior sacral foramen, and opening 1.5 cun beside the median sacral crest. Stab 0.8–1.0 cun straight. It is mainly used for dysuria, frequent micturition, enuresis, diarrhea, constipation, lumbosacral pain, etc.

17. 委中 在膝后区，腘横纹中点。直刺 1.0 ～ 1.5 寸。主治腰痛、下肢痿痹、下肢挛急等。

Weizhong It is located in the posterior knee area and the midpoint of the popliteal transverse striation. Stab 1.0–1.5 cun straight. It is mainly used for treating low back pain, flaccidity of lower limbs, convulsion of lower limbs, etc.

八、足少阴肾经
8 Foot shaoyin kidney meridian

（一）经脉循行
8.1 Meridian circulation

足少阴肾经循行见图 12–9。

The kidney meridian of Foot Shaoyin is shown in Figure 12–9.

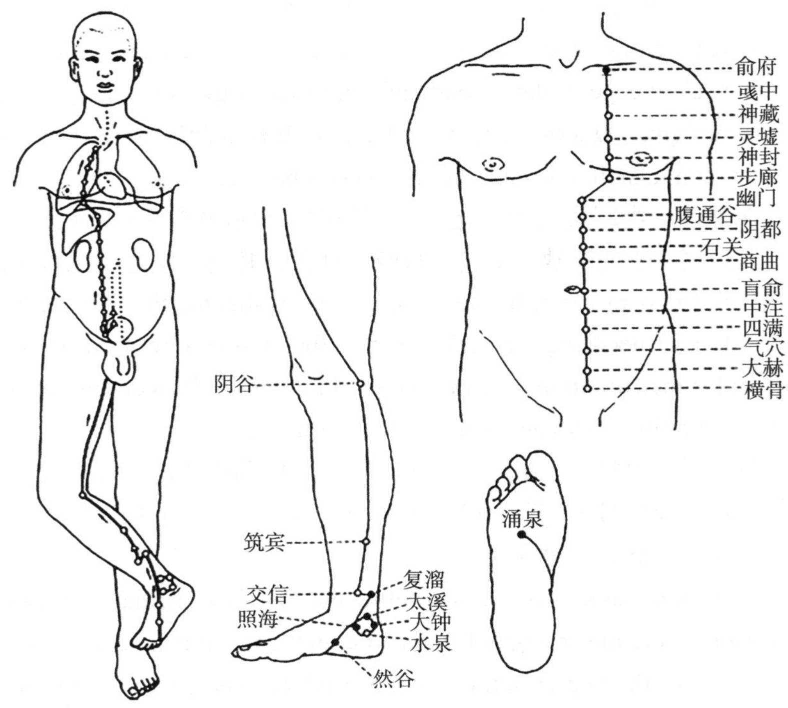

图 12–9 足少阴肾经循行及腧穴示意图

Figure 12–9 Schematic diagram of kidney meridian circulation and acupoints of foot Shaoyin

（二）常用腧穴
8.2 Common acupoints

足少阴肾经分布有 27 个腧穴：涌泉、然谷、太溪、大钟、水泉、照海、复溜、交信、筑宾、阴谷、横骨、大赫、气穴、四满、中注、肓俞、商曲、石关、阴都、腹通谷、幽门、步廊、神封、灵墟、神藏、彧中、俞府。本经腧穴主要治疗口舌咽病症、虚损、黄疸、腹泻，以及肾经循行部位的其他病症。

There are 27 acupoints in Zushaoyin Kidney Meridian: Yongquan, Rangu, Taixi, Dazhong, Shuiquan, Zhaohai, Fuliu, Jiaoxin, Zhubin, Yingu, Henggu, Dahe, Qixue, Siman,

Zhongzhu, Huangshu, Shangqu, Shiguan, Yindu, Futonggu, Youmen, Bulang, Shenfeng, Lingxu, Shencang, Yuzhong and Shufu Acupoints of this meridian mainly treat diseases of mouth, tongue and pharynx, deficiency, jaundice, diarrhea, and other diseases along the kidney meridian.

1. 涌泉　在足底，屈足卷趾时足心最凹陷中（卧位或伸腿坐位，卷足，约当足底第2、3趾蹼缘与足跟连线的前1/3与后2/3交点凹陷中）。直刺0.5～1.0寸，可灸。主治眩晕、厥证、癫、狂、惊风、失眠、足心热等。

Yongquan　It is in the sole of the foot, and the center of the foot is most sunken when bending the foot and rolling the toe (lying position or leg stretching sitting position, rolling the foot, about when the intersection point of the front 1/3 and the back 2/3 of the connecting line between the webbed edge of the second and third toes of the sole and the heel is sunken). Stab 0.5–1.0 cun straight, and moxibustion can be used. It is mainly used for vertigo, syncope, epilepsy, madness, convulsion, insomnia, foot and heart heat, etc.

2. 太溪　在踝区，内踝尖与跟腱之间的凹陷中。直刺0.5～1.5寸，可灸。主治月经不调、遗精、阳痿、小便频数、头痛、目眩、耳聋、耳鸣、腰痛、下肢厥冷等。

Taixi　It is in the depression between the medial malleolus tip and Achilles tendon in the ankle area. Straight needling 0.5–1.5 cun, moxibustion can be used. It is mainly used for treating irregular menstruation, spermatorrhea, impotence, frequent urination, headache, dizziness, deafness, tinnitus, low back pain, cold lower limbs, etc.

3. 照海　在踝区，内踝尖下1寸，内踝下缘边际凹陷中（由内踝尖向下推，至其下缘凹陷中，与申脉内外相对）。直刺0.5～0.8寸，可灸。主治咽喉疼痛、目赤肿痛、月经不调、痛经、带下、下肢痿痹等。

Zhaohai　It is in the ankle area, 1 cun below the tip of the medial malleolus, and in the marginal depression of the lower edge of the medial malleolus (pushing down from the tip of the medial malleolus to the depression of its lower edge, opposite to the inside and outside of Shenmai). Stab 0.5–0.8 cun straight, and moxibustion can be used. It is mainly used for sore throat, red eyes, swelling and pain, irregular menstruation, dysmenorrhea, leukorrhagia, flaccidity of lower limbs, etc.

九、手厥阴心包经
9 Pericardial Meridian of Hand Jueyin

（一）经脉循行
9.1 Meridian circulation

手厥阴心包经循行见图12–10。

The pericardial meridian of hand Jueyin is shown in Figure 12–10.

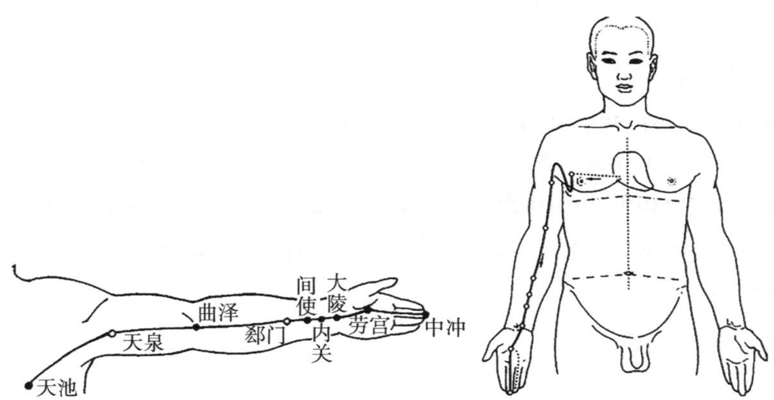

图 12–10 手厥阴心包经循行及腧穴示意图

Figure12–10 Schematic diagram of pericardial meridian circulation and acupoints of hand Jueyin

（二）常用腧穴

9.2 Common acupoints

手厥阴心包经分布有 9 个腧穴：天池、天泉、曲泽、郄门、间使、内关、大陵、劳宫、中冲。本经腧穴主要治疗心、胸、胃、神志病症，以及肾经循行部位的其他病症。

There are 9 acupoints in the pericardial meridian of hand Jueyin: Tianchi, Tian Quan, Quze, Ximen, Jianshi, Neiguan, Daling, Laogong and Zhongchong. Acupoints of this meridian mainly treat diseases of heart, chest, stomach and mind, as well as other diseases along the kidney meridian.

1. 曲泽 在肘前区，肘横纹上，肱二头肌腱的尺侧缘凹陷中（仰掌，屈肘 45°，尺泽尺侧肌腱旁）。直刺 1.0 ～ 1.5 寸，可用三棱针点刺出血。主治心痛、心悸、善惊、肘臂挛痛、热病等。

Quze It is in the anterior elbow area, on the transverse striation of elbow, and in the depression of ulnar edge of biceps brachii tendon (palm upturned, elbow flexion 45, beside ulnar tendon). If you prick 1.0–1.5 cun straight, you can prick bleeding with triangular needles. It is mainly used for heartache, palpitation, convulsion of elbow and arm, fever, etc.

2. 间使 在前臂前区，腕掌侧远端横纹上 3 寸，掌长肌腱与桡侧腕屈肌腱之间。直刺 0.5 ～ 1.0 寸，可灸。主治心痛、心悸、热病、疟疾、癫、狂、痫、肘臂挛痛等。

Jianshi In the anterior area of forearm, 3 cun above the transverse striation at the distal end of carpometacarpal side, between the tendon of palmaris longus and the tendon of flexor carpi radialis. Stab 0.5–1.0 cun straight, and moxibustion can be used. It is mainly used for heartache, palpitation, fever, malaria, epilepsy, mania, epilepsy, elbow and arm convulsion and pain, etc.

3. 内关 在前臂前区，腕掌侧远端横纹上 2 寸，掌长肌腱与桡侧腕屈肌腱之间。直刺 0.5 ～ 1.0 寸，可灸。主治心痛、心悸、胸闷、胃痛、呕吐、呃逆、失眠、眩晕、郁证、癫、狂、痫、肘臂挛痛等。

Neiguan It is closed in the anterior area of forearm, 2 cun above the transverse striation at the distal end of carpometacarpal side, between the tendon of palmaris longus and the tendon of flexor carpi radialis. Stab 0.5–1.0 cun straight, and moxibustion can be used. It is mainly used for treating heartache, palpitation, chest tightness, stomachache, vomiting, hiccup, insomnia, dizziness, depression syndrome, epilepsy, madness, epilepsy, elbow and arm convulsion pain, etc.

十、手少阳三焦经

10 Hand Shaoyang sanjiao meridian

（一）经脉循行

10.1 Meridian circulation

手少阳三焦经循行见图 12–11。

The sanjiao meridian of hand Shaoyang is shown in Figure 12–11.

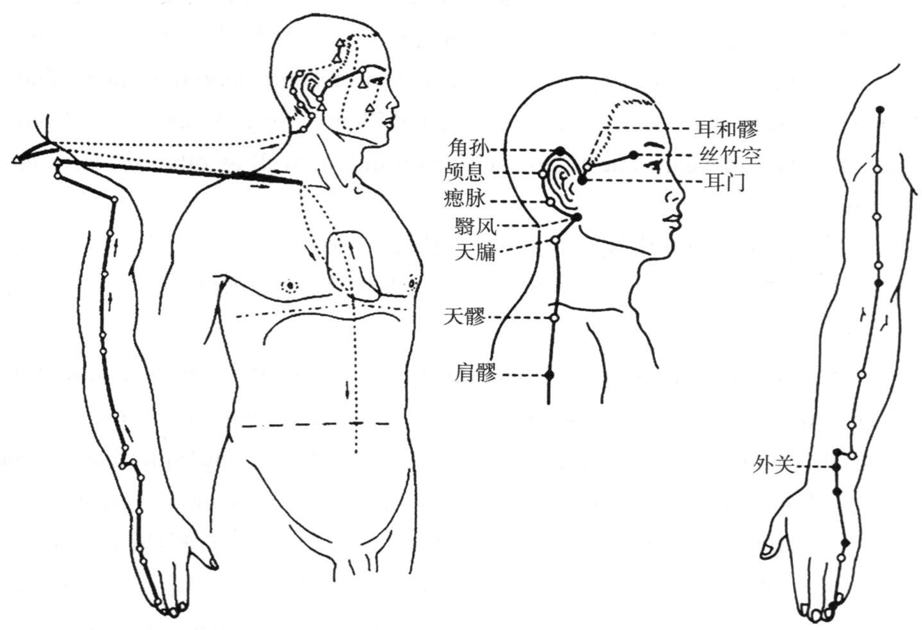

图 12–11 手少阳三焦经循行及腧穴示意图

Figure12–11 Schematic diagram of sanjiao meridian circulation and acupoints of hand Shaoyang

（二）常用腧穴

10.2 Common acupoints

手少阳三焦经分布有 23 个腧穴：关冲、液门、中渚、阳池、外关、支沟、会宗、三阳络、四渎、天井、清冷渊、消泺、臑会、肩髎、天髎、天牖、翳风、瘛脉、颅息、角孙、耳门、耳和髎、丝竹空。本经腧穴主要治疗侧头、耳、目、咽喉、胸胁病，热病，以及三焦经循行部位的其他病症。

There are 23 acupoints distributed in the sanjiao meridian of hand Shaoyang: Guanchong, Shuemen, Zhongzhu, Yangchi, Waiguan, Zhigou, Huizong, Sanyang Luo, Sidu, patio, Qingleng Yuan, Xiaoluo, Yuhui, Jianliao, Tianliao, Tianyou, Yifeng, Chimai, Luxi, Jiaosun, Ermen, Erheliao, Sizhukong. The acupoints of this meridian mainly treat side head, ears, eyes, throat, chest and hypochondriac diseases, fever, and other diseases along the sanjiao meridian.

1. 外关　在前臂后区，腕背侧远端横纹上 2 寸，尺骨与桡骨间隙中点。直刺 0.5 ～ 1.0 寸。主治头痛、颊痛、目赤肿痛、耳鸣、耳聋、热病、上肢痿痹等。

Waiguan　It is closed in the posterior area of forearm, 2 cun above the transverse striation at the distal end of the dorsal wrist, and at the midpoint of the space between ulna and radius. Straight puncture 0.5–1.0 cun. It is mainly used for headache, cheek pain, red eyes, swelling and pain, tinnitus, deafness, fever, flaccidity of upper limbs, etc.

2. 肩髎　在三角肌区，肩峰角与肱骨大结节两骨间凹陷中（屈臂外展时，肩峰外侧缘前后端呈现两个凹陷，后一凹陷即本穴）。直刺 0.8 ～ 1.2 寸。主治肩臂痛、肩重不能举等。

Jianliao　It is located in the deltoid muscle area, in the depression between the acromion angle and the greater tubercle of humerus (when the flexion arm is abducted, there are two depressions at the anterior and posterior ends of the lateral edge of the acromion, and the latter depression is this point). Stab 0.8–1.2 cun straight. It is mainly used for shoulder and arm pain, shoulder weight can't be lifted, etc.

3. 角孙　在头部，耳尖正对发际处。平刺 0.3 ～ 0.5 寸。主治耳部肿痛、痄腮、目赤肿痛、齿痛、偏头痛等。

Jiaosun　The horn sun is on the head, and the tip of the ear is facing the hairline. Flat thorn 0.3–0.5 cun. It is mainly used for treating ear swelling and pain, mumps, red eyes, toothache, migraine, etc.

4. 耳门　在耳区，耳屏上切迹与下颌骨髁突之间的凹陷中（微张口，耳屏上切迹前的凹陷中，听宫直上）。直刺 0.5 ～ 1.0 寸。主治耳鸣、耳聋、聤耳、齿痛等。

Ermen　The auricle is located in the ear area, in the depression between the suprapagal notch and mandibular condyle (slightly open mouth, in the depression before the suprapagal notch, straight up the auditory uterus). Straight puncture 0.5–1.0 cun. Indicates tinnitus, deafness, ear tinnitus, toothache, etc.

十一、足少阳胆经
11 Foot Shaoyang Gallbladder Meridian

（一）经脉循行
11.1 Meridian circulation

足少阳胆经循行见图 12–12。

The gallbladder meridian of Foot Shaoyang follows as shown in Figure 12–12.

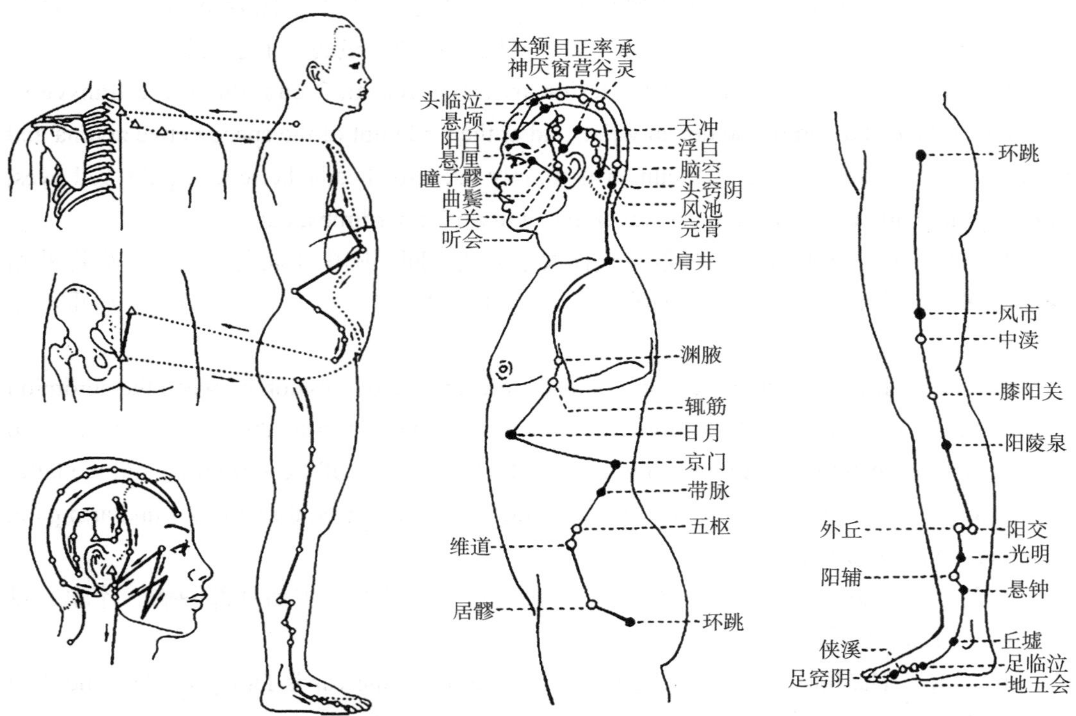

图 12–12 足少阳胆经循行及腧穴示意图

Figure12–12 Schematic diagram of gallbladder meridian circulation and acupoints of foot Shaoyang

（二）常用腧穴
11.2 Common acupoints

足少阳胆经分布有 44 个腧穴：瞳子髎、听会、上关、颔厌、悬颅、悬厘、曲鬓、率谷、天冲、浮白、头窍阴、完骨、本神、阳白、头临泣、目窗、正营、承灵、脑空、风池、肩井、渊腋、辄筋、日月、京门、带脉、五枢、维道、居髎、环跳、风市、中渎、膝阳关、阳陵泉、阳交、外丘、光明、阳辅、悬钟、丘墟、足临泣、地五会、侠溪、足窍阴。本经腧穴主治肝胆病，侧头、目、耳、咽喉、胸胁病，以及胆经循行经过部位的其他病症。

There are 44 acupoints distributed in the gallbladder meridian of Zushaoyang: Tongziliao, Tinghui, Shangguan, jaw–weary, hanging skull, hanging Li, curved temples, rate valley, Tianchong, floating white, head Qiao Yin, bone completion, Ben Shen, Yang Bai, head Lin Qi, eye window, Zhengying, Chengling, brain empty, wind pool, shoulder well, deep armpit, Nojin, sun and moon, Jingmen, belt pulse, five pivots, Wei Dao, residence Liao, Huantiao, wind city, Zhongdu, knee Yang Guan, Yanglingquan, Yangjiao, waiqiu, light, Yangfu, hanging bell, Qiuxu, foot Lin Qi, earth five meetings, xiaxi, foot Qiao Yin. The acupoints of this meridian are mainly used to treat liver and gallbladder diseases, side head, eyes, ears, throat, chest and hypochondriac diseases, and other diseases where the gallbladder meridian runs.

1. 听会　在面部，耳屏间切迹与下颌骨髁突之间的凹陷中（张口，耳屏间切迹前方的凹陷中，听宫直下）。微张口，直刺 0.5 ～ 1.0 寸。主治耳鸣、耳聋、聤耳、面痛等。

Tinghui It is in the depression between the face, the intertragal notch and the mandibular condyle (open mouth, in the depression in front of the intertragal notch, the auditory uterus goes straight down). Open your mouth slightly and stab 0.5–1.0 cun straight. It is mainly used for tinnitus, deafness, tinnitus, facial pain, etc.

2. 上关　在面部，颧弓上缘中央凹陷中。直刺 0.3 ～ 0.5 寸。主治耳鸣、耳聋、齿痛、口㖞、面痛、头痛等。

Shangguan It is closed on the face and in the central depression of the upper edge of zygomatic arch. Stab 0.3–0.5 cun straight. It is mainly used for tinnitus, deafness, toothache, mouth ache, facial pain, headache, etc.

3. 风池　在颈后区，枕骨之下，胸锁乳突肌上端与斜方肌上端之间的凹陷中。向鼻尖方向斜刺 0.8 ～ 1.2 寸。主治头痛、眩晕、目赤肿痛、鼻渊、耳鸣、颈项强痛等。

Fengchi It is in the depression between the upper end of sternocleidomastoid muscle and the upper end of trapezius muscle in the posterior cervical area, under the occipital bone. Stab 0.8–1.2 cun obliquely in the direction of nasal tip. It is mainly used for headache, dizziness, red eyes, swelling and pain, nasal abyss, tinnitus, neck pain, etc.

4. 环跳　在臀区，股骨大转子最凸点与骶管裂孔连线的外 1/3 与内 2/3 交点处（侧卧，伸下腿，上腿屈髋屈膝取穴）。直刺 2.0 ～ 3.0 寸。主治腰腿痛、下肢痿痹、半身不遂等。

Huantiao It is at the intersection of the outer 1/3 and the inner 2/3 of the line connecting the most convex point of the greater trochanter of femur with the sacral canal hiatus (lie on your side, extend your lower leg, bend your hips and knees on your upper leg to select points). Stab 2.0–3.0 cun straight. It is mainly used for treating lumbago and leg pain, flaccidity of lower limbs, hemiplegia, etc.

5. 阳陵泉　在小腿外侧，腓骨头前下方凹陷中。直刺 1.0 ～ 1.5 寸。主治黄疸、胁痛、口苦、下肢痿痹等。

Yanglingquan It is in the depression on the lateral side of the calf and the front and lower part of the fibula head. Stab 1.0–1.5 cun straight. It is mainly used for treating jaundice, hypochondriac pain, bitter taste, flaccidity of lower limbs, etc.

十二、足厥阴肝经

12 Liver Meridian of Foot Jueyin

（一）经脉循行

12.1 Meridian circulation

足厥阴肝经循行见图 12–13。

The liver meridian of foot Jueyin is shown in Figure 12–13.

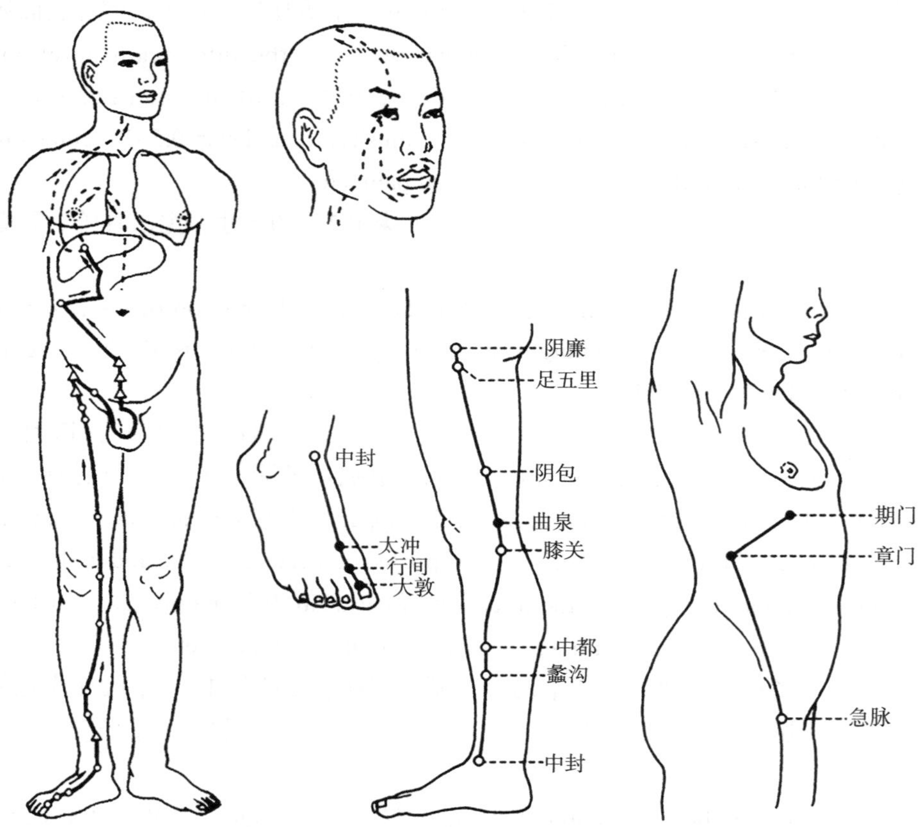

图 12–13　足厥阴肝经循行及腧穴示意图

Figure12–13　Schematic diagram of liver meridian circulation and acupoints of Zujueyin

（二）常用腧穴

12.2 Common acupoints

足厥阴肝经分布有 14 个腧穴：大敦、行间、太冲、中封、蠡沟、中都、膝关、曲泉、阴包、足五里、阴廉、急脉、章门、期门。本经腧穴主要治疗肝胆病，与肝脏有关的胃、心、肺、脾、肾、脑等脏腑病症，以及肝经循行部位的其他病症。

There are 14 acupoints in the liver meridian of Zujueyin: Dadun, Xingjian, Taichong, Zhongfeng, Ligou, Zhongdu, Xiguan, Ququan, Yinbao, Zuwuli, Yinlian, Jimai, Zhangmen and Qimen. Acupoints of this meridian mainly treat hepatobiliary diseases, viscera diseases such as stomach, heart, lung, spleen, kidney and brain related to liver, and other diseases along the liver meridian.

1. 行间 在足背，第 1、2 趾之间，趾蹼缘后方赤白肉际处。直刺 0.5 ～ 0.8 寸。主治头痛、眩晕、目赤肿痛、胸胁胀痛、下肢内侧痛、月经不调、痛经、闭经、崩漏、带下、遗尿、癃闭、小便短赤等。

Xingjian It is on the back of the foot, between the first and second toes, and at the red and white fleshy place behind the webbed edge of the toe. Straight puncture 0.5–0.8 cun. It is mainly used for treating headache, dizziness, red eyes, swelling and pain, chest and hypochondriac pain, inner pain of lower limbs, irregular menstruation, dysmenorrhea, amenorrhea, metrorrhagia, leukorrhagia, enuresis, retention of urine, short and red urine, etc.

2. 太冲 在足背，第 1、2 跖骨间，跖骨底结合部前方凹陷中，或触及动脉搏动。直刺 0.5 ～ 0.8 寸。主治头痛、眩晕、耳鸣、耳聋、面瘫、目赤肿痛、咽喉痛、胁痛、惊风、黄疸、月经不调、痛经、经闭、带下、遗尿、癃闭等。

Taichong It is in the dorsum of foot, between the first and second metatarsals, and in the depression in front of the metatarsal base junction, or touched the arterial pulsation. Straight puncture 0.5–0.8 cun. It is mainly used for treating headache, dizziness, tinnitus, deafness, facial paralysis, red eyes, swelling and pain, sore throat, hypochondriac pain, convulsion, jaundice, irregular menstruation, dysmenorrhea, amenorrhea, leukorrhagia, enuresis, retention of urine, etc.

第三节 奇经八脉及其常用腧穴
Section 3 The eight veins of strange meridians and their common acupoints

一、督脉
1 Du Meridian

（一）经脉循行
1.1 Meridian circulation

督脉循行见图 12–14。

The circulation of Du meridian is shown in Figure 12–14.

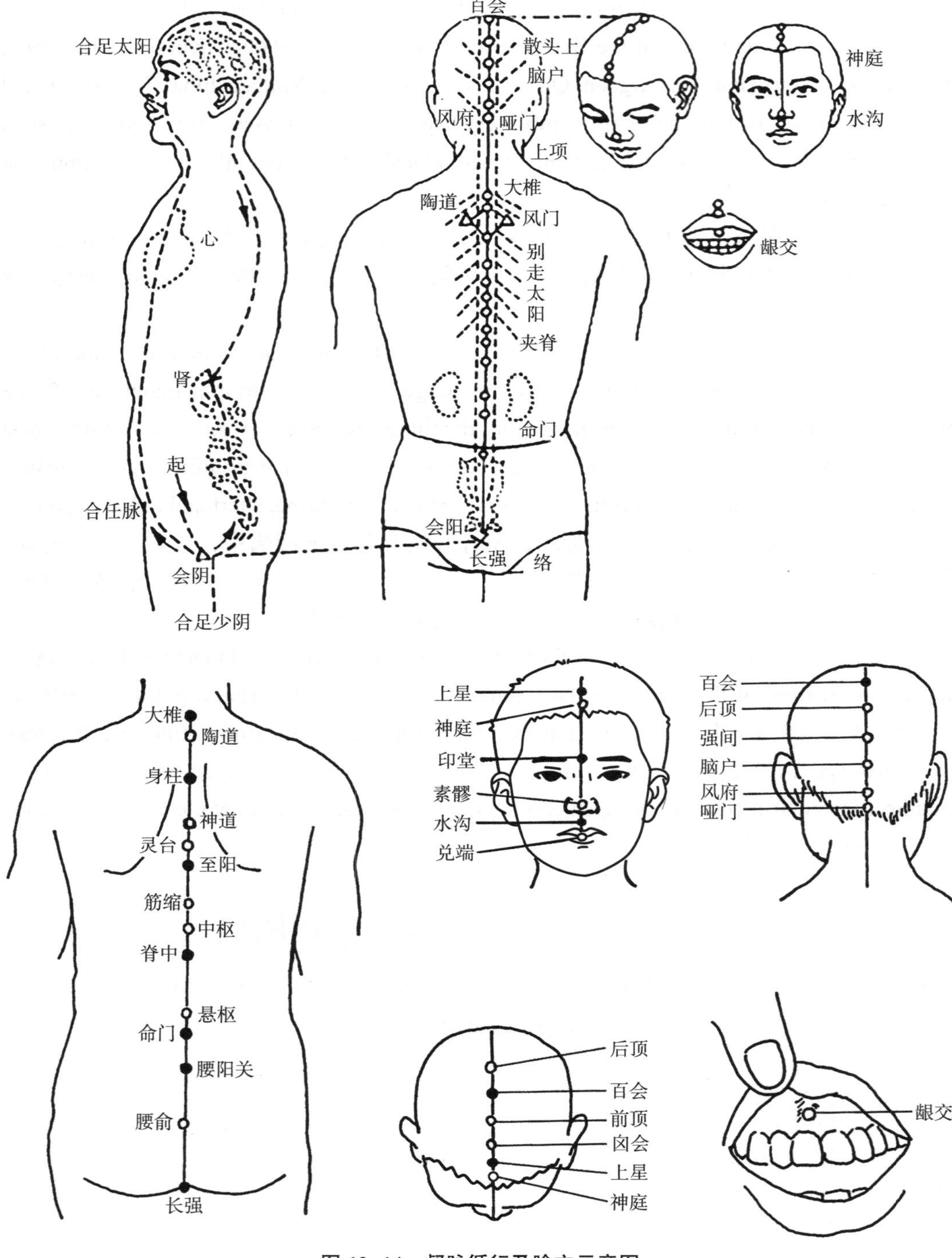

图 12–14 督脉循行及腧穴示意图

Figure12–14 Schematic diagram of Du meridian circulation and acupoints

（二）常用腧穴

1.2 Common acupoints

督脉分布有29个腧穴，均为单穴：长强、腰俞、腰阳关、命门、悬枢、脊中、中枢、筋缩、至阳、灵台、神道、身柱、陶道、大椎、哑门、风府、脑户、强间、后顶、百会、前顶、囟会、上星、神庭、素髎、水沟、兑端、龈交、印堂。督脉腧穴主要治疗神志病、热病，腰骶、背项、头部病症及相应的内脏疾病。

There are 29 acupoints distributed in Du Meridian, all of which are single points: Changqiang, Yaoshu, Yaoyangguan, Mingmen, Xuanshu, Jizhong, Zhongshu, Jinsuo, Zhiyang, Lingtai, Shinto, Shenzhu, Taodao, Dazhui, Yamen, Fengfu, Naohu, Qiangjian, Houding, Baihui, Qianding, Xinhui, Shangxing, Shenting, Suliao, Shuigou, Duiduan, Yinjiao, Yintang. Du meridian acupoints are mainly used to treat mental diseases, fever, lumbosacral diseases, dorsal neck diseases, head diseases and corresponding visceral diseases.

1. 命门 在脊柱区，第2腰椎棘突下凹陷中，后正中线上。向上斜刺0.5～1.0寸。主治腰痛、下肢痿痹、遗精、阳痿、早泄、月经不调、带下、遗尿、尿频、泄泻等。

Mingmen It is in the spinal region, in the depression under the spinous process of the second lumbar spine, and on the posterior midline. Obliquely prick 0.5–1.0 cun upward. It is mainly used for treating low back pain, flaccidity of lower limbs, spermatorrhea, impotence, premature ejaculation, irregular menstruation, leukorrhagia, enuresis, frequent micturition, diarrhea, etc.

2. 大椎 在脊柱区，第7颈椎棘突下凹陷中，后正中线上。向上斜刺0.5～1.0寸。主治热病、疟疾、咳嗽、气喘、颈项强痛、肩背疼痛、癫痫、惊风、风疹等。

Dazhui It is in the spinal region, in the depression under the spinous process of the 7th cervical vertebra, and on the posterior midline. Obliquely prick 0.5–1.0 cun upward. It is mainly used for treating fever, malaria, cough, asthma, neck pain, shoulder and back pain, epilepsy, convulsion, rubella, etc.

3. 百会 在头部，前发际正中直上5寸。平刺0.5～1.0寸，可灸。主治头痛、眩晕、中风失语、癫、狂、痫、失眠、健忘、脱肛、阴挺、久泻等。

Baihui It is in the head, and the front hairline is 5 cun straight. Plain needling 0.5–1.0 cun can be moxibustion. It is mainly used for treating headache, dizziness, apoplexy, aphasia, epilepsy, madness, epilepsy, insomnia, forgetfulness, rectocele, yin stiffness, chronic diarrhea, etc.

4. 水沟 在面部，人中沟上1/3与中1/3交点处。向上斜刺0.3～0.5寸。主治晕厥、中风、口㖞、癫、狂、痫、闪挫腰痛、脊膂强痛、消渴、黄疸、遍身水肿等。

Shuigou It is on the face, at the intersection of the upper 1/3 and the middle 1/3 of the middle ditch. Stab 0.3–0.5 cun obliquely upward. It is mainly used for treating syncope, stroke, facial paralysis, epilepsy, madness, epilepsy, wrenched lumbus pain, strong spinal pain, thirst, jaundice, edema all over the body, etc.

5. 印堂 在额部，当两眉头中间。针刺时提捏局部皮肤，平刺 0.3 ～ 0.5 寸。主治头痛、眩晕、失眠、惊风、产后血晕、鼻渊、鼻衄、目痛等。

Yintang It is on the forehead, between the two eyebrows. When acupuncture, pinch the local skin and prick it flat for 0.3–0.5 cun. It is mainly used for headache, dizziness, insomnia, convulsion, postpartum blood halo, nasal running, epistaxis, eye pain, etc.

二、任脉

2 Ren Meridian

（一）经脉循行

2.1 Meridian circulation

任脉循行见图 12–15。

The circulation of Ren meridian is shown in Figure 12–15.

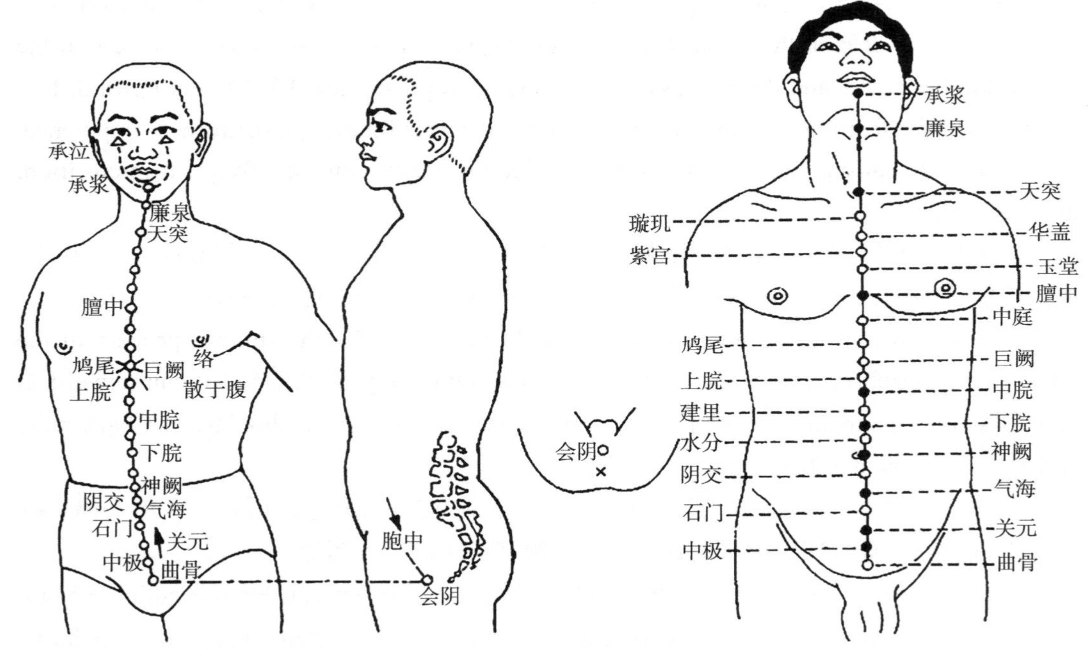

图 12–15 任脉循行及腧穴示意图

Figure12–15 Schematic diagram of Ren meridian circulation and acupoints

（二）常用腧穴

2.2 Common acupoints

任脉分布有 24 个腧穴，均为单穴：会阴、曲骨、中极、关元、石门、气海、阴交、神阙、水分、下脘、建里、中脘、上脘、巨阙、鸠尾、中庭、膻中、玉堂、紫宫、华盖、璇玑、天突、廉泉、承浆。任脉腧穴主要治疗腹、胸、颈、头面的局部病症及相应的内脏器官病症。

There are 24 acupoints distributed in Ren Meridian, all of which are single points: perineum, Qugu, Zhongji, Guanyuan, Shimen, Qihai, Yinjiao, Shenque, Shuifen, Xiawan, Jianli, Zhongwan, Shangwan, Juque, dovetail, atrium, Shanzhong, Yutang, Zigong, Huagai, Xuanji, Tiantu, Lianquan and Chengjiang. Renmai Acupoints mainly treat local diseases of abdomen, chest, neck, head and face and corresponding diseases of internal organs.

1. 关元 在下腹部，脐中下 3 寸，前正中线上。直刺 1.0 ～ 2.0 寸，需排尿后进行针刺。多用灸法。孕妇慎用。主治阳痿、遗精、遗尿、癃闭、尿频、月经不调、痛经、闭经、崩漏、带下、不孕、腹痛、泄泻、虚劳羸瘦、中风脱证等。

Guanyuan It is in the lower abdomen, 3 cun below the umbilicus, on the anterior midline. Stab 1.0–2.0 cun straight, and needling should be carried out after urination. Moxibustion is widely used. Use with caution for pregnant women. It is mainly used for treating impotence, spermatorrhea, enuresis, retention of urine, frequent micturition, irregular menstruation, dysmenorrhea, amenorrhea, metrorrhagia, leukorrhagia, infertility, abdominal pain, diarrhea, asthenia, emaciation, stroke, etc.

2. 气海 在下腹部，脐中下 1.5 寸，前正中线上。直刺 1.0 ～ 2.0 寸。多用灸法。孕妇慎用。主治腹痛、泄泻、便秘、遗尿、遗精、阳痿、闭经、痛经、崩漏、带下、阴挺、虚劳羸瘦、中风脱证等。

Qihai It is in the lower abdomen, 1.5 cun below the umbilicus, on the anterior midline. Stab 1.0–2.0 cun straight. Moxibustion is widely used. Use with caution for pregnant women. It is mainly used for abdominal pain, diarrhea, constipation, enuresis, spermatorrhea, impotence, amenorrhea, dysmenorrhea, metrorrhagia, leukorrhagia, yin stiffness, asthenia, emaciation, stroke and so on.

3. 神阙 在脐区，脐中央。一般不针，宜灸。主治腹痛、泄泻、痢疾、脱肛、水肿、中风脱证等。

Shenque It is in the umbilical area and the center of the umbilical area. Generally, moxibustion is suitable instead of acupuncture. It is mainly used for abdominal pain, diarrhea, dysentery, rectocele, edema, stroke and so on.

4. 中脘 在上腹部，脐中上 4 寸，前正中线上（剑胸结合与脐中连线的中点处）。直刺 1.0 ～ 1.5 寸。主治胃痛、呕吐、呕逆、腹胀、泄泻、便秘、痰多咳喘等。

Zhongwan It located in the upper abdomen, 4 cun above the middle umbilicus, on the anterior midline (at the midpoint of the connecting line between the sword chest and the middle umbilicus). Stab 1.0–1.5 cun straight. It is mainly used for treating stomachache, vomiting, vomiting, abdominal distension, diarrhea, constipation, cough and asthma with excessive phlegm, etc.

5. 膻中　在胸部，横平第 4 肋间隙，前正中线上。平刺 0.3 ～ 0.5 寸。主治胸闷、气短、胸痛、心悸、咳嗽、气喘、呃逆、呕吐、产后乳少、乳痈等。

Danzhong　It is in the chest, horizontally leveling the 4th intercostal space and on the anterior midline. Flat thorn 0.3–0.5 cun. It is mainly used for treating chest tightness, shortness of breath, chest pain, palpitation, cough, asthma, hiccup, vomiting, postpartum hypogalactia, breast carbuncle, etc.

三、冲脉
3 Chong meridian

（一）经脉循行
3.1 Meridian circulation

冲脉循行见图 12–16。

The circulation of Chong meridian is shown in Figure 12–16.

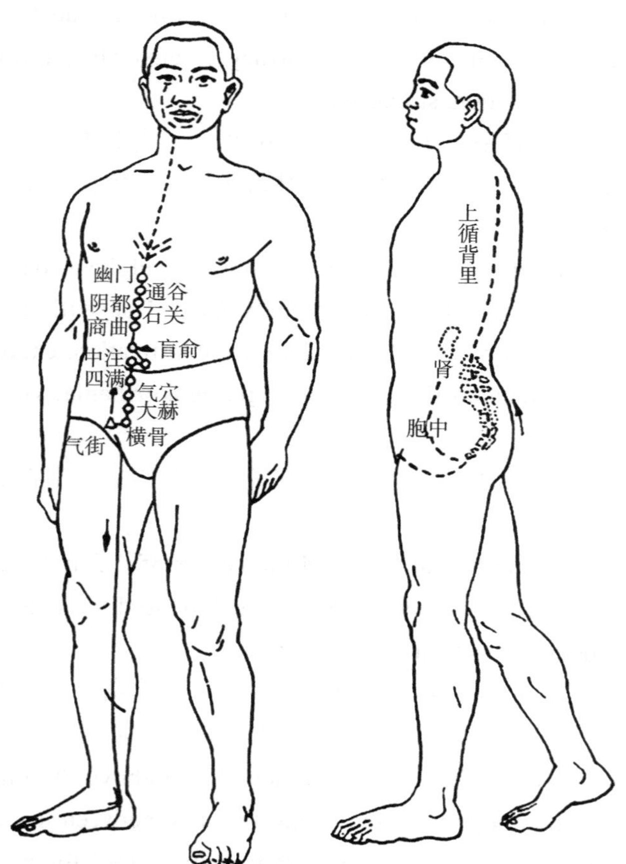

图 12–16　冲脉循行示意图

Figure 12–16　Schematic diagram of pulse circulation

（二）常用腧穴

3.2 Common acupoints

冲脉无所属腧穴，交会腧穴有任脉会阴、阴交，足阳明胃经气冲，足少阴肾经横骨、大赫、气穴、四满、中注、肓俞、商曲、石关、阴都、腹通谷、幽门。

Chong meridian has no acupoints, but intersection acupoints include Ren meridian Huiyin, Yinjiao, foot Yangming stomach meridian Qichong, foot Shaoyin kidney meridian Henggu, Dahe, Qi point, Siman, Zhongzhu, Huangshu, Shangqu, Shiguan, Yindu, Futonggu and Youmen.

四、带脉

4 Dai meridian

（一）经脉循行

4.1 Meridian circulation

带脉循行见图 12–17。

The circulation with veins is shown in Figure 12–17.

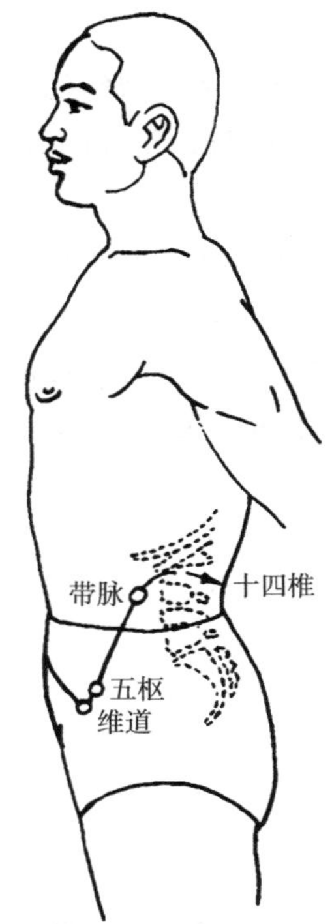

图 12–17 带脉循行示意图

Figure 12–17 Schematic diagram of vein circulation

（二）常用腧穴
4.2 Common acupoints

带脉无所属腧穴，交会腧穴有足少阳胆经的带脉、五枢、维道。

There are no acupoints to which Dai meridian belongs, and there are Daimai, Wushu and Wei Dao of Foot Shaoyang Gallbladder Meridian at the intersection acupoints.

五、阴维脉
5 Yinwei meridian

（一）经脉循行
5.1 Meridian circulation

阴维脉循行见图 12–18。

The circulation of Yinwei meridian is shown in Figure 12–18.

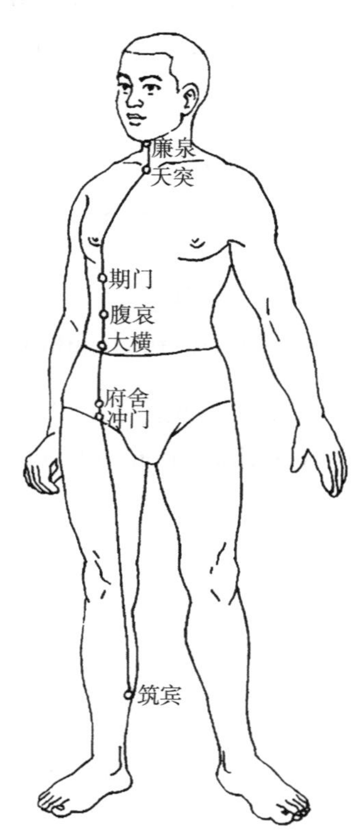

图 12–18　阴维脉循行示意图
Figure 12–18　Schematic diagram of Yin Wei pulse circulation

（二）常用腧穴
5.2 Common acupoints

阴维脉无所属腧穴，交会腧穴有足少阴肾经筑宾，足太阴脾经冲门、府舍、大横、腹哀，足厥阴肝经期门，任脉天突、廉泉。

Yinwei meridian has no acupoints, and the intersection acupoints include Zushaoyin Kidney Meridian Zhubin, Zutaiyin Spleen Meridian Chongmen, Fushe, Daheng, Fu Ai, Zueyin Liver Menstruation Gate, Ren Meridian Tiantu and Lianquan.

六、阳维脉
6 Yangwei meridian

（一）经脉循行
6.1 Meridian circulation

阳维脉循行见图 12–19。

The circulation of Yangwei meridian is shown in Figure 12–19.

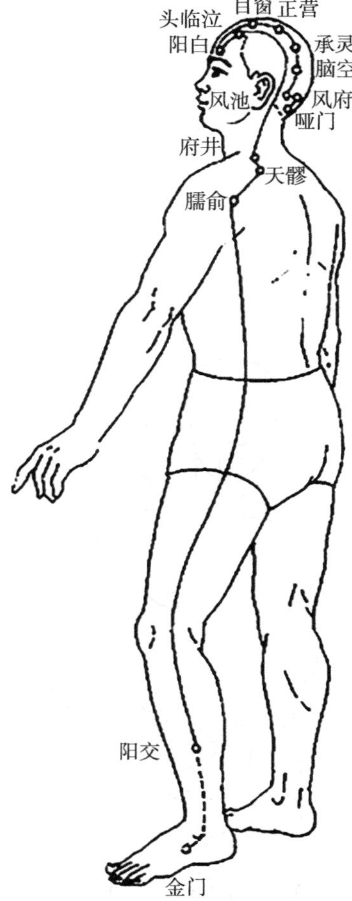

图 12–19　阳维脉循行示意图

Figure12–19　Schematic diagram of Yang Wei pulse circulation

（二）常用腧穴

6.2 Common acupoints

阳维脉无所属腧穴，交会腧穴有足太阳膀胱经金门，足少阳胆经阳交，手太阳小肠经臑俞，手少阳三焦经天髎，足少阳胆经肩井、本神、阳白、头临泣、目窗、正营、承灵、脑空、风池，足阳明胃经头维，督脉风府、哑门。

Yangwei meridian has no acupoints, and the intersection acupoints include foot sun bladder meridian Jinmen, foot shaoyang gallbladder meridian Yangjiao, hand sun small intestine meridian Yu Shu, hand shaoyang sanjiao meridian Tianliao, Zushaoyang gallbladder meridian shoulder well, Ben Shen, Yang Bai, Tou Lin Qi, Mu Chuang, Zhengying, Chengling, Naokong, Fengchi, Zuyangming stomach meridian Touweimo, Du Mai Fengfu and Yamen.

七、阴跷脉
7 Yinqiao meridian

（一）经脉循行
7.1 Meridian circulation

阴跷脉循行见图 12–20。
The circulation of Yinqiao meridian is shown in Figure 12–20.

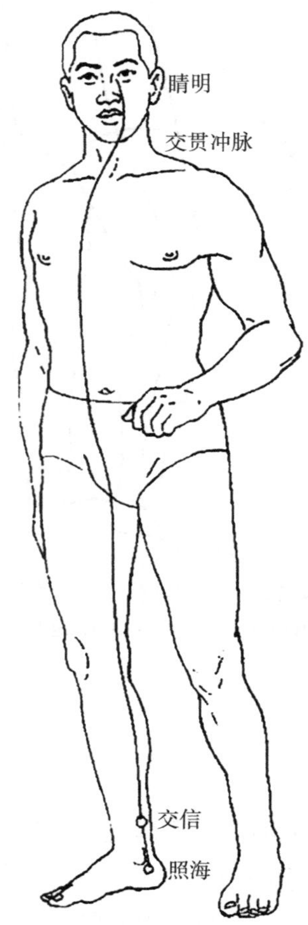

图 12–20　阴跷脉循行示意图
Figure12–20　Schematic diagram of Yin Qiao pulse circulation

（二）常用腧穴
7.2 Common acupoints

阴跷脉无所属腧穴，交会腧穴有足少阴肾经照海、交信，足太阳膀胱经睛明。
Yinqiao meridian has no acupoints, and the intersection acupoints include foot Shaoyin

kidney meridian Zhaohai and Jiaoxin, and foot Taiyang bladder meridian Jingming.

八、阳跷脉
8 Yangqiao meridian

（一）经脉循行
8.1 Meridian circulation

阳跷脉循行见图 12–21。
The circulation of Yangqiao meridian is shown in Figure 12–21.

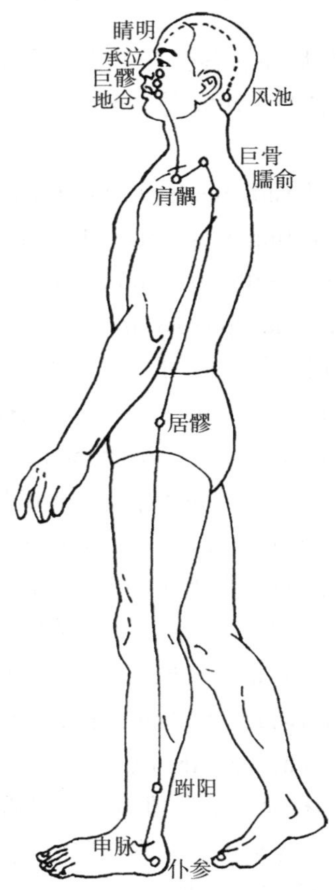

图 12–21　阳跷脉循行示意图
Figure12–21　Schematic diagram of Yang Qiao pulse circulation

（二）常用腧穴
8.2 Common acupoints

阳跷脉无所属腧穴，交会腧穴有足太阳膀胱经申脉、仆参、跗阳、睛明，足少阳胆经居髎，手太阳小肠经臑俞，手阳明大肠经肩髃、巨骨，手少阳三焦经天髎，足阳明胃经地仓、巨髎、承泣。

Yangqiao meridian has no acupoints, but the intersection acupoints include Shenmai, Pushen, Tarsal Yang and Jingming of Foot Taiyang Bladder Meridian, Juliao of Foot Shaoyang Gallbladder Meridian, Yu Shu of Hand Taiyang Small Intestine Meridian, Shoulder Ju and Jugu of Hand Yangming Large Intestine Meridian, Tianliao of Hand Shaoyang Sanjiao Meridian, Dicang, Juliao and Chengqi of Foot Yangming Stomach Meridian.

第四节　常用经外奇穴
Section 4　Commonly used strange points outside meridian

1. 四神聪　在头部，百会前后左右各旁开 1 寸，共 4 穴。取穴时先取百会穴，可用拇指同身寸在其前后左右各量取 1 寸处取穴。平刺 0.5 ～ 0.8 寸。主治头痛、眩晕、失眠、健忘、癫、狂、痫等。

Sishencong　It opens 1 cun beside the head, front, back, left and right sides of Baihui, with a total of 4 points. When selecting acupoints, take Baihui acupoint first, and take 1 cun from the front, back, left and right with your thumb. Flat puncture 0.5–0.8 cun. Indicates headache, dizziness, insomnia, amnesia, epilepsy, madness, epilepsy, etc.

2. 太阳　在头部，眉梢与目外眦之间，向后约一横指的凹陷中。直刺或斜刺 0.3 ～ 0.5 寸，或点刺出血。主治头痛、目疾、口㖞、面痛等。

Taiyang　It is in a depression about one horizontal finger backward between the head, brow and the outer canthus of the eye. Straight prick or oblique prick 0.3–0.5 cun, or prick bleeding. It is mainly used for headache, eye disease, mouth ache and facial pain.

3. 耳尖　在耳区，在外耳轮的最高点（折耳向前时，耳郭上方的尖端处）。直刺 0.1 ～ 0.2 寸，或点刺出血。主治目疾、头痛、咽喉肿痛等。

Erjian　It is in the ear area, at the highest point of the external helix (the tip above the auricle when folding the ear forward). Straight prick 0.1–0.2 cun, or prick bleeding. It is mainly used for eye diseases, headache, sore throat, etc.

4. 夹脊　在脊柱区，第 1 胸椎至第 5 腰椎棘突下两侧，后正中线旁开 0.5 寸，一侧 17 穴，左右共 34 穴。直刺 0.5 ～ 1.5 寸。上胸部腧穴治疗心肺及上肢疾病，下胸部腧穴治疗胃肠疾病，腰部腧穴治疗腰腹及下肢疾病。

Jiaji　It is located in the spinal region, from the first thoracic vertebra to the lower sides of the spinous process of the fifth lumbar vertebra, with 0.5 cun beside the posterior midline, 17 points on one side and 34 points on the left and right sides. Straight puncture 0.5–1.5 cun. The upper chest acupoints are used to treat heart, lung and upper limb diseases, the lower chest acupoints are used to treat gastrointestinal diseases, and the waist acupoints are used to treat waist, abdomen and lower limb diseases.